AIR POLLUTANTS AND
THE RESPIRATORY TRACT

LUNG BIOLOGY IN HEALTH AND DISEASE

Executive Editor

Claude Lenfant
Former Director, National Heart, Lung, and Blood Institute
National Institutes of Health
Bethesda, Maryland

The opinions expressed in these volumes do not necessarily represent the views of the National Institutes of Health.

AIR POLLUTANTS AND THE RESPIRATORY TRACT

Edited by

W. Michael Foster
Duke University
Durham, North Carolina, U.S.A.

Daniel L. Costa
U.S. Environmental Protection Agency
Research Triangle Park, North Carolina, U.S.A.

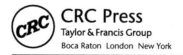
CRC Press
Taylor & Francis Group
Boca Raton London New York

CRC Press is an imprint of the
Taylor & Francis Group, an **informa** business

CRC Press
Taylor & Francis Group
6000 Broken Sound Parkway NW, Suite 300
Boca Raton, FL 33487-2742

First issued in paperback 2019

© 2011 by Taylor & Francis Group, LLC
CRC Press is an imprint of Taylor & Francis Group, an Informa business

No claim to original U.S. Government works

ISBN-13: 978-0-8247-2373-6 (hbk)
ISBN-13: 978-0-367-39290-1 (pbk)

A CIP record for this book is available from the British Library.

Library of Congress Cataloging-in-Publication Data available on application

**Visit the Taylor & Francis Web site at
http://www.taylorandfrancis.com**

**and the CRC Press Web site at
http://www.crcpress.com**

Introduction

The concern about pollution and its health effects is not new. Some 1500 years ago, Actios of Antiochenus (500–575), a Byzantine Greek writer and physician to Emperor Justinian, made the following statement:

> Irritations of the eyes, which are caused by smoke, over-heating dust, or similar injury, are easy to heal; the patient being advised first of all to avoid the irritating causes . . . For the disease ceases without any use of any kind of medicine, if only a proper way of living be adopted.

—From Tetrabiblon

Of course, this is a perfect and simple prescription. Well, maybe it was 1500 years ago!

Today, it is an unfortunate adage that pollution is part of our life, wherever we may be, except perhaps in the wilderness. Even the wilderness is shrinking and therefore the "irritating" causes of health ailments are more and more difficult to avoid. Pollution has become a critical cause of respiratory tract injury, sometimes suddenly and acutely, but more often insidiously and chronically.

It is only six years since the series of monographs Lung Biology in Health and Disease presented the first edition of *Air Pollutants and the*

Respiratory Tract, edited by Drs. David Swift and William M. Foster. The goal of this first volume was to review the history and current knowledge of the effects of ambient air pollution upon the human respiratory system.

Today, I am pleased to present a second and new edition of the volume edited by Drs. William M. Foster and Daniel Costa with the same title but entirely different content reflecting research advances that have occurred since the first publication. This new volume focuses on responses of the cardio-respiratory system to respiratory irritants. Understanding these responses, modulated by exogenous and endogenous determinants, will pave the way to compensatory interventions, not to say therapeutic ones. At the same time we must not abandon the search of finding "the proper way of living."

As the Editor of this series of monographs, I thank Drs. Foster and Costa and all the authors for this contribution to our understanding of lung injury.

Claude Lenfant, MD
Gaithersburg, Maryland

Preface

It is the tension between creativity and skepticism that has produced the stunning and unexpected findings of science.

—Carl Sagan (1935–1997)

The surface of the respiratory tract represents the largest interface between humans and their environments. This surface is constantly exposed to a spectrum of gaseous contaminants and particulates dispersed in the respired air. Despite improvements in air quality in recent decades, epidemiological studies continue to associate air pollutants with increases in human morbidity and mortality. Not surprisingly, the cardio-pulmonary system is often the initial target of these inhaled toxic agents. Consequently, intensive research efforts have attempted to define the specific constituents of air pollution responsible for the adverse health effects and to understand their underlying mechanisms.

We are honored to have developed and edited the second edition to *Air Pollutants and the Respiratory Tract* for the Lung Biology in Health and Disease series. We are pleased by the final compendium of review papers submitted by our colleagues for this volume. This edition continues as a reference source for environmental scientists with updates and expansions of the initial treatise, but it also introduces new areas that have become the focus of research in air pollution. Hence, a strong emphasis has been placed on the responses of the cardio-pulmonary system to respiratory irritants, air toxics, and especially to particulate matter.

The chapter topics have been selected in support of our current paradigm:

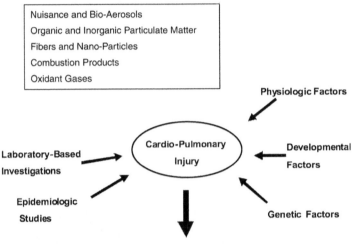

Nuisance and Bio-Aerosols
Organic and Inorganic Particulate Matter
Fibers and Nano-Particles
Combustion Products
Oxidant Gases

Physiologic Factors

Cardio-Pulmonary Injury

Laboratory-Based Investigations

Developmental Factors

Epidemiologic Studies

Genetic Factors

Health Risk and Regulatory Standards

whereby laboratory-based studies (i.e., animal, in vitro, and human volunteers) and epidemiologic investigations have characterized cardio-pulmonary injury resulting from air pollutant exposures. These air pollutants range from nuisance dusts, bio-aerosols, fibers, nano-particles, and organic and inorganic combustion products, to the classic air pollutants—particulate matter and oxidant gases. Individual susceptibility and vulnerability have become prime themes in many studies over the last decade. Hence, several chapters address some of the many elements that contribute to the vulnerability of pulmonary and cardiac tissues, including physiological (e.g., dosimetry), nutritional, developmental (e.g., maturational and aging), and genetic factors. The final chapter summarizes many historic and present-day regulatory considerations involved in improving air quality, using concepts from the preceding chapters in the context of public health. This chapter also discusses some of the unresolved and controversial issues related to particulate matter, which many air pollution scientists believe to be the number one air pollution issue of today.

We trust this edition will provide the scientific community with valuable insights into basic health implications of ambient air pollutants, with comprehensive reviews of the existing science base across study disciplines and issues. In addition, we hope the volume will be a useful resource and teaching guide for clinical scientists and health professionals, as well as to graduate education programs in the environmental health sciences.

W. Michael Foster
Daniel L. Costa

Contributors

William D. Bennett   Center for Environmental Medicine, Asthma, and Lung Biology, University of North Carolina–Chapel Hill, Chapel Hill, North Carolina, U.S.A.

James C. Bonner   National Institute of Environmental Health Sciences and CIIT Centers for Health Research, Research Triangle Park, North Carolina, U.S.A.

James S. Brown   National Center for Environmental Assessment, Office of Research and Development, U.S. Environmental Protection Agency, Research Triangle Park, North Carolina, U.S.A.

Harriet A. Burge   Harvard School of Public Health, Harvard University, Boston, Massachusetts, U.S.A.

Douglas W. Dockery   Department of Environmental Health Exposure, Epidemiology and Risk Program, Harvard School of Public Health, Boston, Massachusetts, U.S.A.

Stephen H. Gavett   National Health and Environmental Effects Research Laboratory, U.S. Environmental Protection Agency, Research Triangle Park, North Carolina, U.S.A.

Terry Gordon   School of Medicine, New York University, Tuxedo, New York, U.S.A.

Urmila P. Kodavanti   Pulmonary Toxicology Branch, Experimental Toxicology Division, National Health and Environmental Effects Research Laboratory, ORD, U.S. Environmental Protection Agency, Research Triangle Park, North Carolina, U.S.A.

Marian Kollarik   Johns Hopkins University Asthma and Allergy Center, Baltimore, Maryland, U.S.A.

Joellen Lewtas   University of Washington, Seattle, Washington, U.S.A.

Morton Lippmann   Nelson Institute of Environmental Medicine, School of Medicine, New York University, Tuxedo, New York, U.S.A.

Janice L. Peake   Center for Health and the Environment, University of California, Davis, California, U.S.A.

Annette Peters   GSF—National Research Center for Environment and Health, Neuherberg, Germany

Kent E. Pinkerton   Center for Health and the Environment, University of California, Davis, California, U.S.A.

Jeffrey G. Sherman   Center for Health and the Environment, University of California, Davis, California, U.S.A.

Ira B. Tager   Division of Epidemiology, School of Public Health, University of California, Berkeley, California, U.S.A.

Bradley J. Undem   Johns Hopkins University Asthma and Allergy Center, Baltimore, Maryland, U.S.A.

Dianne M. Walters   National Institute of Environmental Health Sciences and CIIT Centers for Health Research, Research Triangle Park, North Carolina, U.S.A.

David B. Warheit   DuPont Haskell Laboratory, Newark, Delaware, U.S.A.

William P. Watkinson   Pulmonary Toxicology Branch, Experimental Toxicology Division, National Health and Environmental Effects Research

Laboratory, ORD, U.S. Environmental Protection Agency, Research Triangle Park, North Carolina, U.S.A.

Viviana J. Wong   Center for Health and the Environment, University of California, Davis, California, U.S.A.

Contents

1

Air Pollution and Health Effects: Evidence from Epidemiologic Studies

ANNETTE PETERS

GSF—National Research Center for
    Environment and Health,
Neuherberg, Germany

DOUGLAS W. DOCKERY

Department of Environmental Health
Exposure, Epidemiology and Risk Program,
Harvard School of Public Health,
Boston, Massachusetts, U.S.A.

I. Introduction

Much of the central information for identifying and quantifying the adverse effects of air pollution exposures in the community has come from epidemiologic studies. They have been largely responsible for documenting the effects of air pollution in the community and have provided the basis for regulatory decisions and public health policy.

In this review, we illustrate the contributions of epidemiological studies to our understanding of the health effects of air pollution. We have not attempted to be comprehensive in summarizing the hundreds of air pollution epidemiologic studies that have been published in the past decade. Rather, we highlight specific studies which we feel have been particularly innovative, informative, and influential in advancing the state of knowledge.

Samet and Jaakkoia (1) suggest that epidemiologic studies of the health effects of air pollution have three objectives: (1) to determine if a specific air pollutant poses a hazard to public health; (2) to quantify the

1

exposure–response function between air pollutants and a specific health outcome, and (3) to examine responses of potentially susceptible populations to air pollution exposures. There is general consensus that, at high enough concentrations, any air contaminants would be hazardous to public health. Indeed, the criteria air pollutants have been identified as hazardous by legislation or regulation. The focus of air pollution epidemiology, then, has been on defining the exposure–response function at concentrations normally seen in the community and identifying subsets of the population who are more susceptible to their effects.

II. What Have Epidemiologic Studies Taught Us?
A. Mortality

In the past 15 years, we have seen epidemiology move to the forefront in documenting the effects of ambient air pollution at the modest concentrations commonly observed in developed countries. This understanding has been driven by analyses showing that mortality was related to short-term exposures of a few days (acute) and longer-term exposures of years (chronic) to ambient air pollution.

1. Acute Mortality

In the early 1990s, a series of time series studies showing that daily ambient air pollution concentrations were associated with increased daily deaths in London (3a), Philadelphia (2), and Steubenville (3). These methods now have been applied in hundreds of individual cities. Meta-analyses in which the results of published city-specific risk estimates are combined have found that daily mortality increases by approximately 1% for each $10 \, \mu g/m^3$ increase in daily mean PM_{10} (4,5).

An alternative to meta-analyses is a pooled multicity analysis in which data from multiple cities are analyzed simultaneously using a common approach. The national mortality morbidity air pollution study (NMMAPS) of 90 urban areas of United States (6) found that each increase of $10 \, \mu g/m^3$ in PM_{10} was associated with an increase of 0.2% in daily deaths. The air pollution and health effect association study (APHEAS) in 29 European cities found a consistent increase of 0.6% in daily mortality associated with each increase of $10 \, \mu g/m^3$ (7). These multicenter studies indicated that the dose–response function for PM_{10} is linear and no threshold can be established. PM_{10} was the air pollutant most strongly associated with the increase in mortality in both the NMMAPS and APHEA study. Evidence for effect modification as observed in these large multicenter studies between centers may indicate that the pollution mix, the frailty of the studied population, or other factors such as socioeconomic factors might be responsible for differences in city-specific estimates.

Does reduced ambient air pollution lead to reduced mortality? In 1986–87, a strike led to the 13-month shut down of a steel mill in Utah Valley, and a decrease in mean PM_{10} concentrations. Total mortality during this period decreased by 3% (8). A study in Dublin showed that, after a reduction of $36 \, \mu g/m^3$ in mean particle concentrations measured as black smoke due to a ban on coal burning in 1990, total mortality decreased overall by 6% (9). These studies indicated that ambient particulate air pollution contributes to reversible total mortality in urban areas.

2. Life Shortening (Reduced Survival)

If acute exposures to ambient air pollution are associated with acutely increased daily mortality, how much is life expectancy affected by repeated exposures. That is, is there a detectable effect of cumulative exposures to air pollution of extended periods of time (years to a lifetime). The Harvard six cities studies (HSCS) were designed in the 1970s to provide estimates for the impact of living in areas with elevated pollution concentrations. Mortality over a 14–16 year follow-up was found to increase linearly with city-mean $PM_{2.5}$ concentrations across the six cities (10). When published in 1993, individuals living in Steubenville, Ohio were found to have a 27% increased risk for mortality compared to those living in Topeka, Kansas, which corresponds to 13% higher risk of mortality per $10 \, \mu g/m^3$ in mean $PM_{2.5}$ (10). These results were supported by an analysis of more than 500,000 adults in the American cancer society cancer prevention study (II) living in 50 cities across the United States who were followed over a 16-year period (11). Each $10 \, \mu g/m^3$ increase in mean $PM_{2.5}$ was associated with a 4% increase in total mortality (12).

These studies carefully controlled for major personal characteristics which are predictive of mortality such as age, gender, race, smoking, obesity, and occupational exposures. However, concerns were raised as to the role of residual confounding for factors on which no personal information were collected (13). The development of methods to consider spatial correlations, as well as the collection of proxy data for the regions, showed that the associations were robust against these potential biases (14,15).

In a pilot analysis of study, participants in a long-term follow-up study of cancer incidence in the Netherlands, individual black smoke, and NO_2 concentrations were estimated based on regional air pollution measurements, on estimated impacts of urbanicity and on proximity.to major roads (16). Each $10 \, \mu g/m^3$ increase in black smoke was associated with a 37% increase in long-term mortality (16).

Figure 1 summarizes the effect estimates of the American cancer society study (ACSS) (12), the HSCS (10), and the study from the Netherlands (16). While the ACSS had to rely on available monitoring often for large areas, the HSCS set up monitors to characterize its population exposure. The study from the Netherlands combined regional and local

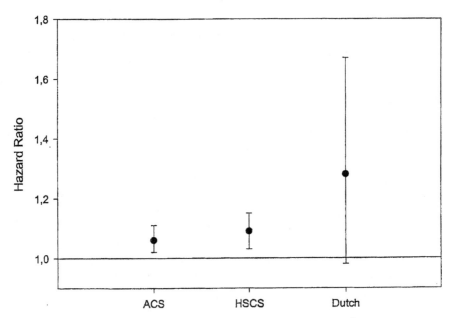

Figure 1   Hazard ratios estimated of the effect of $10\,\mu g/m^3$ PM$_{2.5}$ on total mortality from three cohort studies: The ACSS, the HSCS, and the study from the Netherlands.

exposure assessment (17), thereby considering not only background levels of ambeint particles, but also local traffic related exposures. As air pollution exposure assessment improves, also the effect estimates increase.

3.   Cause-Specific Mortality

Analyses for cause-specific mortality based on death certificates indicate that both short- and long-term mortality is primarily due to death in subjects with underlying respiratory and cardiovascular disease (12,18). In studies of the chronic effects of air pollution, cardiopulmonary deaths were often combined to provide sufficient power. Collectively, they convincingly showed that the observed associations were attributable largely to these major causes of death. Attempts to further analyze the association of air pollution with specific subgroups of diagnoses must be viewed with caution as there is substantial potential for misclassification and crossclassification of cause on death certificates. Nevertheless, these analyses offer important insights for future research.

Links of death data with other administrative data on hospital admissions have provided a useful tool to identify susceptible subgroups within the population and offer the opportunity to follow these susceptible subgroups for mortality (19–21). These studies have consistently found air pollution mortality to be increased among patients with preexisting respiratory and cardiovascular disease. A recent report on the ACS cohort indicated that persons with underlying ischemic disease, dysrhythmia, or congestive heart failure might be especially at risk when chronically exposed to elevated concentrations of particulate matter (22). A finding which in the initial analyses was surprising was the association between chronic exposure to particles and lung cancer deaths (12), although lung cancer has been associated with motor vehicle air pollution in other studies (23,24). This raises the suspicion that chronic exposure to particles might contribute to the development of lung cancer in addition to exacerbating existing disease by respiratory infections in prevalent lung cancer cases.

4. Morbidity

If people are dying on days with high ambient air pollution concentrations, then we should expect to see increased emergency department visits, hospital admissions, and increased symptom reports (25). A large number of studies have assessed this coherence of the association of air pollution with multiple measures of both respiratory and cardiovascular diseases (Fig. 2).

B. Respiratory Diseases
1. Hospital Admissions and Emergency Room Visits

Time series studies of hospital admissions for respiratory diseases indicated that admissions for chronic obstructive lung disease, asthma, and pneumonia were more frequent on days with high air pollution concentrations (18). These associations were observed in association with particuiate matter, although ozone and NO_2 were also implicated. Emergency room visits provide a second data source for morbidity studies as they capture the urgent cases and exclude scheduled admissions. Studies of emergency department visits have demonstrated an association between air pollutants and serious asthma episodes (26,27).

2. Symptom Exacerbation and Medication Use

Small cohort studies in asthmatic patients and individuals with chronic respiratory symptoms have suggested that ambient air pollution concentrations are associated with an increased frequency of lower and upper respiratory tract symptoms (28–32). The results vary with respect to the symptoms being evaluated. These variations in the observations might be attributable to the underlying diseases as well as to the difference in pollution mix. Increased medication intake was associated with ambient air pollution in some studies, which itself potentially could have reduced the observed air pollution associated health effects. Chronically elevated concentrations of ambient air pollution also have the potential to influence the prevalence

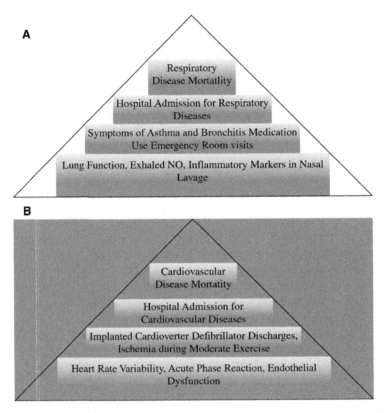

Figure 2 Summary of evidence for respiratory (A) and cardiovascular (B) disease exacerbation in association with ambient air pollution.

of symptoms in children (33–35). Studies conducted in central and eastern Europe indicated that elevated concentrations of SO_2 and particles during the 1980s were associated with elevated prevalence of bronchitis but not an increase in asthma in school children (36,37). The prevalence of bronchitis declined markedly during the 1990s as air pollution concentrations decreased and air quality improved (38). On the other hand, traffic air pollution has been associated with increased respiratory symptom reporting and increased prevalence of allergic symptoms in children (39).

C. Lung Function Changes

Measurements of peak expiratory flow rate have been used to characterize respiratory health on a daily basis. Peak expiratory flow rates have been shown to decrease in association with measures of ambient air pollution in numerous studies (28–32,40). A more reliable data derive from supervized lung function tests such as the forced vital capacity (FVC) and the forced expiratory volume after 1 sec (FEV1). While repeated supervized lung function measures have been applied in air pollution studies (41), these studies are rare. However, supervized lung function measurements have been applied in studies assessing chronic exposure to ambient air pollution. Lung function and growth of lung function in children have been shown to be reduced in association with ambient air pollution (42–45).

D. Other Physiologic Measures

Several other physiological measures have been employed in epidemiologic studies. Some investigators have measured indirect indicators of pulmonary inflammation following particle exposures. Exhaled NO, a biomarker for inflammatory responses in the lung, has been reported to increase following exposures to elevated ambient particulate air pollution (46–48). Other approaches such as nasal lavage (49,50) and induced sputum (51) are based on the correlatioh between inflammatory response in the upper and lower airways.

E. Cardiovascular Diseases

1. Hospital Admissions

Beginning in the middle 1990s, several studies have showed that hospital admissions for cardiovascular diseases were more frequent on days with high air pollution concentrations (52–60). Particulate matter and ozone were implicated; more recent findings from Europe also suggest an association with SO_2 at very low levels (61). Studies that analyzed specific diagnoses suggested that admissions for ischemic heart disease, congestive heart failure, and dysrhythmia were more frequent on days with high ambient air pollution concentrations (54,58,62–65).

Evidence that elevated concentrations of particuiate air pollution might trigger myocardial infarction (MI) indicates an immediate onset of MI at high ambient air pollution concentrations (64,66). One of the studies (66) suggested that elevated concentrations of fine particles in the air may transiently elevate the MI risk up to one day following the exposure. It has been proposed that the onset of MI is triggered by the disruption of a vulnerable but not necessarily stenotic atherosclerotic plaque in response to hemodynamic stress; thereafter, hemostatic and vasoconstrictive forces determine whether the resultant thrombus becomes occlusive (67).

In a case-crossover study, Checkoway and colleagues investigated 362 cases of sudden cardiac arrest among individuals without any evidence of cardiovascular disease prior to the event. No association was found between ambient PM_{10} concentrations and sudden cardiac arrest; the risk estimates were negative, and not statistically significant (68,69). Sudden cardiac death has been associated with the conventional risk factors for ischemic heart disease such as smoking, hypertension, and diabetes, but it also occurs in apparently healthy individuals with low risk factor profiles (70). Major disturbances in cardiac rhythm, such as ventricular fibrillation or tachyarrhythmia, are thought to be responsible for sudden cardiac death (71). Genetic factors are largely felt to be responsible for these unexpected events (70).

Ambient concentrations of $PM_{2.5}$ have been associated with ventricular fibrillation and an increased number of therapeutic interventions in patients with implanted cardioverter defibrillators (72,73). A pilot study showed associations between $PM_{2.5}$ as well as NO_2 and therapies for tachyarrhythmia with a 2 day lag (72). However, a larger study of 195 patients with implanted cardioverter defibrillators reported an association between mean $PM_{2.5}$ concentrations on the same and previous days and arrhythmia (73).

Acceleration of heart rates and diminished heart rate variability in association with air pollution have been documented in elderly persons (74–77), in random samples of the population (78), and in occupational cohorts (79). Some of the studies on heart rate variability reported an immediate response within hours (77,79), or on the same day (75,76), whereas effects on heart rate seemed to accumulate in association with prolonged elevated air pollution concentration (74,78). In a quasi-experimental study, volunteers exposed to passive smoke in a smoking area for 2 hr showed decreased heart rate variability compared to 2 hr exposures in a clean room in a cross-over design (80).

Consistent with these observations, the Finnish subgroup of the ULTRA study showed ischemic reactions during a submaximal exercise test in association with ambient particulate matter in patients with coronary artery disease (81). Specifically, a 3-fold risk for ST-segment depressions was associated with each $10\,\mu g/m^3$ increase in $PM_{2.5}$ 2 days earlier. In addition, evidence for an effect of ultrafine particles also was found with a 2-day delay.

While epidemiologic evidence is accumulating that combustion-related particulate air pollution is an important environmental risk factor for cardiopulmonary mortality, other recent studies are providing incomplete but intriguing results suggesting that particle-induced pulmonary and systemic inflammation, accelerated atherosclerosis, and altered cardiac autonomic function may be part of the pathophysiological pathways, linking particulate air pollution with cardiovascular mortality (82). It has been shown that particles deposited in the alveoli lead to activation of cytokine production by alveolar macrophages (83) and epithelial cells (84), to recruitment of inflammatory cells (85), and to bone marrow stimulation (86,87). Increases in plasma viscosity (88), fibrinogen (89,90), and C-reactive protein (91) have been observed in samples of randomly selected healthy adults in association with particulate air pollution. Endothelial dysfunction has been induced by controlled particle exposures (92) and small increases in blood pressure have been observed in association with elevated concentrations of ambient particles (93,94).

F. Who Is Susceptible to Air Pollution?

Overall, the risk estimates reported in studies assessing the short-term health effects of entire populations are small. Subjects with pre-existing cardiopulmonary disease have been shown to be at increased risk for acute mortality associated with air pollution (19–21). Furthermore, studies indicate that acute air pollution related mortality is not restricted to the frailest members of the population, who were about to die by a few days (harvesting) (95,96).

Recent studies of air pollution effects on cardiovascular diseases have indicated that air pollution worsens the risk factor profiles of individuals and therefore increases the risk for an acute event to occur. In light of a newly proposed concept for the development of acute coronary artery events in vulnerable patients (97,98), the recent evidence for the impact of air pollution on piaque vulnerability, prothrombotic states, and a vulnerable myocardium prone to arrhythmia supports the potentially causal link between ambient air pollution and acute cardiovascular disease. It is therefore conceivable that elevated ambient air pollution concentrations transiently elevate the risk for the occurrence of acute events. This elevated transient risk would consequently be of more importance in already compromised, often elderly individuals than in healthy individuals. Evidence for higher risk estimates in subjects with pre-existing heart disease as well as in elderly subjects has indeed been found, especially for the association between air pollution and all-cause mortality (99).

Similar thinking has evolved for subjects with pre-existing respiratory disease who on days with high air pollution concentrations are at particularly high risk of being hospitalized with pneumonia or dying of it (18). Current research is attempting to evaluate the relative importance of intrinsic personal risk factors such as age, chronic diseases, or genetic predispositions and of modifiable risk factors such as medications, smoking, diet, and physical activity.

Fetal development appears to be another vulnerable period in life. It has been implicated by studies showing that elevated exposure to ambient air pollution results in preterm birth (100) and reduced birth weight (101), and possibly also in a higher frequency of birth defects (102). Children also have been identified as being susceptible to air pollution (103). This might be due to their developing immune systems, their higher exposures to air pollution whiie playing outdoors (42) and secondarily to higher particle deposition efficiency (see Chapter 2: Particulate Dosimetry in the Respiratory Tract).

G. Attributing Health Effects to Specific Air Pollutants?

Episodes of high air pollution are commonly associated with adverse health. A particular problem for air pollution epidemiology is the identification of the air pollutant specifically associated with these observed health effects. The most commonly applied method for estimating the independent effect of multiple predictors, for example multiple air pollutants, is by multiple regression analyses. However, this requires independence of the predictors (air pollutants).

Air pollution is necessarily a mixture of contaminants whose day-to-day concentrations are determined more by dilution and transport (wind speed and direction) than by variations in local source emissions. However, the proportion of locally produced and regionally distributed air pollution might vary depending on meteorological conditions and season. Across locations, the correlation between various gaseous pollutants such as CO, SO_2, NO_2, and O_3 might vary as well as their correlation with particle mass (PM_{10} and $PM_{2.5}$) or particle number concentrations (ultrafine particles). Furthermore, the population average exposure might also depend on the proximity between the pollution sources and housing, workplaces, or schools. For example, pollutants such as NO_2, CO, and ultrafine particles might have relatively high importance in cities with a high population density and dominance of traffic-related pollution, such as Rome, Italy. In contrast, regionally distributed pollutants such as $PM_{2.5}$ might most adequately characterize population average exposures in cities on the east coast of the United States with lower population densities such as Boston, Massachusetts. The former statement does not claim that the health effects are different between cities, but that the signal extracted by similar epidemiological studies might vary (64,66).

This weakness is addressed by consideration of studies from different locations. The most direct method to control for multiple pollutants is by restriction, i.e., by selecting locations or conditions in which one air pollutant is missing or at low concentration. Thus, if an air pollution association is observed in multiple locations with varying mixtures of pollutants, then the information of the strength of the association across these multiple locations can be used to define the relative importance of individual air pollutants.

For example, the early mortality time series analyses in Steubenville, Ohio (3) and Philadelphia, Pennsylvania (2) found increased daily mortality associated with both particulate and sulfur dioxide. Multiple regression analyses suggested stronger associations with particulate air pollution. More compelling evidence for the effects of particles independent of sulfur dioxide came from daily mortality analyses in Utah Valley (8), which showed equivalent particle and mortality associations in a location with effectively no detectable sulfur dioxide air pollution. This is analogous to a controlled experiment in which the experimental subjects were exposed to particles but not sulfur dioxide.

Conceptually, one could imagine effectively conducting a series of such epidemiologic analyses which would identify communities with and without specific air pollutants for comparison. An alternative might be to analyze daily mortality in a pooled analysis over a large number of cities, assessing the role of the varying multiple pollutants by multiple regression analyses. This has been the approach used in the multicity APHEA and NMMAPS studies. These two large, multicenter studies both identified PM_{10} as being most consistently associated with daily mortality. For chronic health effects, particulate mass has also been identified as being consistently associated with decreased survival (10,12). In this manner, epidemiologicai studies have put demonstrated evidence for a possibly crude but relatively simple measure of ambient air pollution to be assessed for control purposes.

While the multicenter approach can provide some insight into the relative contributions of different air pollutants based on differences in the composition of the air pollution mix between cities, it is subject to the weakness of all between-city comparisons. There are many differences between cities other than air pollution, such as baseline chronic disease rates, climate, race, and ethnicity, which may explain differences in response. More importantly, the existing multicity studies have been limited by the air pollution data routinely available in the study cities. Without adequate exposure data, it is impossible to assess whether individual pollutants are associated with health effects.

Individual epidemioiogic studies suffer from an inability to differentiate effects of correlated air pollutants. However, by combing evidence from multiple studies or, more strongly, by pooling data from multiple locations, it is possible to provide insight into the specific components of air pollution responsible for the observed health effects. The main limitation of such epidemiologic assessments is the incomplete data on community exposures to the multiple components of the air pollution mix.

Several particle properties have been hypothesized to be responsible for the observed health effects. Among them are the transition metal content, large surface areas, and others (see Chapter 3: Bio-Availability of Particle-Associated Air Pollutants and Relationship to Cardiopulmonary Injury). Particulate mass measured as PM_{10} or $PM_{2.5}$ could therefore be surrogated measures for the physicochemical characteristics of the particles that elicit the health effects. Epidemiological studies to further identify these physicochemical characteristics would require innovative measurements, a long time frame in order to allow time-series analyses, and possibly even the use of multiple locations in order to allow for the evaluation of chronic health effects. Epidemiological studies apportioning $PM_{2.5}$ concentrations to different sources (104) are an alternative route to gain insight into both relevant particle properties as well as to inform regulatory strategies for particulate pollution control.

III. Summary

One important limitation of epidemiologic studies is that they cannot establish causality and can only suggest mechanisms and pathways of action. Thus, understanding of the associations between air pollution exposure and health outcomes observed in epidemiologic studies requires complementary information from controlled human, animal, and cellular experimental studies.

On the other hand, epidemiology has been able to demonstrate associations with air pollution that have been undetectable in experimental studies. Most notably, the epidemiologic evidence for mortality effects of ambient particulate air pollution has proven to be robust and compelling. Moreover, the evidence that the mortality effects of air pollution are seen most strongly in individuals with pre-existing respiratory and cardiovascular conditions has led to highly productive experimental studies using compromised animal models. Nevertheless, by assessing health effects of air pollution in the full range of people in the population, even the frailest, epidemiology will continue to provide insights into the characteristics that put people at increased risk of responding to ambient air pollution exposures.

Epidemiologic studies have been central in establishing the specific role of particles as a particularly toxic component of the air pollution mix. In addition, the evidence that ambient particles produce such dear effects in epidemiologic studies has led to highly productive experimental studies with controlled exposures to concentrated ambient particles. Nevertheless, particles are themselves a mixture of constituents with varying toxicity, degrees of aging, and multiple sources. By assessing response to specific particle characteristics and constituents, epidemiology will continue to provide leading indicators of the role of specific constituents and particle sources in determining adverse health effects.

References

1. Samet JM, Jaakkola JJK. The epidemiologic approach to investigating outdoor air pollution. In: Samet JM, Holgate ST, Koren HS, Maynard RL, eds. Air Pollution and Health. London: Academic Press, 1999:431–460.
2. Schwartz J, Dockery DW. Increased mortality in Philadelphia associated with daily air pollution concentrations. Am Rev Respir Dis 1992; 145:600–604.
3. Schwartz J, Dockery DW. Particulate air pollution and daily mortality in Steubenville, Ohio. Am J Epidemiol 1992; 135:12–19.

3a. Schwartz J, Marcus A. Mortality and air pollution in London: a time series analysis. Am J Epidemiol 1990; 131:185–194.

4. Dockery DW, Pope CA III. Acute respiratory effects of particulate air pollution. Annu Rev Public Health 1994; 15:107–132.

5. Levy JI, Hammitt JK, Spengler JD. Estimating the mortality impacts of particulate matter: what can be learned from between-study variability? Environ Health Perspect 2000; 108(2):109–117.

6. Dominici F, MCDermott A, Daniels M, Zeger SL, Samet JM. Revised Analyses of the National Morbidity, Mortality, and Air Pollution Study (NMMAPS), Part II: Mortality Among Residents of 90 Cities. Revised Analyses of Time-series Studies of Air Pollution and Health. Boston: Health Effects Institute, 2003:9–24.

7. Katsouyanni K, Touioumi G, Samoli E, Gryparis A, Le Tertre A, Monopolis Y, et al. Confounding and effect modification in the short-term effects of ambient particles on total mortality: results from 29 European cities within the APHEA2 project. Epidemiology 2001; 12(5):521–531.

8. Pope CA III, Schwartz J, Ransom MR. Daily mortality and PM10 pollution in Utah Valley. Arch Environ Health 1992; 47(3):211–217.

9. Clancy L, Goodman P, Sinclair H, Dockery DW. Effect of air-pollution control on death rates in Dublin, Ireland: an intervention study. Lancet 2002; 360(9341):1210–1214.

10. Dockery DW, Pope AC, Xu X, Spengler JD, Ware JH, Fay ME, et al. An association between air pollution and mortality in six U.S. cities. N Engl J Med 1993; 329:1753–1759.

11. Pope CA III, Thun MJ, Namboodiri MN, Dockery DW, Evans JS, Speizer FE, et al. Particulate air pollution as predictor of mortality in a prospective study of U.S. adults. Am J Respir Crit Care Med 1995; 151:669–674.

12. Pope CA III, Burnett RT, Thun MJ, Calle EE, Krewski D, Ito K, et al. Lung cancer, cardiopulmonary mortality, and long-term exposure to fine particulate air pollution. JAMA 2002; 287(9):1132–1141.

13. Lipfert FW. Clean air skepticism. Science 1997; 278(5335):19–20.

14. Jerrett M, Burnett RT, Willis A, Krewski D, Goldberg MS, DeLuca P, et al. Spatial analysis of the air pollution-mortality relationship in the context of ecologic confounders. J Toxicol Environ Health A 2003; 66(16–19): 1735–1777.

15. Krewski D, Burnett RT, Goldberg MS, Hoover BK, Siemiatycki J, Jerrett M, et al. Overview of the reanalysis of the Harvard six cities study and american cancer society study of particulate air pollution and mortality. J Toxicol Environ Health A 2003; 66(16–19):1507–1551.

16. Hoek G, Brunekreef B, Goldbohm S, Fischer P, van den Brandt PA. Association between mortality and indicators of traffic-related air pollution in the Netherlands: a cohort study. Lancet 2002; 360(9341):1203–1209.

17. Hoek G, Fischer P, Van Den BP, Goldbohm S, Brunekreef B. Estimation of long-term average exposure to outdoor air pollution for a cohort study on mortality. J Expo Anal Environ Epidemiol 2001; 11(6):459–469.

18. Schwartz J, Zanobetti A, Bateson TF. Mortality and morbidity among eldery residents of cities with daily PM measurements. Revised Analyses of

Time-Series Studies of Air Pollution and Health. Boston: Health Effects Institute, 2003:25–58.

19. Goldberg MS, Burnett RT, Baiiar JC III, Tamblyn R, Ernst P, Flegel K, et al. Identification of persons with cardiorespiratory conditions who are at risk of dying from the acute effects of ambient air particles. Environ Health Perspect 2001; 109(suppl 4):487–494.

20. Kwon HJ, Cho SH, Nyberg F, Pershagen G. Effects of ambient air pollution on daily mortality in a cohort of patients with congestive heart failure. Epidemiology 2001; 12(4):413–419.

21. Sunyer J, Schwartz J, Tobias A, Macfariane D, Garcia J, Anto JM. Patients with chronic obstructive pulmonary disease are at increased risk of death associated with urban particle air pollution: a case-crossover analysis. Am 2000; 151(1):50–56.

22. Pope CA III, Burnett RT, Thurston GD, Thun MJ, Calle EE, Krewski D, et al. Cardiovascular mortality and long-term exposure to particulate air pollution: epidemiological evidence of general pathophysiological pathways of disease. Circulation 2004; 109(1):71–77.

23. Nyberg F, Gustavsson P, Jarup L, Bellander T, Berglind N, Jakobsson R, et al. Urban air pollution and lung cancer in Stockholm. Epidemiology 2000; 11(5):487–495.

24. Nafstad P, Haheim LL, Wisloff T, Gram F, Oftedai B, Holme I, et al. Urban air pollution and mortality in a cohort of Norwegian men. Environ Health Perspect 2004; 112(5):610–615.

25. Bates DV. Health indices of the adverse effects of air pollution. The question of coherence. Environ Res 1992; 59:336–349.

26. Bates DV, Baker Anderson M, Sizto R. Asthma attack periodicity: a study of hospital emergency visits in Vancouver. Environ Res 1990; 51(1):51–70.

27. Norris G, YoungPong SN, Koenig JQ, Larson TV, Sheppard L, Stout JW. An association between fine particles and asthma emergency department visits for children in Seattle. Environ Health Perspect 1999; 107(6):489–493.

28. Pope CA III, Dockery DW. Acute health effects of PM10 pollution on symptomatic and asymptomatic children. Am Rev Respir Dis 1992; 145: 1123–1128.

29. Neas LM, Dockery DW, Ware JH, Spengier JD, Ferris BG Jr, Speizer FE. Concentration of indoor particulate matter as a determinant of respiratory health in children. Am J Epidemiol 1994; 139:1088–1099.

30. Peters A, Dockery DW, Heinrich J, Wichmann HE. Short-term effects of particulate air pollution on respiratory morbidity in asthmatic children. Eur Respir J 1997; 10:872–879.

31. Delfino RJ, Zeiger RS, Seltzer JM, Street DH, McLaren CE. Association of asthma symptoms with peak particulate air pollution and effect modification by anti-inflammatory medication use. Environ Health Perspect 2002; 110(10): A607–A617.

32. Roemer W, Hoek G, Brunekreef B. Pollution effects on asthmatic children in Europe, the PEACE study. Clin Expl Allergy 2000; 30(8):1067–1075.

33. Braun-Fahrlander C, Vuille JC, Sennhauser FH, Neu U, Kunzle T, Grize L, et al. Respiratory health and long-term exposure to air pollutants in Swiss

school children. SCARPOL team. Swiss study on childhood allergy and respiratory symptoms with respect to air pollution, climate and pollen. Am J Respir Crit Care Med 1997; 155(3):1042–1049.

34. Dockery DW, Cunningham J, Damokosh Al, Neas LM, Spengier JD, Koutrakis P, et al. Health effects of acid aerosols on North American children: respiratory symptoms. Environ Health Perspect 1996; 104(5): 500–505.

35. Peters JM, Avol E, Navidi W, London SJ, Gauderman WJ, Lurmann F, et al. A study of twelve southern California communities with differing levels and types of air pollution. I. Prevalence of respiratory morbidity. Am J Respir Crit Care Med 1999; 159(3):760–767.

36. Nowak D, Heinrich J, Jorres R, Wassmer G, Berger J, Beck E, et al. Prevalence of respiratory symptoms, bronchial hyperresponsiveness and atopy among adults: West and East Germany. Eur Respir J 1996; 9(12):2541–2552.

37. Mutius EV, Martinez FD, Fritzsch C, Nicolai T, Roell G, Thiemann HH. Prevalence of asthma and atopy in two areas of West and East Germany. Am J Respir Crit Care Med 1994; 149:358–364.

38. Heinrich J, Grate V, Peters A, Wichmann H-E. Gesundheitliche Wirkungen von Feinstaub: Epidemiologie der Langzeiteffekte. Umweltmed Forsch Prax 2002; 7(2):91–99.

39. Gehring U, Cyrys J, Sedlmeir G, Brunekreef B, Bellander T, Fischer P, et al. Traffic-related air pollution and respiratory health during the first 2 yrs of life. Eur Respir J 2002; 19(4):690–698.

40. Pope CA III, Dockery DW, Spengler JD, Raizenne ME. Respiratory health and PM10 pollution. A daily time series analysis. Am Rev Respir Dis 1991; 144:668–674.

41. Dockery DW, Ware JH, Ferris BG, Speizer FE, Cook NR, Herman SM. Change in pulmonary function in children associated with air pollution episodes. J Air Poll Contr Assn 1982; 32:937–942.

42. Gauderman WJ, Gilliland GF, Vora H, Avol E, Stram D, Mcconnell R, et al. Association between air pollution and lung function growth in southern California children: results from a second cohort. Am J Respir Crit Care Med 2002; 166(1):76–84.

43. Peters JM, Avol E, Gauderman WJ, Linn WS, Navidi W, London SJ, et al. A study of twelve Southern California communities with differing levels and types of air pollution. II. Effects on pulmonary function. Am J Respir Crit Care Med 1999; 159(3):768–775.

44. Braun Fahrlander C, Kunzli N, Domenighetti G, Carell CF, Ackermann Liebrich U. Acute effects of ambient ozone on respiratory function of Swiss school children after a 10-minute heavy exercise. Pediatr Pulmonol 1994; 17:169–177.

45. Raizenne M, Neas LM, Damokosh Al, Dockery DW, Spengler JD, Koutrakis P, et al. Health effects of acid aerosols on North American children: pulmonary function. Environ Health Perspect 1996; 104(5):506–514.

46. Fischer PH, Steerenberg PA, Snelder JD, Van Loveren H, Van Amsterdam JG. Association between exhaled nitric oxide, ambient air pollution and

respiratory health in school children. Int Arch Occup Environ Health 2002;
75(5):348–353.

47. Koenig JQ, Jansen K, Mar TF, Lumley T, Kaufman J, Trenga CA, et al.
Measurement of offline exhaled nitric oxide in a study of community exposure
to air pollution. Environ Health Perspect 2003; 111(13): 1625–1629.

48. Adamkiewicz G, Ebelt S, Syring M, Slater J, Speizer FE, Schwartz J, et al.
Association between air pollution exposure and exhaled nitric oxide in an
elderly population. Thorax 2004; 59(3):204–209.

49. Hauser R, Elreedy S, Hoppin JA, Christiani DC. Upper airway response in
workers exposed to fuel oil ash: nasal lavage analysis. Occup Environ Med
1995; 52(5):353–358.

50. Steerenberg PA, Bischoff EW, de Klerk A, Verlaan AP, Jongbloets LM, Van
Loveren H, et al. Acute effect of air pollution on respiratory complaints,
exhaled NO and biomarkers in nasal lavages of allergic children during the
pollen season. Int Arch Allergy Immunol 2003; 131(2):127–137.

51. Hiltermann JT, Lapperre TS, van Bree L, Steerenberg PA, Brahim JJ, Sont
JK, et al. Ozone-induced inflammation assessed in sputum and bronchial
lavage fluid from asthmatics: a new noninvasive tool in epidemiologic
studies on air pollution and asthma. Free Radic Bid Med 1999; 27(11–12):
1448–1454.

52. Burnett RT, Dales R, Krewski D, Vincent R, Dann T, Brook JR. Associations
between ambient particulate sulfate and admissions to Ontario hospitals for
cardiac and respiratory diseases. Am J Epidemiol 1995; 142(1):15–22.

53. Schwartz J, Morris R. Air pollution and hospital admissions for cardiovascular disease in Detroit, Michigan. Am J Epidemiol 1995; 142(1):23–35.

54. Poloniecki JD, Atkinson RW, de LA, Anderson HR. Daily time series for
cardiovascular hospital admissions and previous day's air pollution in
London, UK. Occup Environ Med 1997; 54(8):535–540.

55. Schwartz J. Air pollution and hospital admissions for cardiovascular disease
in Tucson. Epidemiology 1997; 8(4):371–377.

56. Burnett RT, Cakmak S, Brook JR, Krewski D. The role of particulate size and
chemistry in the association between summertime ambient air pollution and
hospitalization for cardiorespiratory diseases. Environ Health Perspect 1997;
105(6):614–620.

57. Schwartz J. Air pollution and hospital admissions for heart disease in eight
U.S. counties. Epidemiology 1999; 10(1):17–22.

58. Prescott GJ, Cohen GR, Elton RA, Fowkes FG, Agius RM. Urban air pollution and cardiopulmonary ill health: a 14.5 year time series study. Occup
Environ Med 1998; 55(10):697–704.

59. Zanobetti A, Schwartz J, Gold DR. Are there sensitive subgroups for the
effects of airborne particles? Environ Health Perspect 2000; 108(9):841–845.

60. Schwartz J. Is there harvesting in the association of airborne particles with
daily deaths and hospital admissions? Epidemiology 2001; 12(1):55–61.

61. Sunyer J, Ballester F, Tertre AL, Atkinson R, Ayres JG, Forastiere F, et al.
The association of daily sulfur dioxide air pollution levels with hospital
admissions for cardiovascular diseases in Europe (The Aphea-II study).
Eur Heart J 2003; 24(8):752–760.

62. Hoek G, Brunekreef B, Fischer P, van Wijnen J. The association between air pollution and heart failure, arrhythmia, embolism, thrombosis, and other cardiovascular causes of death in a time series study. Epidemiology 2001; 12(3):355–357.

63. Zanobetti A, Schwartz J, Dockery DW. Airborne particles are a risk factor for hospital admissions for heart and lung disease. Environ Health Perspect 2000; 108(11):1071–1077.

64. D'lppoliti D, Forastiere F, Ancona C, Agabiti N, Fusco D, Michelozzi P, et al. Air pollution and myocardial infarction in Rome: a case-crossover analysis. Epidemiology 2003; 14(5):528–535.

65. Wong TW, Lau TS, Yu TS, Neller A, Wong SL, Tarn W, et al. Air pollution and hospital admissions for respiratory and cardiovascular diseases in Hong Kong. Occup Environ Med 1999; 56(10):679–683.

66. Peters A, Dockery DW, Muller JE, Mittleman MA. Increased particulate air pollution and the triggering of myocardial infarction. Circulation 2001; 103:2810–2815.

67. Muller JE, Abela GS, Nesto RW, Tofler GH. Triggers, acute risk factors and vulnerable plaques: the lexicon of a new frontier. [Review] [29 refs]. J Am Coll Cardiol 1994; 23(3):809–813.

68. Checkoway H, Levy D, Sheppard L, Kaufman J, Koenig J, Siscovick D. A case-crossover analysis of fine particulate matter air pollution and out-of-hospital sudden cardiac arrest. Cambridge, MA, USA: Health Effects Institute 2000; 99:1–34.

69. Levy D, Sheppard L, Checkoway H, Kaufman J, Lumley T, Koenig J, et al. A case-crossover analysis of particulate matter air pollution and out-of-hospital primary cardiac arrest. Epidemiology 2001; 12(2):193–199.

70. Spooner PM, Albert C, Benjamin EJ, Boineau R, Elston RC, George AL Jr, et al. Sudden cardiac death, genes, and arrhythmogenesis: consideration of new population and mechanistic approaches from a National heart, lung, and blood institute workshop, Part II. Circulation 2001; 103(20):2447–2452.

71. Spooner PM, Albert C, Benjamin EJ, Boineau R, Elston RC, George AL Jr, et al. Sudden cardiac death, genes, and arrhythmogenesis: consideration of new population and mechanistic approaches from a National heart, lung, and blood institute workshop, Part I. Circulation 2001; 103(20):2361–2364.

72. Dockery, D. W., Luttmann-Gibson, H., Rich, D. Q., Schwartz, J., Gold, D.R., Koutrakis, P., Link, M.S., Verrier, R. L., and Mittleman, M. A. Particulate Air Pollution and Non-fatal Cardiac Events Part II: Association of Particulate Air Pollution with Arrhythmias Recorded By Implanted Cardioverter Defibrillators. Health Effects Institute Research Report 124, 2005.

73. Dockery DW, Luttmann-Gibson H, Rich DQ, Schwartz J, Gold DR, Koutrakis P. Association of Particulate Air Pollution with Arrhythmias Recorded By Implanted Cardioverter Defibrillators. Health Effects Institute Research Report. In press.

74. Pope CA III, Dockery DW, Kanner RE, Villegas GM, Schwartz J. Oxygen saturation, pulse rate, and particulate air pollution. Am J Respir Crit Care Med 1999; 159:365–372.

75. Pope CA III, Verrier RL, Lovett EG, Larson AC, Raizenne ME, Kanner RE, et al. Heart rate variability associated with particulate air pollution [see comments]. Am Heart J 1999; 138(5 Pt 1):890–899.

76. Liao D, Creason J, Shy C, Williams R, Watts R, Zweidinger R. Daily variation of particulate air pollution and poor cardiac autonomic control in the elderly. Environ Health Perspect 1999; 107(7):521–525.

77. Gold DR, Litonjua A, Schwartz J, Lovett E, Larson A, Nearing B, et al. Ambient pollution and heart rate variability. Circulation 2000; 101(11): 1267–1273.

78. Peters A, Perz S, Doring A, Stieber J, Koenig W, Wichmann HE. Increases in heart rate during an air pollution episode. Am J Epidemiol 1999; 150(10): 1094–1098.

79. Magari SR, Hauser R, Schwartz J, Williams PL, Smith TJ, Christiani DC. Association of heart rate variability with occupational and environmental exposure to particulate air pollution. Circulation 2001; 104(9):986–991.

80. Pope CA III, Eatough DJ, Gold DR, Pang Y, Nielsen KR, Nath P, et al. Acute exposure to environmental tobacco smoke and heart rate variability. Environ 2001; 109(7):711–716.

81. Pekkanen J, Peters A, Hoek G, Tiittanen P, Brunekreef B, de Hartog J, et al. Particulate air pollution and risk of ST-segment depression during repeated submaximal exercise tests among subjects with coronary heart disease: the exposure and risk assessment for fine and ultrafine particles in ambient air (ULTRA) study. Circulation 2002; 106(8):933–938.

82. Peters A, Pope CA III. Cardiopulmonary mortality and air pollution [comment]. Lancet 2002; 360(9341):1184–1185.

83. Crystal RG. Alveolar Macrophages. In: Crystal RG, West JB, eds. The Lung. New York: Raven Press, Ltd., 1991:527–535.

84. Dye JA, Adler KB, Richards JH, Dreher KL. Role of soluble metals in oil fly ash-induced airway epithelial injury and cytokine gene expression. Am J Physiol 1999; 277(3 Pt 1):L498–L510.

85. Driscoll KE, Carter JM, Hassenbein DG, Howard BW. Cytokines and particle-induced inflammatory cell recruitment. Environ Health Perspect 1997; 105(suppl 5):1159–1164.

86. Tan WC, Qiu D, Liam BL, Ng TP, Lee SH, van Eeden SF, et al. The human bone marrow response to acute air pollution caused by forest fires. Am J Resp Crit Care Med 2000; 161(4 Pt 1):1213–1217.

87. Terashima T, Wiggs B, English D, Hogg JC, van Eeden SF. Phagocytosis of small carbon particles (PM10) by alveolar macrophages stimulates the release of polymorphonuclear leukocytes from bone marrow. Am J Respir Crit Care Med 1997; 155(4):1441–1447.

88. Peters A, Döring A, Wichmann HE, Koenig W. Increased plasma viscosity during air pollution episode: a link to mortality? Lancet 1997; 349: 1582–1587.

89. Pekkanen J, Brunner EJ, Anderson HR, Tiittanen P, Atkinson RW. Daily concentrations of air pollution and plasma fibrinogen in London. Occup Environ Med 2000; 57(12):818–822.

90. Schwartz J. Air pollution and blood markers of cardiovascular risk. Environ Health Perspect 2001; 109(suppl 3):405–409.
91. Peters A, Fröhlich M, Doring A, Immervoll T, Wichmann HE, Hutchinson WL, et al. Particulate air pollution is associated with an acute phase response in men. Eur Heart J 2001; 22(14):1198–1204.
92. Brook RD, Brook JR, Urch B, Vincent R, Rajagopalan S, Silverman F. Inhalation of fine particulate air pollution and ozone causes acute arterial vasoconstriction in healthy adults. Circulation 2002; 105(13):1534–1536.
93. Ibald-Mulli A, Stieber J, Wichmann HE, Koenig W, Peters A. Effects of air pollution on blood pressure: a population-based approach. Am J Public Health 2001; 91(4):571–577.
94. Linn WS, Gong H, Clark KW, Anderson KR. Day-to-day particulate exposure and health changes in Los Angeles area residents with severe lung disease. J Air Waste Manag Assoc 1999; 49:108–115.
95. Schwartz J. Harvesting and iong term exposure effects in the relation between air pollution and mortality. Am J Epidemiol 2000; 151(5):440–448.
96. Zeger SL, Dominici F, Samet J. Harvesting-resistant estimates of air pollution effects on mortality. Epidemiology 1999; 10(2):171–175.
97. Naghavi M, Libby P, Falk E, Casscells SW, Litovsky S, Rumberger J, et al. From vulnerable plaque to vulnerable patient: a call for new definitions and risk assessment strategies: Part II. Circulation 2003; 108(15):1772–1778.
98. Naghavi M, Libby P, Falk E, Casscells SW, Litovsky S, Rumberger J, et al. From vulnerable plaque to vulnerable patient: a call for new definitions and risk assessment strategies: Part I. Circulation 2003; 108(14):1664–1672.
99. Bateson TF, Schwartz J. Who is sensitive to the effects of particulate air pollution on mortality?: a case-crossover analysis of effect modifiers. Epidemiology 2004; 15(2):143–149.
100. Ritz B, Yu F, Chapa G, Fruin S. Effect of air pollution on preterm birth among children born in southern California between 1989 and 1993. Epidemiology 2000; 11(5):502–511.
101. Ritz B, Yu F. The effect of ambient carbon monoxide on low birth weight among children born in southern California between 1989 and 1993. Environ Health Perspect 1999; 107(1):17–25.
102. Ritz B, Yu F, Fruin S, Chapa G, Shaw GM, Harris JA. Ambient air pollution and risk of birth defects in southern California. Am J Epidemiol 2002; 155(1):17–25.
103. Schwartz J. Air pollution and children's health. Pediatrics. 2004; 113(4 suppl): 1037–1043.
104. Laden F, Neas LM, Dockery DW, Schwartz J. Association of fine particulate matter from different sources with daily mortality in six U.S. cities. Environ Health Perspect 2000; 108(10):941–947.

2

Particulate Dosimetry in the Respiratory Tract

WILLIAM D. BENNETT

Center for Environmental Medicine,
Asthma, and Lung Biology, University of
North Carolina–Chapel Hill,
Chapel Hill, North Carolina, U.S.A.

JAMES S. BROWN

National Center for Environmental
Assessment, Office of Research and
Development, U.S. Environmental
Protection Agency, Research Triangle Park,
North Carolina, U.S.A.

I. Introduction

Particulate air pollution has been linked to acute increases in mortality and morbidity primarily in the elderly, children, and those with pre-existing respiratory and cardiovascular disease (1,2). In the toxicological paradigm of

Exposure → Dose → Response

any, or all three of these factors may vary among individuals as they relate to ambient particulate air pollution. On the one hand, individuals can have variable *exposures* to ambient air pollution, e.g., depending on their activity

The U.S. Environmental Protection Agency (EPA) through its Office of Research and Development partially funded this chapter under EPA Cooperative Agreement CR829522 to the Center for Environmental Medicine, Asthma, and Lung Biology at the University of North Carolina-Chapel Hill. The views expressed in this chapter are those of the authors and do not necessarily reflect the views or policies of the EPA and no official endorsement should be inferred.

patterns. Susceptible individuals may also be predisposed towards an enhanced biological *response* to the particulate matter, e.g., a preinflamed or a developing lung, so that they have a different dose–response curve compared to healthy, young adults. On the other hand, individuals may also receive a variable *dose* of particulate matter to their lungs or other body organs that may enhance their susceptibility. In other words, susceptible individuals may be at a higher dose on the dose–response curve for ambient particulate toxicity. The dose of inhaled particulate matter is a function of both (1) deposition on lung surfaces as well as (2) clearance from those surfaces. Either or both processes may be altered in susceptible populations, leading to an enhanced dose. In the following chapter, we provide a general summary of the mechanisms associated with particle deposition and clearance in the normal lung and, in many cases, provide the reader with more detailed references on these mechanisms. We also emphasize the particle size dependence, coarse vs. fine vs. ultrafine, associated with these mechanisms. For each of these variables, i.e., particle deposition and clearance, we then illustrate how they may be modulated by individual susceptibility factors (e.g., age, gender, and pre-existing disease), physical activity, and coexposure to ambient gaseous pollutants.

II. Structure of the Respiratory Tract

The basic structure of the respiratory tract is illustrated in Fig. 1 (3). Air enters and exits the respiratory tract through the extrathoracic airways, i.e., the nose and mouth. During rest, the majority of inhaled air passes through the nose, which conditions the temperature and humidity of inhaled air. The distribution of respired air through the nose vs. the mouth changes as a function of activity (4–6). With heavy exercise as much as 70% of each breath may be respired through the mouth. As will be discussed later in this chapter, the partitioning of airflow between the nose and mouth ultimately affects the amount of inhaled particulate reaching the intrathoracic airways.

Weibel (7) provided a simplified description of intrathoracic airway structures. In this model, which begins with the trachea, the lung consists of 23 symmetric and dichotomously branching generations (z) of the airways. The number of airways in the z th generation of the lung is 2^z. Generations 0–16 compose the tracheobronchial region or conducting airways through which air is transported to and from the distal airways. The tracheobronchial region consists of bronchi ($0 \leq z \leq 8$) and bronchioles ($9 \leq z \leq 16$). Rings of cartilage maintain the shape and size of the bronchi and bronchioles to about the 12th generation. Cartilage tapers off toward the end of the tracheobronchial region and is completely gone by respiratory bronchioles ($z = 17$), where the pulmonary region begins. At the beginning of the pulmonary region, the airways are partially alveolated and are fully alveolated with the onset of the 20th generation.

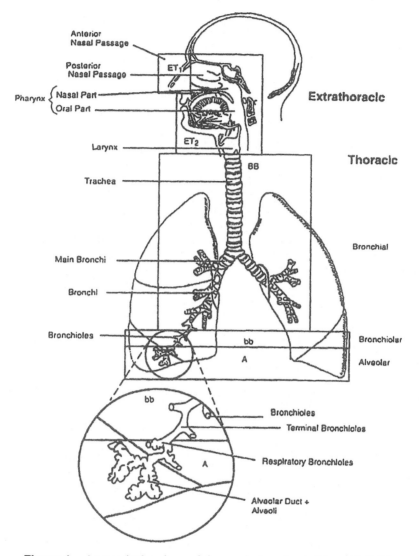

Figure 1   Anatomical regions of the respiratory tract. (From Ref. 3.)

Movement of air in the lung occurs by the combined actions of convection and diffusion. In the bronchi, convective motion of the air predominates. In the bronchioles, the total cross-sectional area of the airways rapidly increases, linear velocities decrease, and diffusion becomes an increasingly important mechanism of gas transport. The movement of air in the pulmonary zone of the lung is predominately by diffusion.

However, the diffusion coefficient (D) of respired air is $0.25 \, \text{cm}^2/\text{sec}$, whereas an extremely small $0.01 \, \mu\text{m}$ particle diameter only has a D of $5.8 \times 10^{-4} \, \text{cm}^2/\text{sec}$ at body temperature. Hence, the diffusion rate of the respired gases is at least 20 times faster that even a $0.01 \, \mu\text{m}$ particle. Thus, convective air flow remains an important transport mechanism for inspired aerosols in the pulmonary zone despite the low linear velocities.

III. Particle Deposition in the Respiratory Tract

The quantity and location of particle deposition in the respiratory tract depends on factors related to both the exposed individual and the inhaled particles. The mechanisms of deposition are, in large part, determined by the physical (size, shape, and density) and chemical (hygroscopicity and charge) characteristics of the inhaled particles (8). The general properties of particles, aerosol distributions, and particle kinetics in air are the topic of several texts (9,10). Particle deposition is also affected by biological factors such as breathing pattern (volume and rate), route of breathing (mouth vs. nose), and the anatomy of the airways.

A. Mechanisms of Particle Deposition

Particle deposition in the respiratory tract occurs primarily by three mechanisms: diffusion, impaction, and sedimentation. Impaction and sedimentation depend on a particle's aerodynamic diameter (d_{ae}), which is the size of a sphere of unit density that has the same terminal settling velocity as the particle of interest. Impaction occurs when a particle, due to its inertia, is unable to follow a change in flow direction, e.g., at airway bifurcations, and strikes an airway surface. Sedimentation occurs by the gravitational settling of particles to an airway wall. The deposition efficiencies for impaction and sedimentation in a region of the respiratory tract region are $d_{ae}^2 u$ (where u is the mean linear velocity within an airway) and $d_{ae}^2 t$ (where t is the mean residence time within an airway), respectively. More generally, since cross-sectional areas are not always known, the deposition efficiency for impaction is considered as a function of $d_{ae}^2 Q$ (where Q is inspiratory flow). Diffusive deposition takes place when a particle reaches an airway surface by random Brownian movement. Diffusion or more specifically a particle's diffusion coefficient, D, is a function of the physical diameter (d_p) of a particle. Particle density does not affect the diffusion coefficient. Diffusive deposition efficiency in a region of the respiratory tract is a function of $(Dt)^{0.5}$, where t is time in the region. The combined processes of diffusive and sedimentary deposition are important for particles in the range of $0.1–1 \, \mu\text{m}$. Impaction and sedimentation predominate above and diffusion predominates below this range (6,11).

Figure 2a–c illustrates the intrathoracic deposition of unit density (1 g/cm³) particles as a function of deposition mechanism for 5,1, and 0.1 μm diameter particles, respectively. As illustrated in this figure, impaction ocurs in the large proximal airways where linear velocities are high, whereas sedimentation and diffusion mainly occur in the smaller distal airways where residence time is long and the distance to an airway surface is short. Data in Fig. 2a–c were calculated using a mathematical particle deposition model (12) for a tidal volume of 750 mL (15 breaths/min) and Weibel's lung morphology scaled to a 3.4 L functional residual capacity (FRC). This mathematical model and others determine aerosol deposition in the lung based on the behavior of particles in air (13–20). In these models, particle diffusion and sedimentation occur on both inspiration and expiration, whereas impaction is generally considered an inspiratory event. Using physical models, however, Kim et al. (21) have demonstrated and mathematically described expiratory deposition by impaction. The inertial deposition of fine particles during expiration may be particularly important in the diseased lung (22) and may even occur in the healthy lung.

Other mechanisms of deposition are interception and electrostatic charge on particles.

Most important for fibers, interception will not be addressed here. Experimental and modeling analyses of fiber deposition are available elsewhere (23,24). Several studies have also examined the effect of particle charge on deposition in the lung (25–27).

B. Total Respiratory Deposition

Total or whole lung particle deposition refers to the fraction of inhaled particles deposited in the lung on a breath-by-breath basis. Experimentally, a lung deposition fraction for particles greater than a micron is most frequently measured by laser photometry (28). The deposition of ultrafine particles has most commonly been measured using condensation particle counting techniques (29,30). Empirical equations for whole lung deposition as a function of particle size and breathing pattern have been derived from analysis of numerous experimental studies (11). These individual factors (particle size and breathing pattern) account for much of the intra- and intersubject variability in particle deposition.

Particle size is one of the most basic parameters governing particle behavior and deposition in the lung. Particles between 0.3 and 0.7 μm diameter have minimal intrinsic mobility, i.e., they are large enough that their diffusive mobility is minimal but yet small enough that their sedimentation and impaction are also minimal (31,32). As a consequence, particles in this size range also have minimal deposition in the lung. Above and below this range of minimum deposition, the efficiency of deposition increases (11). Most environmental aerosols are polydisperse, i.e., they are composed of

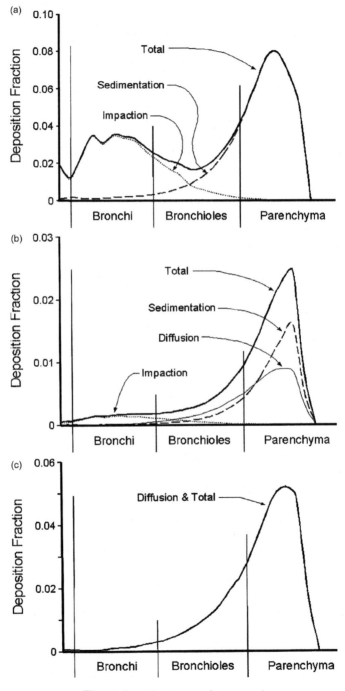

Figure 2   (*Caption on facing page*)

numerous sized particles. The distribution of particle sizes in an aerosol is typically log normal and may be described in terms of a median particle diameter and a geometric standard deviation (GSD) (9,10). Urban aerosols are commonly trimodal, comprised of three overlapping log normal distributions (nuclei, accumulation, and coarse modes) (33). Each mode of a typical urban aerosol is polydisperse with a GSD of between 1.7 and 2.15. By contrast, most experimental studies of particle deposition in the lung have used monodisperse particles (GSD < 1.15). Due to these differences between real world and experimental aerosol size distributions, deposition data for a given median particle diameter cannot be directly compared. The deposition of polydisperse aerosols in the lung may, however, be simulated by considering a series of monodisperse aerosols. The validity of this type of simulation has been tested in a physical model (34). In general, the deposition of a polydisperse aerosol in the lung is expected to be greater than that of a monodisperse aerosol for median particle diameters between 0.04 and 2 μm (13). For median particle diameters above 2 μm and below 0.04 μm, the polydisperse aerosol is expected to have less deposition than a monodisperse aerosol.

Hygroscopicity is the propensity for a particle to absorb water in a humid environment, thereby increasing its diameter. In the environment, hygroscopic aerosols include sulfates, nitrates, some organics, and aerosols laden with sodium or potassium (35). At near 100% relative humidity, the diameter of hygroscopic salt (NaCl) particles in the lung can increase by 3–6 times (36–38). For nonhygroscopic aerosols, minimal deposition in

---

Figure 2 (*Facing page*) (a) Predicted intrathoracic deposition of 5 μm diameter particles for a 750 mL tidal volume and 15 breaths per minute in Weibel's symmetric morphology scaled to a lung volume of 3375 mL. The respiratory tract regions are designated as bronchi, bronchioles, and parenchyma and refer to generations 1–8, 9–15, and 16–23, respectively. Deposition in the proximal airways occurs by impaction which increases with particle size and linear flow velocity. Sedimentation predominates in the distal airways where linear velocities are low and particle residence times are high. (b) Predicted intrathoracic deposition of 1 μm diameter particles. Details regarding breathing conditions, lung morphology, and respiratory regions are provided in (a). Note that the magnitude of the ordinate is decreased relative to (a), the total intrathoracic deposition (area under the curve) for the 5 μm particles was nearly six times greater than the 1 μm particles illustrated here. Impaction of 1 μm particles is minimal. Particle deposition occurs mainly in the distal lung by sedimentation and to a lesser extent by diffusion. (c) Predicted intrathoracic deposition of 0.1 μm diameter particles. Details regarding breathing conditions, lung morphology, and respiratory regions are provided in (a). The deposition of these particles occurs mainly in the distal airways by diffusion. The total intrathoracic deposition of these particles is approximately 2.4 times greater than that for the 1 μm diameter particles in (b).

the human lung occurs for 0.5 μm diameter particles (31,32). However, 0.5 μm diameter salt particles (dry) will grow in the lung to nearly 3 μm diameter particles which deposit to a far greater extent in the lung (36). For salt particles, the inhaled dry particle size having minimal deposition is actually only 0.08 μm because these particles grow into 0.5 μm particles (37,38). Hence, the effect of particle growth on deposition depends on the inhaled particle size. If the inhaled particles are less than 0.1 μm, an increase in particle diameter will decrease their diffusive mobility, thereby decreasing deposition efficiency (38). For inhaled particles greater than 0.5 μm, an increasing d_{ae} will increase deposition. Since deposition by sedimentation and impaction increases as a function of d_{ae}^2, a small increase in particle diameter can dramatically increase whole lung deposition. For particles between 0.1 and 0.5 μm, deposition will only be minimally affected unless growth beyond a diameter of 0.7 μm is achieved. The effects of particle growth and deposition in the lung have been modeled extensively (39,15,40).

Limited in vivo data suggest that a relatively small charge (50 electronic units) may increase the deposition of 0.5 μm particle by as much as 25% (relative increase) (41). In general, the level of charge must be increased with increasing particle size to achieve similar effects on deposition (27,41). For instance, 50 electronic units has a negligible influence on the deposition of 1 μm particles (27). However, relative increases in 1 μm particle deposition of 2.6- and 4-fold are predicted at 200 and 500 electronic units, respectively (27). Aerosols produced by nebulization carry a charge (9). As a source of experimental variability, nebulized aerosols may have increased deposition in the lung relative to charge neutralized aerosols. Charge on aerosols in either the workplace or urban environment has not been investigated but may affect respiratory deposition.

Breathing patterns vary between and within individuals with changes in tidal volumes, breathing rates, and the route of inhalation. The distribution of respired air through the nose vs. the mouth changes as a function of activity (4–6). Tidal volumes and breathing rates are also subject to changes with activity level (6), i.e., minute ventilation increases with activity. Stahlhofen et al. (11) performed a large cross-laboratory analysis and provided empirical equations for lung deposition as a function of breathing pattern and the route of inhalation for particles sizes from 0.005 to 15 μm. For a constant breathing period, deposition increases with increasing tidal volume. Under this scenario, as tidal volume is increased so too are respiratory flows which leads to increased impaction for $d_{ae} > 1$ μm. Additionally, increasing tidal volume causes a larger fraction of the breath and associated particles to reach the distal airways where deposition by both sedimentation and diffusion are enhanced. For a constant flow rate, the deposition of all particle sizes increases with tidal volume in large part due to the increase in residence time (42). For a fixed tidal volume, decreasing respiratory flows increases residence time and the deposition of fine and ultrafine particles ($d_{ae} < 3\,\mu m$). For coarse particles, $d_{ae} > 3\,\mu m$, decreasing respired flows (e.g., from 500 to 250 mL/sec) reduce the deposition efficiency from impaction and can cause a small reduction in total deposition. However, with further reductions in flow and associated increases in residence time, particle sedimentation quickly overcomes the drop in deposition by impaction. Some more recent data are available for multiple breathing patterns and particles sizes within the same subjects. Jaques and Kim (43) conducted an extensive particle deposition study in young healthy adults with six breathing patterns and the count median diameters (CMD) of 40, 60, 80, and 100 nm. The effect of breathing pattern on fine and coarse particle (d_{ae} of 1, 3, and 5μm) deposition has also been recently reported (44).

In most studies, particle deposition has been measured with fixed breathing patterns, i.e., each subject inhaled aerosol at the same tidal volume and breathing rate. Since particle deposition depends on breathing conditions, controlled breathing patterns were adopted as a necessary means of controlling intersubject variability. However, in reality, breathing patterns vary as a function of age, race, gender, activity, and respiratory health (6,45–48). Hence, for estimating the respiratory dose to an individual, it is important to know that individual's natural breathing pattern for the exposure conditions. Bennett et al. (45) measured deposition fraction of fine particles in healthy adults breathing at rest for realistic spontaneous breathing patterns determined by respiratory inductance plethysmography. They found that the fractional deposition of fine particles was best predicted by variability in (1) the breathing period *(T)* during aerosol inhalation, (2) airway resistance, and (3) expiratory reserve volume (ERV). Slower breathing increases deposition in the lung by time-dependent mechanisms, i.e., sedimentation or diffusion, consistent with deposition by sedimentation in the peripheral airspaces of the lung. Decreased caliber of the airways, i.e., increased airway resistance, affects deposition fraction by (1) decreasing the distances that particles have to settle or diffuse before depositing, and (2) increasing velocities and decreasing stopping distances for particles that inertially impact in the airways. Finally, increases in the FRC or the ERV in a given individual tends to decrease deposition fractions (49). This effect may be due to both a decrease in aerosol penetration into the lung periphery and/or an increase in mean airspace size with increased lung volume.

C. Regional Respiratory Deposition

Experimental data on the regional deposition of inhaled particles in man are available for the nose, mouth, tracheobronchial airways, and alveolar region. Deposition in the nose and mouth have been directly measured or calculated based on nose-in, mouth-out and mouth-in, nose-out breathing maneuvers. However, deposition in the tracheobronchial airways and alveolar region cannot be directly measured in vivo. The assumptions implicit in tracheobronchial and alveolar deposition data are relatively good for the healthy lung but not for the diseased lung. The potential limitations and error in regional deposition data should be recognized and are discussed further below.

The nose is a more effective filter than the mouth for preventing penetration of particles to the lower respiratory tract. Heyder et al. (49) showed that total deposition of 0.5–3μm particles is greater for nose than mouth breathing, i.e., a greater deposition efficiency for the nose vs. mouth. Very large (>5 μm aerodynamic diameter) and very small (<0.01 μm) particles are deposited very efficiently in the nose by inertial impaction and diffusion, respectively, during nasal breathing (17,50). For fine and coarse particles, the deposition efficiency of the nose has been shown to be proportional to the product d_{ae}^2 and the mean inspiratory flow rate (51,52). Kesavanathan et al. (53) recently showed in adults that nasal deposition efficiency for fine and coarse particles was increased with (1) increased flow rate, (2) increased ellipticity of nostril dimensions, and (3) decreased minimal cross-sectional area of the nasal passage measured by acoustic rhinometry. Interestingly, they also noted that African-Americans had less ellipticity of nostril dimensions than European-Americans, and thus there was a tendency for the latter to have greater nasal deposition efficiency. In contrast to these data for fine and coarse particle uptake by the nose, Cheng et al. (50) showed that ultrafine particle deposition in the nose decreased with increasing flow rate in adults. They also found that the intersubject variability in particle deposition was correlated with variation of nasal dimensions, also measured by acoustic rhinometry.

Though the mouth is less efficient than the nose at removing inhaled particles, Chan and Lippman (54) also showed that mouth deposition of fine and coarse particles is proportional to the square of particle aerodynamic size and flow rate. Also like nasal deposition, ultrafine particle deposition in the mouth increases with both decreasing particle size and flow rate (50). Based on data showing an increasing extrathoracic deposition with decreasing subject height (55), there is also likely a dependence on mouth size. Bowes and Swift (56) also showed that normal mouth breathing tends to give higher deposition of coarse particles than when the same subject breathes through a mouthpiece. Emmett and Aitken (57) showed that most of the extrathoracic deposition of coarse particles during mouth breathing occurs in the larynx. While losses in this region may still protect the lower respiratory tract, the larynx is also high in irritant receptor density and may be responsible for cough or neurally mediated bronchospasm responses associated with ambient particulate matter.

Most of the available data on tracheobronchial and alveolar deposition have been acquired using radiolabeled aerosols. In radioaerosol studies, the site of deposition is typically inferred from particle retention at

24-hr postinhalation under the premise that mucus clearance of the bronchial airways is complete by this time (58–62). However, when deposition and clearance are modeled in an asymmetric lung morphology, particle ($d_{ae} = 0.1$, 1, 2, and 7 μm) retention of 10–16% is predicted in the ciliated airways at 24 hr postinhalation (63). Using 24-hr retention as an index of regional deposition is even more problematic in the diseased lung, since even when deposition patterns are matched, whole lung and central airway clearance rates are reduced in obstructed patients relative to normals (64,65). Estimates of deposition in the tracheobronchial airways by 24-hr retention measurements may also be erroneously high in some studies due to leaching of the radiolabel from particles in the lung.

The tracheobronchial region consists of relatively large airways and small airways, i.e., the bronchi and bronchioles, respectively (Fig. 1). Relative to the bronchioles, linear velocities in the bronchi are high and residence time is short. Deposition in the bronchi occurs mainly by impaction and by diffusion, whereas deposition in the bronchioles occurs due to sedimentation and diffusion. In general, the deposition efficiency of fine and coarse particles in the tracheobronchial (TB) region increases in a sigmoidal fashion with log (d_{ae}) from a few percent at $d_{ae} = 1$ μm to nearly 100% at $d_{ae} = 10$ μm (11). Due to deposition in the extrathoracic airways (particularly during nasal breathing), however, the deposition fraction of particles in the TB region begins to decrease above d_{ae} of 5 μm for a relatively high inspiratory flow of 500 mL/sec (1000 mL tidal volume). With decreasing d_p below 0.1 μm, deposition in the TB region also increases (11,66,67). Other indices of large central airway deposition vs. peripheral deposition are the central-to-peripheral ratio (C/P) (60,62,64) and penetration index (PI) (68,69). Unlike 24-hr retention data, which rely on the function of pulmonary clearance mechanisms for data interpretation, this method is based on the premise that there are more large airways distributed toward the interior (hilar) regions of lung images than the exterior areas of these images. As indicated by a reduction in PI, hygroscopic growth shifts particle deposition proximally within central airways (69,70).

More recently, a bolus technique has been used to estimate tracheobronchial and alveolar deposition (66,71,72). The bolus technique of determining the deposition site assumes that: (1) inhaled air moves as a plug through the airways, (2) the filling and emptying of parallel pathways is uniform and synchronous, and (3) the structure of the lung is generally symmetric. However, even in young healthy adults, there is some asymmetry in filling and emptying of the lung as demonstrated by a "volumetric shift" in a bolus between inspiration and expiration (73). Using a radiolabelled aerosol, left–right asymmetry in the pattern of bolus deposition in the lung has also been reported (74,75). The effects of asynchronous filling and emptying on inhaled boluses increase with bronchoconstriction (76) and respiratory disease (77,78). A further limitation of the regional deposition data derived from this bolus technique was the adoption of rigid volume definitions of respiratory regions (upper airways, 0–50 mL; tracheobronchial region; 50–150 mL; alveolar region, > 150 mL) (66,72). Further, identical bolus volumetric penetrations into the lung were used for all subjects regardless of their size. As a general rule, an individual's anatomic dead space in milliliters is roughly equal to their height in centimeters. Similarly, lung volume in adults is known to depend on height, gender, race, and age (6,79). Even for a matched height and age, women have smaller lungs and airway dimensions than men (6,79,80). Hence, the utility of regional data based on the bolus technique could have been enhanced by adjusting bolus penetrations and regional volume definitions to anatomical dead space. As the data exist, estimates of tracheobronchial deposition are artificially increased (due to inclusion of respiratory bronchioles and alveoli) with decreasing anatomical dead space, e.g., the tracheobronchial region (50–150 mL) includes more anatomically distal airways in women than in men.

Sedimentation and diffusion mainly occur in the smaller distal airways where residence time is long and the distance to an airway surface is short. Across all particle sizes, alveolar deposition increases with increasing tidal volume and decreasing flow, i.e., alveolar deposition is favored by slow-deep inhalations. In general, the deposition efficiency for most particle sizes less than d_{ae} of 3–4 μm and natural breathing patterns is greater for the alveolar region than the TB region of the lung (see Fig. 2a–c). For d_{ae} greater than 3–4 μm, the efficiency of deposition due to impaction in the TB region can exceed the efficiency of sedimentation in the alveolar region. Due to deposition in the extrathoracic airways (particularly during nasal breathing) and TB region, the deposition fraction of particles in the alveolar region decreases for d_{ae} > 3 μm for a relatively high inspiratory flow of 500 mL/sec (1000 mL tidal volume) (11). For a more modest flow (250 mL/sec), deposition fraction of particles in the alveolar region decreases at a slightly larger d_{ae} of between 3 and 5 μm (11). Hence, the proximal removal of particles dramatically affects deposition in the alveolar region.

Despite generally higher deposition efficiencies in the alveolar vs. tracheobronchial regions of the lung for coarse, fine, and ultrafine particles under resting breathing conditions, the actual surface concentrations are much higher in the large airways due to the smaller surface areas associated with these airway generations. Figure 3 illustrates the predicted dose rate per airway surface area as a function of airway generation based on the same model predictions shown in Fig. 2a–c for each particle size. This dose rate is based on the particle deposition fraction, the minute ventilation of the subjects, and a representative ambient particulate concentration of 100 μg/m³. Certainly, such an ambient concentration is more likely for the coarse mode than the ultrafine mode particles. Yet, these predictions illustrate that, while deposition efficiencies for these three particle sizes are higher in the lung parenchyma (Fig. 2a–c), the highest surface

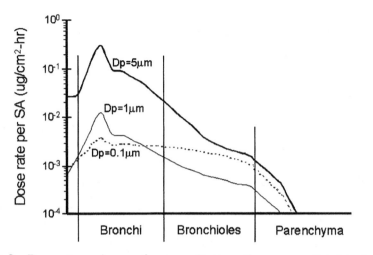

Figure 3   Dose rate per lung surface area. Data are the mass predicted to deposit per lung surface area per hour of exposure to $100\,\mu g/m^3$ of particles having the sizes specified in the figure. Details regarding breathing conditions, lung morphology, and respiratory regions are provided in Fig. 2a. The deposition fractions for these particles are illustrated in Fig. 2a–c.

concentration of deposited particles occurs in the large, bronchial airways, as much as 3 orders of magnitude higher than what occurs in the parenchyma. From this dosimetry perspective, it might be expected, then, that the epithelium of the bronchial airways is most susceptible to toxicological effects from inhaled, ambient particulate matter. Furthermore, these surface dose estimates may provide some linkage to in vitro studies where particulate matter is distributed on small surfaces of airway epithelial cells to assess various toxicological responses.

D. Effect of Physical Activity on Particle Deposition

When individuals increase their ventilation during exercise, the total number of particles inhaled obviously increases, but the fractional deposition may also be altered depending on the change in breathing pattern that occurs. During exercise, both tidal volume and breathing frequency increase. As discussed previously, fractional deposition of particles of all sizes increases with increased tidal volume but decreases with increased frequency of breathing. Thus, it may be expected that the change in deposition fraction with exercise will vary among individuals, depending on the relative influences of these two variables for a given subject. The lung deposition fractions of fine particles during moderate exercise and mouth breathing are unchanged between rest and exercise (81,82). Heyder et al. (83) found that the deposition fraction for 1–7 µm particles increased by 33% for spontaneous breathing following exercise vs. spontaneous breathing at rest, but their subjects increased their ventilation following exercise primarily by increasing tidal volume rather than breathing frequency. These studies suggest that the total deposited dose of particles will generally increase in direct proportion to the increase in minute ventilation associated with exercise. One of the difficulties with all these studies, however, is that neither spontaneous breathing on a mouthpiece nor controlled breathing conditions truly reflect spontaneous breathing conditions associated with either rest or exercise (45). Several investigators have shown that spontaneous mouthpiece breathing is much different from unencumbered breathing (i.e., without mouthpiece) at rest and for various levels of activity (84,85). In addition, individuals typically breathe through their nose while at rest, switching to oronasal breathing as ventilation increases (4,5). The role of the nose in filtering particles is diminished as airflow is diverted from the nose to the mouth during exercise, bringing more particles to the lower respiratory tract. Thus, it is likely that particle deposition within the lower respiratory tract actually increases in greater proportion to the increase in ventilation with exercise.

As discussed previously, the changes in ventilation, i.e., breathing pattern and flow rate, associated with exercise may alter the regional deposition of particles. Coarse particle deposition increases in the tracheobronchial and extrathoracic regions during exercise due to the increased flow rates and associated impaction. A rapid-shallow breathing pattern during exercise may result in more bronchial airway vs. alveolar deposition, while a slow-deep pattern will shift deposition to deeper lung regions (86). Bennett et al. (81) showed, for 2.6 µm particles, that moderate exercise shifted deposition from the lung periphery towards extrathoracic and larger, bronchial airways. Similarly, Morgan et al. (82) showed that even for fine particles (0.7 µm) tracheobronchial deposition was enhanced with exercise. Again, this shift in deposition toward the bronchial airways results in a much greater dose per unit surface area of tissue in those regions (Fig. 3). As discussed previously, during resting breathing, particles deposit preferentially in the basal regions of the lung. Morgan et al. (82) found that the apical-to-basal distribution of fine particles increased with exercise, i.e., a shift towards increased deposition in the lung apices. This shift may be less likely for larger particles, however, whose deposition in large airway bifurcations may preclude their transport to these more apical regions (81).

E. Effect of Gender on Particle Deposition

Because males and females have different conducting airway sizes (87) and ventilatory parameters (88), it might be expected that there would be gender differences in total and regional deposition of particles. For a fixed breathing pattern, whole lung deposition in adult females is significantly increased relative to males across a large range of inhaled particle sizes, e.g., 0.04, 2, 3, and 5 μm (43,45,72). In these studies, men and women were breathing at the same tidal volume and frequency. From the analysis of detailed deposition patterns measured by the serial-bolus mouth-delivery method, Kim and Hu (72) and Jaques and Kim (43) found a marked enhancement in deposition in the very shallow region (lung penetration depth <150 mL) of the lungs in females. This enhanced local deposition for both ultrafine and coarse particles was attributed to a smaller size of the upper airways, particularly the larynx. Though it also may be that females, having a generally smaller anatomic dead space than males (87), bring more of the fixed bolus volume of particles into the deep lung where they deposit in alveoli. Contrary to the gender differences in large airway caliber the alveolar dimensions are not different between males and females (89). Using particles in the 2.5–7.5 μm size range, Pritchard et al. (90) indicated that, for comparable particle sizes and fixed inspiratory flow rates, females had higher extrathoracic and tracheobronchial deposition and smaller alveolar deposition than males. Again, these differences were attributed to gender differences in large airway size but they were also obtained for fixed inspiratory flow conditions.

Since males and females have different minute ventilations and associated breathing patterns, Bennett et al. (45) also measured fine particle deposition in males and females as they breathed the aerosol with a pattern previously determined by respiratory inductance plethysmography in each individual at rest (47), i.e., their normal resting breathing pattern. Under these more realistic conditions, there was still a tendency for a greater deposition fraction in females compared to males that could be attributed to slightly higher airway resistances in the females. But, because males had greater minute ventilations than females, the deposition rate (i.e., deposition per unit time) was greater in males than in females (about 30%). However, in terms of deposition per unit area of lung tissue, there was much less of a difference between the genders, though still a tendency for males to receive a higher dose. In summary, it appears that females may have increased deposition per unit surface area in the largest airways, and particularly the larynx, due to their smaller caliber, but less deposition per unit surface area in the deeper lung due to smaller minute ventilations.

F. Effect of Age of Particle Deposition

While few deposition data are available, both lung growth and changes in breathing patterns with age from child to adult may affect the fractional deposition of inhaled particles. The dimensions (diameters and lengths) of the airways are thought to increase during childhood as a function of height (91). Less is known about development of the alveolated airspaces, but they appear to remain relatively constant during childhood, increasing only slightly in size as the lung matures to its adult size (92). Breathing patterns also change with increasing age; i.e., tidal volumes increase and respiratory rates decrease (47,93). Based on these data, particle deposition models predict less deposition in the pulmonary region but greater tracheobronchial deposition in children as compared to adults, resulting in little difference in total deposition fraction between children and adults for nearly all inhalable particles (14). A recent study by Schiller-Scotland et al. (94), however, found higher deposition (about 50%) of fine particles (1–3 μm) in children (age 3–14) compared to adults for spontaneous breathing on a mouthpiece. The reported minute ventilation of these children was much higher than might be expected (93), breathing more deeply than normal on the mouthpiece apparatus (85,93) and thus contributing to an increased deposition fraction in these children (45). In contrast, Bennett and Zeman (95) measured deposition fraction of inhaled, fine ($d_{ae} = 2\mu m$) particles in children as they breathed the aerosol with a pattern previously determined by respiratory inductance plethysmography in each individual at rest (47,93), i.e., that child's "real" resting breathing pattern. Among the children, variation in deposition fraction was not dependent on subject age or height, but was highly dependent on intersubject variation in tidal volume. Unlike the Schiller-Scotland et al. (94) study they found no difference in deposition fraction for the children vs. adults for these fine particles. This finding and the modeling results (14) are in part explained by the smaller tidal volume and faster breathing rate of children relative to adults for natural breathing conditions. On the other hand, the rate of deposition normalized to lung surface area tended to be greater (35%) in the children vs. the combined group of adolescents and adults for resting breathing of these particles (95). This increase in deposition rate per surface area in the children was due to their higher minute ventilation in relation to their lung volume. Furthermore, within children (age 6–14), there is a dependence of minute ventilation and tidal volume on body size (96). These most recent data suggest that for a given height and age, children with higher body mass index (BMI) have larger minute ventilations and tidal volumes at rest than those with lower BMI. These differences in breathing patterns as a function of BMI translated into increased deposition of fine particles in the heaviest children.

There are limited data on the regional deposition of particles within the respiratory tract of children. As discussed previously, the first line of defense for protecting the lower respiratory tract from inhaled particles is the nose and mouth, and the mode of breathing, i.e., oral vs. nasal, influences the quantity of particles penetrating to the lung. In limited studies, it has been shown that children (age 7–16) tended to have more oral breathing both at rest and during exercise and also displayed more variability than adults (97,98). In contrast to adults, there is little data on the uptake of particles for oral or nasal breathing in children. Theoretical calculations by Xu and Yu (20) predict enhanced deposition of particles (greater than 2 μm) in the head region for children when compared to adults. Studies of fine particle deposition in physical models of the nose, scaled to adult vs. children sizes, predict that deposition efficiency in the nose is a function of pressure drop across the nose (99). Consequently, these model analyses suggest that, when properly scaled physiological flows are used in the calculation of nasal deposition, children, who have higher nasal resistance than adults, should have higher nasal deposition compared to adults. Surprisingly, the one study reporting measures of nasal deposition in children, found lower nasal deposition efficiencies for fine particles (1–3 μm MMAD) as compared to adults, despite their higher nasal resistances (100).

As adults age, even under healthy conditions, changes in breathing patterns and airway structure may also influence deposition in the lung. Using respiratory inductance plethysmography to measure spontaneous breathing patterns, Tobin et al. (47) found no difference in tidal volume and frequency between young (mean age 29) and old (mean age 69) subjects with normal lung function. The impact of airway caliber on particle deposition may be more important with increasing age in adults. Even in the non-diseased lung, loss of lung recoil with age may lead to a narrowing of small airways in the lung (101). On the other hand, alveolar dimensions tend to increase with age due to loss of lung tissue (102). Bennett et al. (45), however, showed there was no effect of age on the whole lung deposition fraction of fine particles (2 μm) for realistic spontaneous breathing conditions in adults with normal lung function aged 18–80. Across all subjects, the deposition fraction was found to be independent of age, depending solely on breathing pattern and airway resistance. In those same adults breathing with a fixed pattern, they did observe a mild decrease in the whole lung deposition of fine particles as a function of age, which could be attributed to increased peripheral airspace dimensions in the elderly.

G. Effect of Respiratory Tract Disease on Particle Deposition

The mechanisms of deposition in the diseased lung are the same as in the healthy lung. Yet to a greater extent than either age or gender effects, airway structure and breathing patterns with lung disease are considerably varied from normal. Changes in airway geometry, especially associated with obstructive lung disease, may have a dramatic effect on total deposition efficiency. Patients with chronic obstructive pulmonary disease (COPD) breathe at higher resting minute ventilation, using different breathing patterns than individuals with normal lungs (48). Bennett et al. (103) showed that COPD patients receive on average 2.5 times the deposited dose of fine particles (2 μm) at rest than an age-matched healthy cohort. The deposited dose in COPD increased (as much as five times normal) with increasing airway obstruction (as determined by airway resistance measures). While much of the increase in deposited dose was attributable to the airway narrowing in these individuals, some of the increase (about 50% on average) was due to their increased resting minute ventilation compared to healthy individuals. Furthermore, patients characterized as generally chronic bronchitic, rather than emphysematous, had the greatest increase in total deposition. The enlargement of peripheral airspaces associated with emphysema tended to decrease total deposition efficiency. Similar findings under realistic breathing conditions were recently observed for ultrafine particles (< 60 nm) (46), i.e., greater deposition fractions in bronchitic vs. emphysematous and healthy subjects and greater deposited dose in all patients compared to healthy controls. Kim and Kang (104) reported deposition fractions of 1 μm particles inhaled via the mouth by healthy adults and by those with various degrees of airway obstruction, smokers, smokers with small airway disease (SAD), asthmatics, and patients with COPD breathing under the same controlled breathing pattern. Deposition was 16%, 49%, 59%, and 103% greater in smokers, smokers with SAD, asthmatics and people with COPD, respectively, than in healthy adults. Deposition fraction was found to be inversely correlated with percentage predicted forced expiratory volume (FEV1) and forced expiratory flow (FEF25–75%). Increased deposition fractions in COPD (46,105,106) and asthmatics (107) compared to normal have also been observed for ultrafine and coarse particles under controlled breathing conditions. Anderson et al. (105) showed that the largest increase in deposition fraction from normal was greatest for the largest particles studied, 129% for 0.24 μm vs. only 15% for 0.02 μm particles. Regional deposition patterns within the lung are also significantly affected by airway obstruction. Dolovich et al. (68) found that alveolar deposition of 3 μm particles was decreased and tracheobronchial deposition increased for smokers and patients with chronic obstructive lung disease compared to normal that correlated with their degree of obstruction. The same effect has been observed in asthmatics for 3.6 μm particles (108). A shift of particle deposition from alveolar regions, in the normal lung, to the conducting airways in the patient with obstructive lung disease results in a greatly enhanced dose per surface area of lung tissue in this latter group. Smaldone and Messina (22) also showed enhanced airway deposition of fine particles in COPD patients with chronic expiratory flow limitation that was further enhanced by coughing in these individuals. Model and animal experiments suggest that this enhancement of particle deposition is highly localized to airway surfaces immediately downstream to sites of flow limitation (e.g., segmental and subsegmental bronchi) (109,110). In fact, such "hot spots" of particle deposition have been observed in severely obstructed patients by gamma scintigraphy for a variety of particle sizes (111–115). A recent study by Pellegrino et al. (116) clearly illustrated this effect in asthmatics as they were challenged with three increasing doses of methacholine to compare the pattern of fine particle deposition in the lung with the occurrence of expiratory flow limitation (Fig. 4). As maximal expiratory flow was reduced following increasing doses of methacholine, particle deposition became less uniform with increasing occurrence of "hot spots," presumably at sites of airway obstruction and expiratory collapse. While these authors used a Technegas aerosol, the particles associated with this generation technique are generally aggregates of ultrafine particles, forming particles in the fine particle mode (117). Regional deposition of ultrafine particles (< 60 nm) seems less associated with such "hot spots" in COPD patients (46).

As illustrated in Figure 4, when asthmatics with hyperreactive airways develop acute bronchospasm, fine and coarse particle deposition also shifts towards proximal airways, away from the lung periphery (116,118–120). A variety of stimuli, gaseous copollutants or particles themselves, in the ambient pollutant mix may induce bronchospasm in these individuals. As a

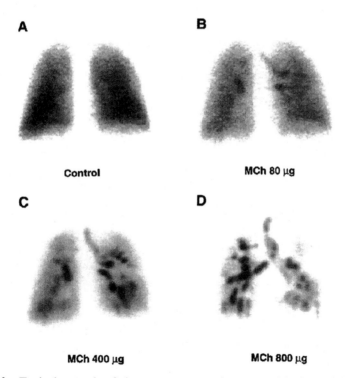

Figure 4   Typical example of planar posteroanterior scans of the lungs in a subject after inhaling Technegas while tidal breathing from FRC on day 1 (control; A) and after increasing doses of methacholine (MCh) (B–D). Note the enhanced distribution of the Technegas in the central areas of the lungs even with the smallest dose of constrictor agent. (From Ref. 116.)

result, the particulate dose to the bronchial airways may be further enhanced (Fig. 3), potentially amplifying the response to an inhaled particulate stimulus. While there are no data in asthmatics illustrating this effect for exposures to realistic ambient pollutant stimuli, the effects of pharmacologic stimuli (e.g., methacholine) support such a claim (118). Foster et al. (121) showed a slight increase in total particle deposition ($d_{ae} = 3 \mu m$) in healthy subjects following acute exposure to ozone but no detectable shift in site of deposition. Presumably, this response might be more pronounced in asthmatics who have more profound bronchial responsiveness to high ozone concentration exposures (122).

Relative to healthy individuals, individuals with obstructive lung diseases also have marked ventilatory inhomogeneity. While the obstructed airways in such patients likely receive an increased particle dose, the preferential ventilation of "healthy" regions within the obstructed lung may also result in an increased surface dose within these alveolar regions (123). Published data on the association between ventilation distribution and fine particle deposition have shown inconsistent results, viz. a positive, negative, or lack of association between these variables. A trend for increasing aerosol ($d_{ae} = 0.78 \mu m$) deposition with increasing ventilation to a region has been reported in normal healthy individuals and asymptomatic smokers (124). On the other hand, increased particle deposition in poorly ventilated lung regions has been reported for aerosols in the $0.5–1.0 \mu m$ size range and attributed to increased residence time in obstructed lung regions (125,126). However, others, using similar sized aerosols, have found no association between ventilation distribution and particle deposition (127). Brown et al. (128) recently found that coarse particle (5 μm) deposition in the peripheral lung regions of cystic fibrosis patients followed ventilation patterns as measured by xenon-133 washout. However, in these same patients, there was increased coarse particle deposition within the bronchial airways of poorly ventilated lung regions. This was in sharp contrast to the association between particle deposition within the airways of healthy subjects, which followed regional ventilation. Their results suggest that airways within poorly ventilated regions may receive a high surface dose of coarse particles, while the parenchyma of these regions will receive less deposition than the parenchyma of well-ventilated lung regions. Similar analyses, i.e., assessing parenchymal vs. tracheobronchial deposition as a function of ventilation, for other particle sizes and disease states have not been done. But preliminary evidence for ultrafine particle deposition suggests that these very small particles follow ventilation patterns fairly closely, primarily depositing in the lung periphery of both healthy and obstructed subjects (46,129).

While particle deposition is modulated by the presence of obstructive lung disease as discussed above, other respiratory tract diseases may also alter total and regional deposition. Cystic fibrosis, like chronic bronchitis and asthma, is associated with increased fine particle deposition in the airways and inhomogeneities of deposition within the lung compared to normal (65,77,130). Patients with restrictive lung disease show no difference from normal for fine and ultrafine particle deposition fractions (105). Studies in an animal model of pulmonary fibrosis suggest inhomogeneous deposition with less deposition in fibrotic regions of the lung. Finally, while there is no human data on particle deposition in pneumonia, Jakab and Green (131) showed in a mouse model of viral pneumonia that subsequently inhaled bacterial particles (3.5 μm) deposited more in noninfected regions of the lungs, likely due to the better ventilation to these areas.

IV. Particle Clearance and Translocation from the Respiratory Tract

A. Mechanisms and Pathways of Clearance

Once deposited on an airway surface, a number of factors affect a particle's clearance from the lung, including site of deposition, particle solubility, and epithelial integrity. Regional deposition of inhaled particles within extrathoracic, tracheobronchial, or alveolar compartments of the respiratory tract was discussed in the previous section. The biological variability and susceptibility factors associated with the regional deposition of particles were also discussed previously. As with deposition, there are a number of factors that can modulate clearance from the respiratory tract that will be discussed further below. Particle solubility refers to solubility within the respiratory tract fluids and cells. A poorly soluble particle is one whose rate of clearance by dissolution is insignificant compared to its rate of clearance as an intact particle. Thus, all particles may clear by solubilization as well as by physical transport, the relative contributions of each will depend on the particle's solubility. The integrity of the airway epithelium can affect both transepithelial absorption of particulate matter as well as the functioning of the mucociliary transport system. The epithelium's integrity can be affected by inflammation associated with airway disease and/or copollutant exposures, resulting in modulation of particle clearance.

The mechanisms and pathways by which a particle clears from an airway surface are dependent on the region of the respiratory tract in which the particle deposits. The various mechanisms associated with each region are outlined in Table 1 and can be categorized as either (1) physical particle transport, by mucociliary action or transepithelial into the lymphatic system, or (2) absorptive, dissolution of material and subsequent clearance into the lymphatics or bloodstream. These mechanisms and pathways may occur simultaneously or with temporal variations as a particle moves from one region to another. This chapter will not detail the biology associated with these mechanisms, except where such details may be relevant to associated alterations in particle clearance.

Table 1 Mechanisms and Pathways of Particle Clearance within the Respiratory Tract

Extrathoracic region (ET)
  Mucociliary transport
  Sneezing
  Nose wiping and blowing
  Dissolution and absorption into blood
  Swallowing
Tracheobronchial region (TB)
  Mucociliary transport
  Coughing
  Endocytosis by macrophages/epithelial cells
  Dissolution and absorption into blood/lymph
Alveolar region (A)
  Macrophages, epithelial cells
  Interstitial translocation
  Dissolution and absorption into blood/lymph

Source: Modified from Ref. 132.

Clearance from the extrathoracic region of the respiratory tract primarily refers to particles initially deposited in either the nasal passages or the mouth. Anderson and Proctor (133) have provided a thorough review of nasal physiology and particle clearance pathways in the nose. Poorly soluble particles deposited in the posterior portions of the nasal passages are cleared by mucociliary transport towards the nasopharynx and swallowed. Similar particles depositing in the anterior portion of the nasal passages are cleared forward towards the nasal vestibule, where their removal occurs by sneezing, wiping, or blowing. Soluble material deposited on the nasal epithelium may access underlying cells via diffusion through the mucus, but may also move within the mucociliary transport system [as evidenced by the frequent use of the saccharine test to study nasal mucociliary transport (134)]. Dissolved substances reaching epithelial surfaces may also be subsequently translocated into the bloodstream depending on their molecular size. The nasal passages have a rich vasculature, and uptake of soluble matter into the blood from this region may occur rapidly. Some have suggested that ultrafine or nanoparticles may be transported across the nasal epithelium, possibly via olfactory nerves, finding their way into brain tissue (135). Quantification of such movement relative to the deposited dose of ultrafines in the nasal passages has not been elucidated, however, so that its toxicological relevance is unclear.

Clearance of poorly soluble particles deposited in the oral passages is by coughing and expectoration or by swallowing into the gastrointestinal tract. Such clearance may be partially dependent on the rate of salivary production and ability to swallow (136). Whether reduced clearance of particulates from the oral cavity has toxicological relevance to inhalation of ambient particulate matter is unclear. Palmer et al. (136) suggested that reduced oral clearance may be a major risk factor for the colonization of potentially pathogenic organisms in the mouth, a well-known risk factor for the development of pneumonia. As such, bacteria associated with ambient particulate matter may be similarly affected.

Within the tracheobronchial region of the lung, insoluble particles will tend to clear more rapidly by mucociliary clearance if they deposit more proximally (i.e., closer to the mouth) in the bronchial tree (11,60). This is presumably due to the fact that (1) they have less distance to travel, and (2) the rates of mucus transport are fastest in the trachea, becoming progressively slower in more distal airways [summarized by Wanner et al. (137)]. Consequently, ambient particles that escape deposition in the extrathoracic airways will tend to deposit more proximally with increasing aerodynamic size above 0.5 μm and therefore be expected to clear the lung more rapidly (11). A thorough review on the physiology of mucociliary clearance has been provided by Wanner et al. (137). Although clearance from the TB region is generally believed to be rapid (hours to days), there is experimental evidence that a fraction of material deposited in the TB region is retained much longer than 24 hr, a period commonly used as the outer range of clearance time for particles within this region (138–140). More recent data suggest that this slow-clearing tracheobronchial compartment is likely associated with bronchioles < 1 mm in diameter (141–143). The mechanism of long-term TB retention is not clear. However, both a less continuous mucus layer with distal progression into the TB region (144), and movement of particles into the sol phase due to surface tension forces in the liquid lining of the small airways (145,146) may play a role in a slow phase of TB clearance. These particles may be engulfed by airway macrophages, the existence and number of which have been observed in a number of species including humans (147). In animal models, a large percentage of particles found in the airways 1–2 hr after inhalation were already within macrophages (148–150). These findings have been interpreted to suggest that particle uptake by airway macrophages plays a role in the slow phase of TB clearance (151), though a direct connection between these two phenomena has not been established. There is no evidence that free, insoluble particles within the TB region clear at a faster (or slower) rate than those within airway macrophages.

It has also been suggested that poorly soluble particles may traverse the tracheobronchial epithelium by endocytotic processes, entering the peribronchial region. Ultrafine particles, because of their small size, may more easily penetrate the airway epithelium and cause cellular damage (152). Using electron microscopy to examine rat tracheal explants treated with fine (0.12 μm) and ultrafine (0.02 μm) TiO_2 particles for 3 or 7 days, Churg et al. (152) found both sized particles in the epithelium at each time point, but in the subepithelial tissues, they were found only at day 7, and the ratio of epithelial to subepithelial particles was greater for fine than ultrafine particles. Whether or not such transepithelial movement within the TB region accounts for a significant transport of insoluble particles in vivo is not clear however, since the action of mucociliary clearance may remove many of these particles over the period of 3 or 7 days. There is evidence that long-term TB retention patterns are nonuniform, with an enhancement at airway bifurcations (153), probably the result of both greater deposition and less effective mucus clearance within these areas. Thus, doses calculated based on uniform surface retention density may be misleading, especially if the material is slow acting toxicologically. In fact, Churg and Stevens (154) found an association between particles retained in certain airway walls and occurrence of lung cancer in those lobes.

It is clear, however, that soluble particles can be absorbed through the airway epithelium into the blood, though likely at a slower rate than from the alveolar compartment (155,156). Bronchial blood flow may have a modulating effect on this clearance, as decreased bronchial blood flow has been shown to result in increased airway retention of soluble particles (157). There is considerable evidence as well that soluble particles are also cleared by mucociliary transport (155,157–160). The relative contribution of their removal by transepithelial absorption vs. mucociliary clearance is likely a function of both the molecular size and water or lipid solubility of the material (159,161–163). Furthermore, the rate of mucociliary transport for soluble particles may be less than that of insoluble particles (160). Consequently, non permeating hydrophilic solutes may remain in contact with the airway epithelium for a longer period than insoluble particles. This may be due to diffusion of a greater portion of the solute into the periciliary sol layer which may be transported less efficiently than the mucus layer during mucociliary clearance.

Finally, clearance from the airways by coughing is important in various lung diseases where mucociliary clearance has been compromised (164). In fact, in some patients, such as those with primary ciliary dyskinesia, clearance of mucus and associated particles from the airways would be insignificant without cough (165). The relative importance of cough clearance in various lung disorders will be discussed further in the section on modulation of clearance mechanisms by lung disease. Leith et al. (164) provide a detailed summary of the mechanisms by which cough may be effective at enhancing mucus clearance, but depth of airway fluid, rheological properties of the fluid, and local airflow characteristics all play a role. While cough and its frequency likely contribute little to clearance of particles under healthy conditions, cough has been shown to transiently stimulate mucociliary clearance in the normal lung (166).

Particles that deposit in the alveolar region of the respiratory tract are generally retained longer (months to years) than those are deposited in the

TB region. Species comparison of alveolar clearance kinetics for relatively insoluble particles using what limited data are available for humans (167,168) suggest that alveolar clearance rates in humans are much slower (an order of magnitude) than other species, particularly rodents (which are commonly used in toxicological testing). Furthermore, there appears to be a particle size dependence for the rate of alveolar clearance, i.e., particles larger than 5 μm clear much slower than fine particles in rats and dogs (169,170). In addition, ultrafine particles (0.02 μm) also clear slower than fine particles (0.2 μm) of the same material (titanium dioxide) in rats (171,172).

Clearance from the alveolar region occurs via a number of mechanisms and pathways, a detailed description of which is provided by Kreyling and Scheuch (151). Most evidence suggest that particle removal by macrophages residing on the alveolar epithelium is the main nonabsorptive clearance process in this region. Alveolar macrophages phagocytize and transport deposited material that they contact by random motion or via directed migration under the influence of chemotactic factors. The factors influencing recognition and interaction between macrophages and particles have been thoroughly reviewed by Valberg and Blanchard (173). Lay et al. (174) showed that by 1-day postinstillation of iron oxide particles (2.6 μm CMD) in humans, more than 90% of lavageable particles were contained in alveolar macrophages, i.e., less than 10% free particles were observed. Similar observations have been made in animals for inhalation of particles (175,176). While some particles may be transported to regional lymph nodes (177,178) or become sequestered in the pulmonary interstitium/epithelium (especially at high particulate lung burdens), the vast majority of particles are thought to eventually leave the lung as intracellular particles within alveolar macrophages, predominantly by the tracheobronchial route (179,180). Thus, particle clearance is intimately linked to egress of alveolar macrophages from the lung while the movement of free particles towards the TB ciliated airways likely plays little role in alveolar clearance. The time for clearance of particle-laden alveolar macrophages via the mucociliary system may depend on the site of uptake in relation to the distal end of the ciliated airways. Macrophage migration towards the mucociliary escalator is unlikely due to random motion, but more likely is controlled by chemotactic and biological mediators (173,181). The relative differences in path length between alveolar structures and the mucociliary escalator (182) may also play a role for the species differences observed in alveolar clearance kinetics. Furthermore, macrophage uptake of particles may also be size dependent (173,183,184) and thus may also affect the observed particle size dependence of alveolar clearance kinetics. For example, it has been suggested that smaller ultrafine particles (< 0.02 μm) of TiO_2 are less effectively phagocytosed than larger ones and as a consequence clear the lung more slowly than fine TiO_2 particles (185).

The importance of insoluble particle transport across the epithelium is also likely species dependent, seemingly accounting for a small portion of transport in rodents but a larger fraction in dogs (151). Without any similar data in humans, one might presume that this pathway is similar in relative importance to that of dogs, given their similar alveolar clearance rates. While particle uptake by epithelial cells may play some roles in this pathway, it is also believed that alveolar macrophages laden with particles migrate from the alveolar epithelial surface into the interstitium (151), at least for fine and coarse insoluble. Ultrafine particles, that may be less easily recognized and phagocytosed by macrophages, were found to more readily enter the pulmonary tissue and translocate to hilar lymph nodes than fine particles of the same material (186). Such particles may be taken up by epithelial cells for transport to the interstitium. The mechanisms associated with epithelial uptake of particles have been reviewed by Churg (187). The role that such transport might play in acute responses to ambient particulate matter is unclear and is likely more important for chronic, occupational particle exposures or "overload" conditions. In such cases, the alveolar macrophages may reach their limits of phagocytosis resulting in a greater mass of free particles that may move across the epithelial barrier (163).

Particle dissolution and eventual transport into the bloodstream can occur in alveolar fluid, for readily soluble materials that are either hydro- or lipophilic, or within alveolar macrophages for less soluble materials. The rate of absorption across the epithelium for materials that dissolve in the alveolar lining fluid is fairly rapid (minutes to hours) and is a function of their molecular size and their water or lipid solubility (161–163,188). Absorption of lipophilic compounds that pass easily through cell membranes is perfusion limited and thus generally occurs very rapidly. However, if lipophilic materials are adsorbed onto insoluble particles, their retention in the lung may be prolonged (189). Such a case was observed with benzo-a-pyrene adsorbed onto inhaled carbon particles (189). Clearance of hydrophilic solutes is limited by diffusion rate and pore sizes associated with intercellular tight junctions (estimated at 0.6–1.5 nm). Diffusional clearance of hydrophilic solutes is inversely related to solute molecular weight. In addition to diffusion through intercellular junctions, transcellular transport of large solutes by pinocytosis in epithelial cells has also been observed (190). Once a particle is phagocytosed by an alveolar macrophage, it may slowly dissolve and be released from the cell to move across the epithelium into the bloodstream. The dissolution rate is inversely related to particle size and directly related to specific surface area (151). Particle dissolution is facilitated by the acidic environment of the phagolysosome (pH 4.3–5.3), especially for metal oxides (191).

Recent interest has focused on ambient ultrafine particles as being especially toxic, particularly as they may be associated with observed cardiovascular effects of ambient particulate matter. Part of the impetus for this attention is based on dosimetric evidence that these particles may easily penetrate the alveolar epithelium into the bloodstream. While soluble material may easily diffuse from airway surfaces into the bloodstream as a function of molecular size (161), the ability for insoluble nanoparticles to do the same is not clear. As discussed above, lung retention of ultrafine insoluble particles (e.g., titanium dioxide) appears to exceed that of fine particles (172) in rats, for either instillation or inhalation, suggesting that such particles, while they may translocate to the interstitium, do not rapidly translocate into the bloodstream. In contrast, Oberdörster et al. (192) recently reported effective translocation of ultrafine elemental carbon (C13) particles to the liver by 1 day after inhalation exposure in rats, though they acknowledge that transport from the GI tract need also be considered. They also suggested that such translocation to blood and extrapulmonary tissues may be different between ultrafine carbon and other insoluble (metal) ultrafine particles. This was borne out by additional studies in rats showing particle translocation of $< 1\%$ of deposited, insoluble iridium particles into secondary organs such as liver, spleen, heart, and brain (193). Nemmar et al. (194) recently reported rapid clearance of instilled albumin nanoparticles (80 nm) from the lungs to the bloodstream of hamsters (25–30% in 5 min), presumably by rapid diffusion across the pulmonary epithelium. By contrast, Peterson et al. (195) compared the clearance of aerosolized Tc99m-DTPA (molecular weight $= 492$ Da molecular size $= 0.6$ nm), Tc99m-human serum albumin (molecular weight $= 69$ KDa, molecular size $= 3.6$ nm) and Tc99m-aggregated albumin (molecular weight $= 383$ KDa, approximate molecular size $= 20$ nm) delivered to the lungs of sheep, the latter tracer similar to that used by Nemmar et al. (194). For the case of aggregated albumin, Peterson et al. (195) found clearance of the tracer was described well by single compartment exponential loss at a rate of 0.04 % per minute over an 80 min period of observation (less than 5% lung clearance during that time). Even the rate constant for the smallest tracer (DTPA) was only 0.4% per minute with less than 10% clearance in 30 min. These aerosol data in sheep are inconsistent with the observations of Nemmar et al. (194), i.e., 25–30% translocation in 5 min after instillation of aggregated albumin in presumably healthy hamsters (a rapid rate of 5–6% per minute).

There are limited data on the kinetics of ultrafine particle clearance from the lungs of humans. A number of investigators have used Technegas (radiolabeled carbon particles) (196–200) as an ultrafine aerosol in these studies. There are two difficulties with the use of Technegas for such experiments. Firstly, while the primary particles associated with this aerosol generation technique may be ultrafine (20 nm or less), they can rapidly aggregate into much larger, fine particles (200 nm), depending on the dilution rate and period of time allowed before inhalation. Secondly, with as little as 0.2% O_2 concentration in the generator, the technique may produce significant portions of Pertechnegas, a soluble form of the aerosol for which the radiolabel Tc99m is not firmly attached to the carbon and can readily diffuse into the bloodstream. Recently, Nemmar et al. (196) detected activity in the blood at 1 min post inhalation of a Technegas aerosol in healthy subjects that reached a maximum between 10 and 20 min. Thin layer chromatography of blood showed that in addition to a species corresponding to oxidized Tc99m, i.e., pertechnetate, there was also a species corresponding to particle-bound Tc99m, yet there was no quantification of this species relative to what was inhaled and deposited in the lung. Nor was there a control inhalation or intravenous injection of pertechnetate to determine if it would bind to circulating proteins in vivo that might correspond to the observed particle bound Tc99m after inhalation. While their gamma camera images showed substantial radioactivity over the liver and other areas of the body, whether this was the soluble or insoluble form of the particles was not clear. Xu et al. (197) reported Pertechnegas contamination of Technegas in their clearance study of patients and healthy volunteers. These investigators noticed the contamination because of thyroid visualization and rapid clearance during the first 20 min after inhalation. The rapid clearance rates (half time of about 10 min) found by Xu et al. (197) are quite similar to the Pertechnegas half times reported by Monaghan et al. (198) and Isawa et al. (199) in healthy subjects. Interestingly, Monaghan et al. (198) provided a whole-body scan illustrating organ uptake of Pertechnegas, which appears remarkably similar to the whole-body scan from Nemmar et al. (196) with high amounts of activity evident in the bladder, stomach, thyroid, and salivary glands. Based on the organ uptake reported by Nemmar et al. (196) and rapid pulmonary clearance rates inferred from their findings, the bulk of the lung clearance that they observed was very likely that of pertechnetate ionized from Pertechnegas and not that of radiolabeled ultrafine particles. In contrast to Nemmar et al. (196), the Technegas pulmonary retention reported by Roth et al. (117) was 95% and by Isawa et al. (200) was 98% at 45 min postinhalation when care was taken to eliminate the soluble form of the aerosol, Pertechnegas. Similarly, after accounting for the soluble portion of Tc99m in an ultrafine aerosol (activity median diameter of 60 nm) generated by sparking electrodes, Brown et al. (46) found in healthy subjects a mean retention of 85% at 24 hr postinhalation. Unlike the findings of Nemmar et al. (196) in humans and Oberdörster et al. (192) in rats, they were also unable to find any accumulation of activity in the region of the liver over a 2 hr period postinhalation. Similarly, Roth et al. (201) found greater than 90% lung retention 24 hr post deposition for a very insoluble indium oxide ultrafine particles (18 and 27 nm) in healthy humans. Based on deposition models, the 10% or less that cleared during that 24 hr period could be explained by tracheobronchial deposition for these particle sizes, suggesting little or no translocation of these insoluble particles into the bloodstream.

B. Effects of Age on Particle Clearance

While there is little evidence for age-related differences in clearance of insoluble or soluble particles from the respiratory tract, the limited data suggest enhanced clearance with age from child to adult, and slowed clearance from young adult to elderly.

Salivary clearance from the oral cavity is often abnormal in the aged and was shown to be related to colonization with pathogenic bacteria (136). They found that salivary clearance was not reduced by aging per se but by iatrogenic sources such as drug therapy for other diseases (e.g., antidepressants that tended to dry the mouth).

In newborn lambs, tracheal mucus velocity was shown to be about 25% of adult values, increasing to those of adults (24 weeks) by 8 weeks of age (202). A similar postnatal increase in mean tracheal mucus velocity was observed in dogs (203). Whether these observations in other mammals apply to humans are not clear. Use of radioactive tracers for assessing clearance, and the associated radiation exposure, has made such studies in healthy infants and children impractical. In adults, tracheal and bronchial clearance rates of insoluble particles have been shown to be reduced in elderly nonsmokers compared to younger nonsmokers (204–206).

Few studies have investigated age effects on alveolar clearance of particles. Antonini et al. (207) demonstrated that advanced age in rats is associated with alterations in lung defense mechanisms and increased susceptibility to pulmonary bacterial infection, slowed pulmonary bacterial clearance, and altered AM function. Similarly, impaired clearance of pneumococcal aerosols by neonatal rats was associated with an age-dependent deficiency in numbers of resident alveolar macrophages (208). Whether or not a similar age-dependent depression in macrophage-mediated clearance of particulate matter in either rats or humans is not clear. In humans, the clearance of water soluble particles (Tc99m-DTPA) from the alveolar epithelium has been shown to be slowed with increasing age (209,210). However, Tankersley et al. (211) recently showed enhanced permeability of soluble particles (Tc99m-DTPA) in terminally senescent mice just before death, suggesting that a disintegration of the epithelial barrier may be a feature of lung homeostatic loss during this period of terminal senescence.

C. Effect of Physical Activity on Particle Clearance

Previous discussion on the effect of exercise on particle deposition illustrated that fine and coarse particles may deposit more proximally in the respiratory tract when ventilation rates are increased. This mouthward shift in particle deposition results in more rapid clearance from the lung (60,81). But additionally, once deposited, exercise has been shown to enhance particle clearance from the bronchial airways (212). Sweeney et al. (213) also showed in hamsters that exercise enhanced clearance of insoluble particles from the alveolar region. Their data may be explained by findings that breathing with an increased tidal volume also increased the rate of insoluble particle clearance from the alveolar region (214). These authors suggested that the distension-related transport of surfactant into proximal airways may have facilitated movement of particle-laden macrophages or uningested particles. On the other hand, Valberg et al. (215) found no effect of CO_2-stimulated hyperpnea on pulmonary clearance of fine particles in dogs, so increased ventilation, per se, may not affect clearance. It may be that endocrine and blood flow changes associated with exercise are required to affect clearance (213). The role of alveolar macrophages in exercise-induced effects on alveolar clearance is unclear. In mice, it has been shown that severe exercise enhances phagocytic function of alveolar macrophages (216), but in trained horses phagocytosis was impaired (217). Finally, the transepithelial transport rates of soluble particles, Tc99m-DTPA, have also been found to increase during exercise (218,219). This enhancement was linked to increases in tidal volume associated with exercise (218). Regionally, this effect was dominated by increased apical lung clearance and attributed to an increase in apical blood flow (219). While enhanced clearance of insoluble particles acts to reduce dose to airway tissue, increased transport of soluble matter into the bloodstream may enhance effects on extrapulmonary organs.

D. Effect of Respiratory Tract Disease on Particle Clearance

A variety of lung diseases affect insoluble and soluble particle clearance at various sites along the respiratory tract. Nasal mucociliary clearance is slowed in those with chronic sinusitis (220), allergic rhinitis (221), as well as those with cystic fibrosis (222).

As discussed previously, differences in deposition of particles used to assess mucociliary clearance (11,60) may occur between normal individuals and those with disease which would in turn, affect the measured clearance. Thus, evaluation of bronchial airway clearance in individuals with lung disease requires careful interpretation of results. A number of investigators have shown that insoluble particles clear more slowly from the airways of patients with chronic obstructive lung disease than from healthy airways (206,223–225). This occurs despite the fact that, due to their obstructive lung disease, particles tend to deposit in more proximal airways in these patients. It seems clear that this slowing is a result of chronic exposure to cigarette smoke and is worse in those with chronic sputum production (206,224). There are also data to suggest that the presence of chronic expiratory flow limitation in the large, bronchial airways of these patients contributes to regional, local impairment at these sites (226,227). As discussed earlier, these sites of flow limitation may also be associated with high, localized deposition of particles (227). Mucociliary clearance also appears to be impaired to a mild degree in stable asthma (228–230), especially once differences in deposition patterns between asthmatics and healthy individuals were considered. During acute exacerbations in these patients, mucociliary clearance is severely impaired but is reversible after hospitalization and associated steroid and bronchodilator treatment (231). Slowed mucociliary clearance is also associated with acute respiratory infections. Camner et al. (232) were able to detect slowed whole lung clearance in patients infected with influenza, a virus at 1 week following onset of symptoms independent of cough. Puchelle et al. (233) showed that chronic bronchitic patients (all exsmokers) with purulent sputum (reflecting ongoing infection) had significantly lower mucociliary clearance rates than patients with nonpurulent sputum. In all these cases of bronchial airway disease discussed above, coughing may serve as an adjunct to particle clearance (234) from the airways but as lung function continues to decline cough, also, may become less effective (235).

Clearance rates of relatively insoluble iron oxide particles from the alveolar region of the lung were found reduced in humans with chronic obstructive lung disease (236,237), with one study showing that the decrease in clearance rate was correlated with the pack years of smoking in their COPD patients (237). In a rat model of emphysema, no difference in alveolar clearance was observed compared to control rats (238), but copresence of inflammation in a hamster model of emphysema did result in prolonged retention of particles (239). Moller et al. (237) also found slowed alveolar clearance in patients with sarcoidosis and idiopathic pulmonary fibrosis. In mice and calves, it has been shown that acute inflammation induced by influenza virus impaired fine, insoluble particle clearance from the deep lung (240–242). This impaired alveolar clearance may be associated with airway lesions disrupting the mucociliary clearance pathway or viral-induced decreased viability and phagocytic function of alveolar macrophages (240,243). Both airway and alveolar macrophages in asthmatics have depressed phagocytic capability (244,245) but how these findings may relate to retarded short-or long-term clearance in asthmatics is unclear. Similarly, Madl et al. (246) showed that macrophage chemotaxis was impaired in a rat model of pulmonary hypertension leading these authors to speculate that such a condition may lead to impaired particle clearance from the lung. The increased retention associated with acute inflammation may also be due to particle translocation into the interstitium through a damaged epithelial barrier. Adamson and Prieditis (247) recently showed that when silica (<0.3 μm) was instilled into lungs of mice having alveolar epithelial damage (as evidenced by increased permeability), particles were found to more readily reach the interstitium and lymph nodes.

Because the integrity of the epithelial surface lining of the lungs may be damaged from lung disease, particles (either insoluble or soluble) may gain greater access to the interstitium, lymph, and bloodstream. Damage to the epithelial barrier is most likely to acutely affect transepithelial transport rates of soluble particles. From bronchial biopsies, Laitinen et al. (248) found various degrees of epithelial damage, from loosening of tight junctions to complete denudation of the airway epithelium, in asthmatics. Consistent with these findings, Ilowite et al. (229) found that asthmatics had increased permeability of the bronchial mucosa to the hydrophilic solute Tc99m-DTPA (Fig. 5). On the other hand, a more recent study in a sheep model showed that the presence of bronchial edema could slow the uptake of soluble DTPA into the blood and enhanced retention in the airways, likely within the expanded interstitial barrier (249). Both a leaky epithelial barrier and expanded interstitial barrier associated with asthma may result in enhanced exposure of submucosal immune and smooth muscle cells to xenobiotic substances. Alveolar epithelial permeability was also shown affected by the presence of lung inflammation. The most common finding has been a clear increase in alveolar permeability induced by cigarette

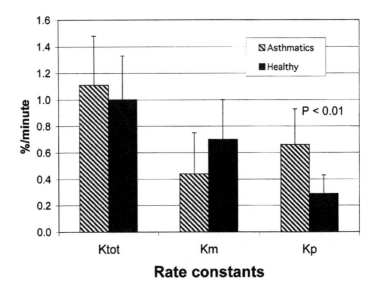

Rate constants

Figure 5 Rate constants for total clearance of hydrophilic solute Tc99m-DTPA (K_{tot}), mucociliary clearance of solute Tc99m-albumin, and calculated clearance of Tc99m-DTPA due to transepithelial absorption. Total clearance rates (K_{tot}) for soluble DTPA are not different between healthy and asthmatic subjects. Because the mucociliary component of DTPA clearance tends to be depressed in the asthmatics (as deduced from Tc99m-albumin clearance, K_m), the rate of transport across the epithelium (K_p) is enhanced in these patients. (Data from Ref. 229.)

smoking (250). This effect appears to be somewhat reversible in that the permeability of exsmokers may return towards normal in those with lesser increase from normal to begin with (251). In fact, Huchon et al. (252) demonstrated that COPD patients who have stopped smoking have normal clearance of Tc99m-DTPA. In general, increased alveolar permeability to Tc99m-DTPA has been found to be associated with any lung syndrome characterized by pulmonary edema. While the transalveolar transport of a small solute like DTPA is very sensitive to even mild acute lung injury (such as that associated with even mild cigarette smoking), increased transport rates of larger molecules (>100 KDa) across the alveolar epithelium require more severe damage like that seen in adult respiratory distress syndrome (ARDS) (195,253). The same study that showed decreased clearance of insoluble cesium oxide particles following influenza infection also showed a virus-induced enhancement of clearance for a soluble cesium chloride (241). Finally, more recently, as evidence of lung complications associated with noninsulin dependent diabetes patients, Lin et al. (254) found impairment of alveolar integrity as shown by increased transport rates of both hydrophilic and lipophilic solutes from the lungs in these patients. Interestingly, diabetics are another group recently shown to have increased susceptibility to particulate air pollution (255).

To summarize the general effects of respiratory disease on particle clearance from the lung, it seems clear that chronic lung inflammation results in prolonged retention of insoluble particles on the airway epithelium. By contrast, as particles solubilize, the particulate matter is more likely to permeate the airway epithelium to interact with interstitial tissue and gain access to the bloodstream. Thus, in patients with compromised lungs, ambient, deposited particles may have longer retention times in the lung with slow dissolution and eventual release of potential toxins. Diffusable toxins may interact with underlying lung tissue and/or penetrate into the bloodstream to produce systemic effects.

E. Effect of Ambient Pollutants on Particle Clearance

Coexposure of ambient particulate matter with other gaseous pollutants or the particles themselves may alter their retention in the lung. Inhaled irritants (e.g., ozone, sulfur dioxide, acid aerosols, and cigarette smoke) have been shown to effect rates of mucociliary clearance in both humans and experimental animals (137,256,257). Acute exposures to these irritants generally tend to enhance mucociliary clearance of particles, especially at low concentrations (256), but chronic exposures generally lead to a retarded clearance as the airway epithelium becomes damaged. One of the best examples of these effects can be seen in the numerous studies regarding cigarette-smoke exposure. Short-term effects of cigarette smoking show speeding to retardation depending on the number of cigarettes smoked (258,259). On the other hand, as discussed previously, chronic exposure to cigarette smoke invariably leads to slowed mucociliary clearance such as that seen in chronic bronchitis (206,223–225). One of the most common gaseous pollutants to exist in combination with particulate matter is ozone. It also has been shown to acutely enhance rates of mucociliary clearance in humans (260) but this acute, irritant effect seems transient (261). As was the case for cigarette smoke, however, long-term exposure and higher doses in animals show that ozone causes mucociliary dysfunction and a slowing of particle clearance (262). Increased uptake of insoluble particles by airway epithelial cells induced by ozone exposure may play a role in this slowed clearance (263). Sulfur dioxide, another common copollutant with particulate matter, also causes impairment of mucociliary clearance following long-term exposure to relatively low levels (264). Relatively high levels of NO_2 are required to impair mucociliary clearance (e.g., 6 ppm for 6-week exposure) (265). Sulfuric acid particles seem to produce variable effects, from accelerated to depressed clearance, depending on particle size, concentration, and relative acidity (266,267). More importantly, for ambient pollutant conditions, when mixtures of gases such as ozone and sulfur dioxide are combined for long exposures, there seems to be an additive effect on the retarding of mucociliary clearance (268,269). In fact when rats were exposed to the "real world" ambient, urban air of Sao Paulo, Brazil for 6 months, they were observed to have decreased rates of mucociliary clearance (270). Once again, this slowing of particle clearance from airway surfaces may prolong retention of potentially harmful toxins to interact with and damage lung tissue.

Alveolar clearance rates for insoluble particles have also been shown to be affected by acute or chronic exposures to ambient pollutants (271). As with mucociliary clearance, the pattern of these effects on alveolar clearance seems to be initial acute speeding followed by chronic depression. Alterations in alveolar macrophage function by these pollutants may play a role in the observed effects since a number of irritants have been shown to impair numbers and phagocytic capability of these cells (272). As discussed previously, prolonged retention of particles is associated with long-term cigarette smoking (263,273). While smoking has been shown to increase numbers of alveolar macrophages, their functionality is compromised by chronic exposure to cigarette smoke (274,275). Acute exposure of animals to ozone or NO_2 also produces a depression of phagocytosis (272) that may translate into increased retention of insoluble particles (271). The integrity of the alveolar epithelium is also disrupted by copollutants so that soluble components of inhaled particles can more easily enter the interstitium and bloodstream. Like cigarette smoke discussed previously, acute exposure of humans to 0.4 ppm ozone and intermittent exercise has been shown to alter epithelial integrity and increase clearance of soluble hydrophilic particles from the alveolar surfaces of the lung (276), an effect

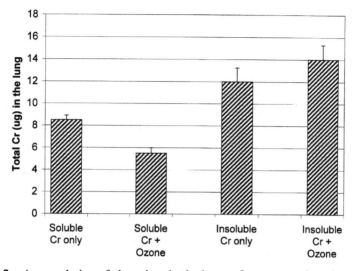

Figure 6   Accumulation of chromium in the lungs of rats over a 2 week period for inhalation in a relatively soluble form, potassium chromate, vs. a more insoluble form, barium chromate ($360\,\mu g/m^3$). In each case of chromium exposure, a group of rats were coexposed to 0.3 ppm ozone. The presence of ozone significantly decreased accumulation of soluble chromium in the lung while it significantly increased accumulation of the insoluble form. (Modified from Ref. 279.)

found in humans to be still present 24 hr postexposure to even low concentrations of ozone (277). Similarly, 0.8 ppm exposure for 2 hr in rats shows increased permeability to macromolecules at all levels of the respiratory tract (277) that persisted in the alveolar region beyond 24 hr postexposure.

In general, coexposure to irritant pollutants results in a disruption of epithelial integrity and macrophage function which, on the one hand, retards mucociliary and alveolar clearance, but also may allow for a more rapid movement of soluble constituents across the epithelial surface into the interstitium and bloodstream. Cohen et al. (279) may have best illustrated these competing effects by showing that coexposure to ozone affected the retention of inhaled chromium in rats differently depending on its solubility (Fig. 6). In its soluble potassium chromate form, ozone decreased the retention of chromium, but when chromium was inhaled as insoluble barium chromate, its retention was increased by ozone coexposure.

V.   Summary

The dose of inhaled particulate matter depends on both (1) deposition on lung surfaces and (2) clearance from those surfaces. Particle deposition in the lung varies with particle size, breathing patterns, and airway geometry. Total deposition efficiency of particles in the respiratory tract increases (1) as particle size increases from 0.5 to 10 μm mass median aerodynamic diameter and (2) as particle size decreases from 0.5 μm to ultrafine 0.01 μm particles. While minimal deposition efficiency occurs in the 0.1–1.0 μm range, it is important to remember that many ambient particles in this size range are hygroscopic, growing to larger sizes as they enter the respiratory tract, enhancing their deposition efficiency. Sites of deposition in the lung shift to more proximal airways as particle size increases from 0.5–10 μm and as particle size decreases in the ultrafine range (0.1–0.04 μm), enhancing local tissue doses in the lung several fold.

Once a particle deposits on an airway surface, a number of factors affect its clearance from the lung, including site of deposition, particle solubility, uptake by macrophages, and epithelial integrity. Insoluble particles will tend to clear more rapidly by mucociliary clearance if they deposit more proximally (i.e., closer to the mouth) in the bronchial tree. Because larger particles tend to deposit more proximally, they would be expected to clear the lung more rapidly. While rapid transepithelial movement of soluble particulate matter constituents into the bloodstream likely occurs, similar clearance of substantial numbers of ultrafine, insoluble particles from the lung is not supported by present data.

Altered dosimetry in susceptible populations may play a role in the observed mortality/morbidity associated with exposure to urban particulate matter. For example, changes in airway geometry and ventilation distribution associated with COPD results in enhanced deposition of particles. Furthermore, the regional deposition patterns in COPD patients are very nonuniform in the lung, i.e., "hotspots" associated with airway deposition, further enhancing dose per surface area several fold in these patients. Insoluble particles clear more slowly from the lungs of COPD patients than from healthy lungs, further enhancing particle dose in COPD compared to normal. While smokers and asthmatics also show a slowed clearance of insoluble particles, they also exhibit a speeding of clearance for soluble particles. This is likely due to a disruption of epithelial integrity which, on the one hand, retards mucociliary clearance, but also allows a more rapid movement of soluble constituents across the epithelial surface into the interstitium and bloodstream. Finally, copollutants such as ozone also enhance movement of soluble particles across the epithelium into the bloodstream. Rapid movement of soluble, toxic particle constituents into the bloodstream may translate into extrapulmonary effects of particulate matter.

Acknowledgments

The authors would like to express appreciation to Kirby Zeman, Ph.D., for his invaluable help in preparing this chapter.

References

1. Schwartz J, Dockery DW. Increased mortality in Philadelphia associated with daily air pollution concentrations. Am Rev Respir Dis 1992; 145:600–604.
2. Pope CA, Dockery DW. Acute health effects of PM10 pollution on symptomatic and asymptomatic children. Am Rev Respir Dis 1992; 145:1123–1128.
3. Raabe OG. Respiratory exposure to air pollutants. In: Swift DL, Foster WM. Air Pollutants and the Respiratory Tract. New York, NY: Marcel Dekker, 1999:39–73.
4. Bennett WD, Zeman KL, Jarabek A. Nasal contribution to breathing with exercise: effect of race and gender. J Appl Physiol 2003; 95:497–503.
5. Niinimaa V, Cole P, Mintz S, Shephard RJ. The switching point from nasal to oronasal breathing. Respir Physiol 1980; 42:61–71.
6. International Commission on Radiological Protection. Human Respiratory Tract Model for Radiological Protection. Oxford: Pergamon Press; ICRP Publication 66. Ann. ICRP 1994; 24(1–3).
7. Weibel ER. Morphology of the Lung. New York: Academic, 1963.
8. Agnew JE. Physical properties and mechanisms of deposition of aerosols. In: Clarke SW, Pavia D, eds. Aerosols and the Lung. London: Butterworth, 1984:49–70.
9. Reist PC. Aerosol Science and Technology. 2nd ed. New York: McGraw-Hill, 1993:Inc.
10. Hinds WC. Aerosol Technology: Properties, Behavior and Measurement of Airborne Particles. 2nd New York: John Wiley & Sons, 1999.
11. Stahlhofen W, Rudolf G, James AC. Intercomparison of experimental regional aerosol deposition data. J Aerosol Med 1989; 2(3):285–308.
12. Martonen TB, Katz IM. Deposition patterns of aerosolized drugs within human lungs: effects of ventilatory parameters. Pharm Res 1993; 10(6):871–878.
13. Diu CK, Yu CP. Respiratory tract deposition of polydisperse aerosols in humans. Am Ind Hyg Assoc J 1983; 44:62–65.
14. Hofmann W, Martonen TB, Graham RC. Predicted deposition of nonhygroscopic aerosols in the human lung as a function of subject age. J Aerosol Med 1989; 2(1):49–68.
15. Martonen TB. Analytical model of hygroscopic particle behavior in human airways. Bull Math Biol 1982; 44:425.
16. Yeh HC, Schum GM. Models of human lung airways and their application to inhaled particle deposition. Bull Math Biol 1980; 42:461–480.
17. Yu CP, Diu CK, Soong TT. Statistical analysis of aerosol deposition in nose and mouth. Am Ind Hyg Assoc J 1981; 42:726–773.
18. Yu CP, Diu CK. A comparative study of aerosol deposition in different lung models. Am Ind Hyg Assoc J 1982; 43:54–65.
19. Yu CP, Diu CK. A probabilistic model for intersubject deposition variability of inhaled particles. Aerosol Sci Technol 1982; 1:355–336.
20. Xu GB, Yu CP. Effects of age on deposition of inhaled aerosols in the human lung. Aerosol Sci Technol 1986; 5:349–357.
21. Kim CS, Iglesias AJ, Garcia L. Deposition of inhaled particles in bifurcating airway models: II. Expiratory deposition. J Aerosol Med 1989; 2(1):15–27.

22. Smaldone GC, Messina MS. Flow limitation, cough, and patterns of aerosol deposition in humans. J Appl Physiol 1985; 59:515–520.

23. Asgharian B, Yu CP. Deposition of inhaled fibrous particles in the human lung. J Aerosol Med 1988; 1:37–50.

24. Myojo T. Deposition of fibrous aerosol in model bifurcating tubes. J Aerosol Sci 1987; 18:337–347.

25. Cohen BS, Xiong JQ, Fang C, Li W. Deposition of charged particles in lung airways. Health Phys 1998; 74:554–560.

26. Chan TL, Yu CP. Charge effects on particle deposition in the human tracheo-bronchial tree. Ann Occup Hyg 1982; 26:65–75.

27. Hashish AH, Bailey AG, Williams TJ. Modeling the effect of charge on selective deposition of particles in a diseased lung using aerosol boli. Phys Med Biol 1994; 39:2247–2262.

28. Gebhart J, Heigwer G, Heyder J, Roth C, Stahlhofen W. The use of light scattering photometry in aerosol medicine. J Aerosol Med 1988; 1:89–112.

29. Schiller CF, Gebhart J, Heyder J, Rudolf G, Stahlhofen W. Deposition of monodisperse insoluble aerosol particles in the 0.005 to 0.2 µm size range within the human respiratory tract. Ann Occup Hyg 1988; 32(suppl 1):41–49.

30. Jaques PA, Kim CS. Measurement of total lung deposition of inhaled ultrafine particles in healthy men and women. Inhal Tox 2000; 12:715–731.

31. Gebhart J. To the relevant diameter of aerosol particles in the 0.1 to 1µm transition range. J Aerosol Sci 1992; 23:S305–S308.

32. Heyder J, Gebhart J, Scheuch G. Interaction of diffusional and gravitational particle transport in aerosols. Aerosol Sci Technol 1985; 4:315–326.

33. Whitby, K. Aerosol formation in urban plumes. Ann N Y Acad Sci 1980; 338:258–275.

34. Rosati JA, Brown JS, Peters TM, Leith D, Kim CS. A polydisperse aerosol inhalation system designed for human studies. J Aerosol Sci 2002; 33:1433–1446.

35. McMurry PH, Litchy M, Huang PF, Cai X, Turpin PJ, Dick WD, Hanson A. Elemental composition and morphology of individual particles separated by size and hygroscopicity with the TDMA. Atmos Environ 1996; 30:101–108.

36. Anselm A, Heibel T, Gebhart J, Ferron G. In-vivo studies of growth factors of sodium chloride particles in the human respiratory tract. J Aerosol Sci 1990; 12:S427–S430.

37. Blanchard JD, Willeke K. Total deposition of ultrafine sodium chloride particles in human lungs. J Appl Physiol 1984; 57:1850.

38. Tu KW, Knutson EO. Total deposition of ultrafine hydrophobic and hygroscopic aerosols in the human respiratory system. Aerosol Sci Technol 1984; 3:453–465.

39. Ferron GA. The size of soluble aerosol particles as a function of the humidity of the air: application to the human respiratory tract. J Aerosol Sci 1977; 8:251.

40. Robinson RJ, Yu CP. Theoretical analysis of hygroscopic growth rate of mainstream and sidestream cigarette smoke particles in the human respiratory tract. Aerosol Sci Tech 1998; 28:21–32.

41. Scheuch G, Gebhart J, Roth C. Uptake of electrical charges in the human respiratory tract during exposure to air loaded with negative ions. J Aerosol Sci 1990; 21:S439–S442.

42. Heyder J, Gebhart J, Rudolf G, Schiller CF, Stahlhofen W. Deposition of particles in the human respiratory tract in the size range 0.005–15 μm. J Aerosol Sci 1986; 5:811–825.

43. Jaques PA, Kim CS. Measurement of total lung deposition of inhaled ultra-fine particles in healthy men and women. Inhal Tox 2000; 12:715–731.

44. Kim CS. Methods of calculating lung delivery and deposition of aerosol particles. Respir Care 2000; 45:695–711.

45. Bennett WD, Zeman KL, Kim CS. Variability of fine particle deposition in healthy adults: effect of age and gender. Am J Resp Crit Care Med 1996; 153(5):1641–1647.

46. Brown JS, Zeman KL, Bennett WD. Ultrafine particle deposition and clearance in the healthy and obstructed lung. Am J Resp Crit Care Med 2002; 166:1240–1247.

47. Tobin MJ, Chadha TS, Jenouri G, Birch SJ, Gazeroglu HB, Sackner MA. Breathing patterns: 1. Normal subjects. Chest 1983; 84:202–205.

48. Tobin MJ, Chadha TS, Jenouri G, Birch SJ, Gazeroglu HB, Sackner MA. Breathing patterns: 2. Diseased subjects. Chest 1983; 84(3):286–294.

49. Heyder J, Armbruster L, Gebhart, et al. Total deposition of aerosol particles in the human respiratory tract for nose and mouth breathing. J Aerosol Sci 1975; 6:311–328.

50. Cheng KH, Cheng YS, Yeh HC, Guilmette RA, Simpson SQ, Yang YH, Swift DL. In vivo measurements of nasal airway dimensions and ultrafine aerosol deposition in the human nasal and oral airways. J Aerosol Sci 1996; 27: 785–801.

51. Pattle RE. The retention of gases and particles in the human nose. In: Davies CN, ed. Inhaled Particles and Vapours: Proceedings of an International Symposium Organized by the British Occupational Hygiene Society. Oxford, UK, New York, NY: Pergamon Press, 1961:302–311.

52. Heyder J, Rudolf G. Deposition of aerosol particles in the human nose. In: Walton WH, McGovern B, eds. Inhaled Particles IV: Proceedings of an International Symposium, Part 1, Edinburgh, United Kingdom, Oxford, United Kingdom, Pergamon Press, Ltd, 1977:107–126.

53. Kesavanathan J, Bascom R, Swift DL. The effect of nasal passage characteristics on particle deposition. J Aerosol Med 1998; 11:27–39.

54. Chan TL, Lippman M. Experimental measurements and empirical modeling of the regional deposition of inhaled particles in humans. Am Ind Hyg Assoc J 1980; 41:379–409.

55. Bennett WD, Zeman KL, Kang CW, Schechter MS. Extrathoracic deposition of inhaled, coarse particles (4.5 μm) in children vs. adults. Ann Occup Hyg 1997; 41(suppl 1):497–502.

56. Bowes SM, Swift DL. Deposition of inhaled particles in the oral airway during oronasal breathing. Aerosol Sci Technol 1989; 11:157–167.

57. Emmett PC, Aitken RJ. Measurements of the total and regional deposition of inhaled particles in the human respiratory tract. J Aerosol Sci 1982; 13: 549–560.

58. Donno MD, Pavia D, Agnew JE, Lopez-Vidriero MT, Clarke SW. Variability and reproducibility in the measurement of tracheobronchial clearance in

healthy subjects and patients with different obstructive lung diseases. Eur Respir J 1988; 1:513–620.

59. Foster WM. Is 24-hour lung retention an index of alveolar deposition? J Aerosol Med 1988;1.

60. Ilowite J, Smaldone GC, Perry R, Bennett WD, Foster WM. The relationship between tracheobronchial clearance rates and sites of initial deposition in man. Arch Env Health 1989; 44:267–273.

61. Lee PS, Gerrity TR, Hass RJ, Lourenco RV. A model for tracheobronchial clearance of inhaled particles in man and a comparison with data. IEEE Trans Biomed Eng 1979; 26:624–630.

62. Smaldone GC, Perry R, Bennett WD, Messina M, Zwang J, Ilowite J. Interpretation of 24 hr lung retention in studies of mucociliary clearance. J Aerosol Med 1988; 1:11–20.

63. Hofmann W, Asgharian B. The effect of lung structure on mucociliary clearance and particle retention in human and rat lungs. Toxicol Sci 2003; 73: 448–456.

64. Smaldone GC, Foster WM, O'Riordan TG, Messina MS, Perry RJ, Langenback EG. Regional impairment of mucociliary clearance in chronic obstructive pulmonary disease. Chest 1993; 103:1390–1396.

65. Regnis JA, Zeman KL, Noone PG, Knowles MR, Bennett WD. Prolonged airway retention of insoluble particles in cystic fibrosis vs. primary ciliary dyskinesia. Exp Lung Res 2000; 26(3):149–162.

66. Kim CS, Jaques PA. Respiratory dose of inhaled ultrafine particles in healthy adults. Phil Trans R Soc Lond A 2000; 358:2693–2705.

67. Smith S, Cheng Y, Yeh HC. Deposition of ultrafine particles in human tracheobronchial airways of adults and children. Aerosol Sci Technol 2001; 35:697–709.

68. Dolovich MB, Sanchis J, Rossman C, Newhouse MT. Aerosol penetrance: a sensitive index of peripheral airways obstruction. J Appl Physiol 1976; 40:468–471.

69. Chan HK, Eberl S, Daviskas E, Constable C, Young I. Changes in lung deposition of aerosols due to hygroscopic growth: a fast SPECT study. J Aerosol Med 2002; 15:307–311.

70. Phipps RP, Gonda I, Anderson SD, Bailey D, Bautovich G. Regional deposition of saline aerosols of different tonicities in normal and asthmatic subjects. Eur Respir J 1994; 7:1474–1482.

71. Kim CS, Hu SC, Dewitt P, Gerrity TR. Assessment of regional deposition of inhaled particles in human lungs by serial bolus delivery method. J Appl Physiol 1996; 81:2203–2213.

72. Kim CS, Hu SC. Regional deposition of inhaled particles in human lungs: comparison between men and women. J Appl Physiol 1998; 84:1834–1844.

73. Brown JS, Gerrity TR, Bennett WD, Kim CS, House DE. Dispersion of aerosol boluses in the human lung: dependence on lung volume, bolus volume, and gender. J Appl Physiol 1995; 79(5):1787–1795.

74. Bennett WD, Scheuch G, Zeman KL, Brown JS, Kim C, Heyder J, Stahlhofen W. Bronchial airway deposition and retention of particles in inhaled boluses: effect of anatomic dead space. J Appl Physiol 1998; 85(2):685–694.

75. Bennett WD, Scheuch G, Zeman KL, Brown JS, Kim C, Heyder J, Stahlhofen W. Regional deposition and retention of particles in shallow, inhaled boluses: effect of lung volume. J Appl Physiol 1999; 86(1):168–173.

76. Siekmeier R, Schiller-Scotland CHF, Gebhart J, Kronenberger H. Pharmacon-induced airway obstruction in healthy subjects: dose dependent changes of inspired aerosol boluses. J Aerosol Sci 1990; 21(S1):S423–S426.

77. Anderson PJ, Blanchard JD, Brain JD, Feldman HA, McNamara JJ, Heyder J. Effect of cystic fibrosis on inhaled aerosol boluses. Am Rev Respir Dis 1989; 140:1317–1324.

78. Brown JS, Gerrity TR, Bennett WD. Effect of ventilation distribution on aerosol bolus dispersion and recovery. J Appl Physiol 1998; 85(6):2112–2117.

79. McDonnell WF, Seal E Jr. Relationships between lung function and physical characteristics in young adult black and white males and females. Eur Respir J 1991; 4(3):279–289.

80. Martin TR, Castile RG, Fredberg JJ, Wohl MER, Mead J. Airway area is related to sex but not lung size in normal adults. J Appl Physiol 1987; 63:2042–2047.

81. Bennett WD, Messina MS, Smaldone GC. The effect of exercise on deposition and subsequent retention of inhaled particles. J Appl Physiol 1985; 59(4):1046–1054.

82. Morgan WKC, Ahmad D, Chamberlain MJ, Clague HW, Pearson MG, Vinitski S. The effect of exercise on the deposition of an inhaled aerosol. Respir Physiol 1984; 56:327–338.

83. Heyder J, Gebhart J, Stahlhofen W, Stuck B. Biological variability of particle deposition in the human respiratory tract during controlled and spontaneous mouth-breathing. Ann Occup Hyg 1982; 26:137–147.

84. Paek D, McCool FD. Breathing patterns during varied activities. J Appl Physiol 1992; 73:887–893.

85. Perez W, Tobin MJ. Separation of factors responsible for change in breathing pattern induced by instrumentation. J Appl Physiol 1985; 59:1515–1520.

86. Valberg PA, Brain JD, Sneddon SL, LeMott SR. Breathing patterns influence aerosol deposition sites in excised dog lungs. J Appl Physiol 1982; 53:824–837.

87. Hart MC, Orzalesi MM, Cook CD. Relation between anatomic respiratory dead space and body size and lung volume. J Appl Physiol 1963; 18(3):519–522.

88. Shea SA, Walter J, Murphy K, Guz A. Evidence for individuality of breathing patterns in resting healthy man. Respir Physiol 1987; 68:331–344.

89. Zeman KL, Bennett WD. Measuring alveolar dimensions at total lung capacity by aerosol-derived airway morphometry. J Aerosol Med 1995; 8(2):135–147.

90. Pritchard JN, Jefferies SJ, Black A. Sex differences in the regional deposition of inhaled particles in the 2.5–7.5 μm size range. J Aerosol Sci 1986; 17:385–389.

91. Phalen RF, Oldham MJ, Beaucage CB, Crocker TT, Mortensen JD. Postnatal enlargement of human tracheobronchial airways and implications for particle deposition. Anat Rec 1985; 212:368–380.

92. Asgharian B, Menache MG, Miller FJ. Modeling age-related particle deposition in humans. J Aerosol Med 2004; 17:213–224.
93. Tabachnik E, Muller N, Toye B, Levison H. Measurement of ventilation in children using the respiratory inductive plethysmograph. J Pediatrics 1981; 99:895–899.
94. Schiller-Scotland CHF, Hlawa R, Gebhart J. Total deposition of monodisperse aerosol particles in the respiratory tract of children. Toxicol Lett 1994; 72:137–144.
95. Bennett WD, Zeman KL. Deposition of fine particles in children spontaneously breathing at rest. Inhal Toxicol 1998; 10:831–842.
96. Bennett WD, Zeman KL. Obesity is associated with increased fine particle deposition in children. Am J Resp Crit Care Med 2002; 165(8):A435.
97. Becquemin MH, Berthalon JF, Bouchikhi A, Malarbet JL, Roy M. Oronasal ventilation partitioning in adults and children: effect on aerosol deposition in airways. Radiat Prot Dosimet 1999; 81:221–228.
98. James DS, Lambert WE, Mermier CM, Stidley CA, Chick TW, Samet JM. Oronasal distribution of breathing at different ages. Arch Environ Health 1997; 52:118–123.
99. Phalen RF, Oldham MJ, Mautz WJ. Aerosol deposition in the nose as a function of body size. Health Phys 1989; 57(suppl 1):299–305.
100. Becquemin MH, Swift DL, Bouchikhi A, Roy M, Teillac A. Particle deposition and resistance in the noses of adults and children. Eur Respir J 1991; 4:694–702.
101. Knudson RJ. Physiology of the aging lung. In: Crystal RG, West JB, eds. The Lung: Scientific Foundations. New York: Raven Press Ltd, 1991:1749–1759.
102. Thurlbeck WM. Morphology of the aging lung. In: Crystal RG, West JB, eds. The Lung: Scientific Foundations. New York: Raven Press Ltd, 1991: 1743–1748.
103. Bennett WD, Zeman KL, Kim C, Mascarella J. Enhanced deposition of fine particles in COPD patients spontaneously breathing at rest. Inhal Tox 1997; 9:1–14.
104. Kim CS, Kang TC. Comparative measurement of lung deposition of inhaled fine particles in normal subjects and patients with obstructive airway disease. Am J Respir Crit Care Med 1997; 155:899–905.
105. Anderson PJ, Wilson JD, Hiller FC. Respiratory tract deposition of ultrafine particles in subjects with obstructive or restrictive lung disease. Chest 1990; 97:1115–1120.
106. Schiller-Scotland CF, Gebhart J, Hochrainer D, Siekmeier R. Deposition of inspired aerosol particles within the respiratory tract of patients with obstructive lung disease. Toxicol Lett 1996; 88(1–3):255–261.
107. Chalupa DC, Morrow PE, Oberdörster G, Speers D, Daigle C, Utell MJ, Frampton MW. Deposition of ultrafine carbon particles in subjects with asthma. Am J Respir Crit Care Med 2002; 165(8):A829.
108. Svartengren M, Anderson M, Bylin G, Philipson K, Camner P. Regional deposition of 3.6 μm particles and lung function in asthmatic subjects. J Appl Physiol 1991; 71:2238–2243.

109. Christensen WD, Swift DL. Aerosol deposition and flow limitation in a compliant tube. J Appl Physiol 1986; 60:630–637.
110. Smaldone GC, Itoh H, Swift DL, Wagner HN. Effect of flow-limiting segments and cough on particle deposition and mucociliary clearance in the lung. Am Rev Respir Dis 1979; 120:747–758.
111. Isawa T, Wasserman K, Taplin GV. Lung scintigraphy and pulmonary function studies in obstructive airway disease. Am Rev Respir Dis 1970; 102: 161–172.
112. Lin MS, Goodwin DA. Pulmonary distribution of an inhaled radioaerosol in obstructive lung disease. Radiology 1976; 118:645–651.
113. Taplin GV, Tashkin DP, Chopra SK, Anselmi OE, Elam D, Calvarese B, Coulson A, Detels R, Rokaw SN. Early detection of chronic obstructive pulmonary disease using radionuclide lung-imaging procedures. Chest 1977; 71(5):567–575.
114. Burch WM, Sullivan PJ, Lomas FE, Evans VA, McLaren CJ, Arnot RN. Lung ventilation studies with Technetium-99m pseudogas. J Nucl Med 1986; 27:842–846.
115. Santolicandro A, Giuntini C. Patterns of deposition of labelled monodisperse aerosols in obstructive lung disease. J Nucl Med All Sci 1979; 23:115–127.
116. Pellegrino R, Biggi A, Papaleo A, Camuzzini G, Rodarte JR, Brusasco V. Regional expiratory flow limitation studied with Technegas in asthma. J Appl Physiol 2001; 91:2190–2198.
117. Roth C, Kreyling WG, Scheuch G, Busch B, Stahlhofen W. Deposition and clearance of fine particles in the human respiratory tract. Ann Occup Hyg 1997; 41(suppl 1):503–508.
118. O'Riordan TG, Walser L, Smaldone GC. Changing patterns of aerosol deposition during methacholine bronchoprovocation. Chest 1993; 103:1385–1389.
119. Backer V, Mortensen J. Distribution of radioactive aerosol in the airways of children and adolescents with bronchial hyper-responsiveness. Clin Physiol 1992; 12:574–585.
120. Svartengren M, Philipson K, Camner P. Individual differences in regional deposition of 6 µm particles in humans with induced bronchoconstriction. Exp Lung Res 1989; 15:139–149.
121. Foster WM, Silver JA, Groth ML. Exposure to ozone alters regional function and particle dosimetry in the human lung. J Appl Physiol 1993; 75: 1938–1945.
122. Kreit JW, Gross KB, Moore TB, Lorenzen TJ, D'Arcy J, Eschenbacher WL. Ozone induced changes in pulmonary function and bronchial responsiveness in asthmatics. J Appl Physiol 1989; 66:217–222.
123. Miller FJ, Anjilvel S, Menache MG, Asgharian B, Gerrity TR. Dosimetric issues relating to particle toxicity. Inhal Tox 1995; 7:615–632.
124. Chamberlain MJ, Morgan WK, Vinitski S. Factors influencing the regional deposition of inhaled particle in man. Clin Sci 1983; 64:69–78.
125. Susskind H, Brill AB, Harold WH. Quantitative comparison of regional distributions of inhaled Tc-99m DTPA aerosol and Kr-81m gas in coal miners' lungs. Am J Physiol Imaging 1986; 1:67–76.

126. Trajan M, Logus JW, Enns EG, Man SFP. Relationship between regional ventilation and aerosol deposition in tidal breathing. Am Rev Respir Dis 1984; 130:64–70.

127. O'Riordan TG, Smaldone GC. Regional deposition and regional ventilation during inhalation of pentamidine. Chest 1994; 105:395–401.

128. Brown JS, Zeman KL, Bennett WD. Regional deposition of coarse particles and ventilation distribution in patients with cystic fibrosis. J Aerosol Med 2001; 14(4):443–454.

129. Brown JS, Zeman KL, Kim CS, Bennett WD. Regional deposition of fine vs. ultrafine particles in the human respiratory tract. Am J Respir Crit Care Med 2000; 161(3):A257.

130. Laube BL, Links JM, LaFrance ND, Wagner HN, Rosenstein BJ. Homogeneity of bronchopulmonary distribution of 99m-Tc aerosol in normal subjects and in cystic fibrosis. Chest 1989; 95:822–830.

131. Jakab GJ, Green GM. Effects of pneumonia on intrapulmonary distribution of inhaled particles. Am Rev Respir Dis 1973; 107:675–678.

132. Schlesinger RB. Deposition and clearance of inhaled particles. In: McClellan RO, Henderson RF, eds. Concepts in Inhalation Toxicology. 2nd ed. Washington, DC: Taylor & Francis, 1995:191–224.

133. Anderson I, Proctor DF. The fate and effects of inhaled materials. Proctor DF, Anderson I, eds. The Nose: Upper Airway Physiology and the Atmospheric Environment. New York: Elsevier Biomedical Press, 1982.

134. Stanley P, MacWilliam L, Greenstone M, MacKay I, Cole P. Efficacy of a saccharin test for screening to detect abnormal mucociliary clearance. Br J Dis Chest 1984; 78:62–64.

135. Oberdörster G, Utell MJ. Ultrafine particles in the urban air: to the respiratory tract—and beyond? Environ Health Perspect 2002; 110(8):A440–A441.

136. Palmer LB, Albulak K, Fields S, Filkin AM, Simon S, Smaldone GC. Oral clearance and pathogenic oropharyngeal colonization in the elderly. Am J Respir Crit Care Med 2001; 164(3):464–468.

137. Wanner A, Salathe M, O'Riordan TG. Mucociliary clearance in the airways (state of the art). Am J Respir Crit Care Med 1996; 154:1868–1902.

138. Stahlhofen W, Gebhart J, Rudolf G, Scheuch G. Measurement of lung clearance with pulses of radioactively-labelled aerosols. J Aerosol Sci 1986; 17:333–336.

139. Smaldone GC, Perry RJ, Bennett WD, Messina MS, Zwang J, Ilowite J. Interpretation of "24 hour lung retention" in studies of mucociliary clearance. J Aerosol Med 1988; 1:11–20.

140. Falk R, Philipson K, Svartengren M, Jarvis N, Bailey M, Camner P. Clearance of particles from small ciliated airways. Exp Lung Res 1997; 23:495–515.

141. Lay JC, Berry CR, Kim CS, Bennett WD. Retention of insoluble particles after local intrabronchial deposition in dogs. J Appl Physiol 1995; 79: 1921–1929.

142. Kreyling WG, Blanchard JD, Godleski JJ, Haussermann S, Heyder J, Hutzler P, Schulz H, Sweeney TD, Takenaka S, Ziesenis A. Anatomic localization of 24- and 96-hr particle retention in canine airways. J Appl Physiol 1999; 87: 269–284.

143. Falk R, Philipson K, Svartengren M, Bergmann R, Hofmann W, Jarvis N, Bailey M, Camner P. Assessment of long-term bronchiolar clearance of particles from measurements of lung retention and theoretical estimates of regional deposition. Exp Lung Res 1999; 25:495–516.
144. Van As A. Pulmonary airway clearance mechanisms. Am Rev Respir Dis 1977; 115:721–727.
145. Gehr P, Schürch S, Berthaiume Y, Im Hof V, Geiser M. Particle retention in airways by surfactant. J Aerosol Med 1990; 3:27–43.
146. Gehr P, Im Hof V, Geiser M, Schürch S. The fate of particles deposited in the intrapulmonary conducting airways. J Aerosol Med 1991; 4:349–362.
147. Brain JD. Macrophages in the respiratory tract. In: Fishman AP, Fisher AB, eds. Handbook of Physiology. Bethesda, MD: American Physiology Society, 1985:447–471.
148. Geiser M, Cruz-Orive LM, Im Hof V, Gehr P. Assessment of particle retention and clearance in the intrapulmonary conducting airways of hamster lungs with the fractionater. J Microsc 1990; 160:75–88.
149. Geiser M, Baumann M, Cruz-Orive LM, Im Hof V, Waber U, Gehr P. The effect of particle inhalation on macrophage number and phagocytic activity in the intrapulmonary conducting airways of hamsters. Am J Respir Cell Mol Biol 1994; 10:594–603.
150. Stirling C, Patrick G. The localisation of particles retained in the trachea in the rat. J Pathol 1980; 131:309–320.
151. Kreyling WG, Scheuch G. Clearance of particles deposited in the lungs. In: Gehr P, Heyder J, eds. Particle–Lung Interactions. New York, NY: Marcel Dekker, 2000:323–376.
152. Churg A, Stevens B, Wright JL. Comparison of the uptake of fine and ultrafine TiO_2 in a tracheal explant system. Am J Physiol 1998; 274: L81–L86.
153. Radford EP, Martell EA. Polonium-210: lead-210 ratios as an index of residence time of insoluble particles from cigarette smoke in bronchial epithelium. Walton WH, McGovern B, eds. Inhaled Particles IV: Proceedings of an International Symposium, Part 2, September 1975. Oxford, United Kingdom: Pergamon Press, Ltd., 1977:567–581.
154. Churg A, Stevens B. Association of lung cancer and airway particle concentration. Environ Res 1988; 45:58–63.
155. Bennett WD, Ilowite JS. Dual pathway clearance of 99m Tc-DTPA from the bronchial mucosa. Am Rev Respir Dis 1989; 139:1132–1138.
156. Oberdörster G, Utell MJ, Morrow PE, Hyde RW, Weber DA. Bronchial and alveolar absorption of inhaled 99mTc-DTPA. Am Rev Respir Dis 1986; 134:944–950.
157. Wagner EM, Foster WM. Interdependence of bronchial circulation and clearance of 99mTc-DTPA from the airway surface. J Appl Physiol 2001; 90: 1275–1281.
158. Matsui H, Randell SH, Peretti SW, Davis CW, Boucher RC. Coordinated clearance of periciliary liquid and mucus from airway surfaces. J Clin Invest 1998; 102:1125–1131.

159. Sakagami M, Byron PR, Venitz J, Rypacek F. Solute disposition in the rat lung in vivo and in vitro: determining regional absorption kinetics in the presence of mucociliary escalator. J Pharm Sci 2002; 91:594–604.

160. Lay JC, Stang MR, Fisher PE, Yankaskas JR, Bennett WD. Airway retention of materials of different solubility following local intrabronchial deposition in dogs. J Aerosol Med 2003; 16(2):153–166.

161. Huchon GJ, Montgomery AB, Lipavsky A, Hoeffel JM, Murray JF. Respiratory clearance of aerosolized radioactive solutes of varying molecular weight. J Nucl Med 1987; 5:894–902.

162. Enna SJ, Schanker LS. Absorption of drugs from the rat lung. Am J Physiol 1972; 223:1227–1231.

163. Oberdöerster G. Lung clearance of inhaled insoluble and soluble particles. J Aerosol Med 1988; 1:289–330.

164. Leith DE, Butler JP, Sneddon SL, Brain JD. Cough. Fishman, ed. Handbook of Physiology, Section 3, The Respiratory System,Vol. 3 Mechanics of Breathing, Part 1. Bethesda, Maryland: American Physiological Society, 1986: 315–336.

165. Camner P, Mossberg B, Afzelius BA. Measurements of tracheobronchial clearance in patients with immotile cilia syndrome and its value in differential diagnosis. Eur J Respir Dis 1983; 64:57–63.

166. Bennett WD, Foster WM, Chapman WF. Cough enhanced mucus clearance in the normal lung. J Appl Physiol 1990; 69(5):1670–1675.

167. Bailey MR, Kreyling WG, Andre S, Batchelor A, Black A, Collier CG, Drosselmeyer E, Ferron GA, Foster P, Haider B, Hodgson A, Metivier H, Moores SR, Morgan A, Muller HL, Patrick G, Pearman I, Pickering S, Ramsden D, Stirling C, Talbot RJ. An interspecies comparison of the lung clearance of inhaled monodisperse cobalt oxide particles—part I: objectives and summary of results. J Aerosol Sci 1989; 20:169–188.

168. Kreyling WG, Andre S, Collier CG, Ferron GA, Metivier H, Schumann G. Interspecies comparison of lung clearance after inhalation of monodisperse, solid cobalt oxide aerosol particles. J Aerosol Sci 1991; 22:509–535.

169. Snipes MB, Clem MF. Retention of microspheres in the rat lung after intratracheal instillation. Environ Res 1981; 24:33–41.

170. Snipes MB, Chavez GT, Muggenburg BA. Disposition of 3-, 7-, and 13-µm microspheres instilled into lungs of dogs. Environ Res 1984; 33:333–342.

171. Ferin J, Oberdörster G, Penney DP, Soderholm SC, Gelein R, Piper HC. Increased pulmonary toxicity of ultrafine particles? I. Particle clearance, translocation, morphology. J Aerosol Sci 1990; 21:381–384.

172. Ferin J, Oberdörster G, Penney DP. Pulmonary retention of ultrafine and fine particles in rats. Am J Respir Cell Mol Biol 1992; 6:535–542.

173. Valberg PA, Blanchard JD. Pulmonary macrophage physiology: origin; motility; endocytosis. In: Parent RC, ed. Treatise on Pulmonary Toxicology: Comparative Biology of the Normal Lung. New York: CRC Press, 1992:681–724.

174. Lay JC, Bennett WD, Kim CS, Devlin RB, Bromberg PA. Retention and intracellular distribution of instilled iron oxide particles in human alveolar macrophages. Am J Respir Cell Mol Biol 1998; 18:687–695.

175. Lehnert BE, Morrow PE. Association of 59iron oxide with alveolar macrophages during alveolar clearance. Exp Lung Res 1985; 9:1–16.
176. Naumann BD, Schlesinger RB. Assessment of early alveolar particle clearance and macrophage function following an acute inhalation of sulfuric acid mist. Exp Lung Res 1986; 11:13–33.
177. Ferin J, Feldstein ML. Pulmonary clearance and hilar lymph node content in rats after particle exposure. Environ Res 1978; 16:342–352.
178. Harmsen AG, Muggenburg BA, Snipes MB, Bice D. The role of macrophages in particle translocation from lungs to lymph nodes. Science 1985; 230: 1277–1280.
179. Bowden DH, Adamson IYR. Pathways of cellular efflux and particulate clearance after carbon instillation to the lung. J Pathol 1984; 143:117–125.
180. Langenback EG, Bergofsky EH, Halpern JG, Foster WM. Supramicron-sized particle clearance from alveoli: route and kinetics. J Appl Physiol 1990; 69:1302–1308.
181. Warheit DB, Overby LH, George G, Brody AR. Pulmonary macrophages are attracted to inhaled particles through complement activation. Exp Lung Res 1988; 14:51–66.
182. Tyler WS, Julian MD. Gross and subgross anatomy of lungs, pleura, connective tissue septa, distal airways, and structural units. In: Parent RC, ed. Treatise on Pulmonary Toxicology: Comparative Biology of the Normal Lung. New York: CRC Press, 1992.
183. Ayhan H, Tuncel A, Bor N, Piskin E. Phagocytosis of monosize polystyrene-based microspheres having different size and surface properties. J Biomater Sci Polym Ed 1995; 7:329–342.
184. Gonzalez O, Smith PL, Goodman SB. Effect of size, concentration, surface area, and volume of polymethacrylate particles on human macrophages in vitro. J Biomed Mater Res 1996; 30:463–473.
185. Oberdörster G. Lung dosimetry: pulmonary clearance of inhaled particles. Aerosol Sci Technol 1993; 18:279–289.
186. Ferin J, Oberdörster G, Soderholm SC, Gelein R. Pulmonary tissue access of ultrafine particles. J Aerosol Med 1991; 4:57–68.
187. Churg A. The uptake of mineral particles by pulmonary epithelial cell. Am J Respir Crit Care Med 1996; 154:1124–1140.
188. Schanker LS, Mitchell EW, Brown RA. Species comparison of drug absorption from the lung after aerosol inhalation or intratracheal injection. Drug Metab Dispos 1986; 14:79–88.
189. Creasia DA, Poggenburg JK, Nettesheim P. Elution of benzo[alpha]pyrene from carbon particles in the respiratory tract of mice. J Toxicol Environ Health 1976; 1:967–975.
190. Chinard FP. The alveolar-capillary barrier: some data and speculations. Microvasc Res 1980; 19:1–17.
191. Kreyling WG, Beisker W, Berg I, Gercken G, Miaskowski U, Neuner M, Schluter T, Heilmann P. Particle clearance functions of alveolar macrophages of different species: intracellular particle dissolution and phagolysosomal pH. Eur Respir J 1992; 4:70.

192. Oberdörster G, Sharp Z, Atudorei V, Elder A, Gelein R, Lunts A, Kreyling W, Cox C. Extrapulmonary translocation of ultrafine carbon particles following whole-body inhalation exposure of rats. J Toxicol Environ Health A 2002; 65(20):1531–1543.

193. Kreyling WG, Semmler M, Erbe F, Mayer P, Takenaka S, Schulz H, Oberdörster G, Ziesenis A. Translocation of ultrafine insoluble iridium particles from lung epithelium to extrapulmonary organs is size dependent but very low. J Toxicol Environ Health A 2002; 65(20):1513–1530.

194. Nemmar A, Vanbilloen H, Hoylaerts MF, Hoet PHM, Verbruggen A, Nemery B. Passage of intratracheally instilled ultrafine particles from the lung into the systemic circulation in hamster. Am J Respir Crit Care Med 2001; 164: 1665–1668.

195. Peterson BT, Dickerson KD, James HL, Miller EJ, McLarty JW, Holiday DB. Comparison of three tracers for detecting lung epithelial injury in anesthetized sheep. J Appl Physiol 1989; 66:2374–2383.

196. Nemmar A, Hoet PHM, Vanquickenborne B, Dinsdale D, Thomeer M, Hoylaerts MF, Vanbilloen H, Mortelmans L, Nemery B. Passage of inhaled particles into the blood circulation in humans. Circulation 2002; 105: 411–414.

197. Xu JH, Moonen M, Johansson A, Bake B. Dynamics of "Technegas" deposited in the lung. Nucl Med Commun 2001; 22:383–387.

198. Monaghan P, Provan I, Murray C, Mackey DWJ, Van der Wall H, Walker BM, Jones PD. An improved radionuclide technique for the detection of altered pulmonary permeability. J Nucl Med 1991; 32:1945–1949.

199. Isawa T, Teshima T, Anazawa Y, Miki M, Mahmud AM. Inhalation of pertechnegas: similar clearance from the lung to that of inhaled pertechnetate aerosol. Nucl Med Commun 1995; 16:741–746.

200. Isawa T, Teshima T, Anazawa Y, Miki M, Motomiya M. Technegas inhalation lung imaging. Nucl Med Commun 1991; 12:47–55.

201. Roth C, Scheuch G, Stahlhofen W. Clearance measurements with radioactively labelled ultrafine particles. Ann Occup Hyg 1994; 38(suppl 1): 101–106.

202. Phipps RJ, Abraham WM, Mariassy AT, Torrealba PJ, Sielczak MW, Ahmed A, McCray M, Stevenson JS, Wanner A. Developmental changes in the tracheal mucociliary system in neonatal sheep. J Appl Physiol 1989; 67:824–832.

203. Whaley SL, Muggenburg BA, Seiler FA, Wolff RK. Effect of aging on tracheal mucociliary clearance in dogs. J Appl Physiol 1987; 62:1331–1334.

204. Puchelle E, Zahm JM, Bertrand A. Influence of age on bronchial mucociliary transport. Scand J Respir Dis 1979; 60:307–313.

205. Incalzi RA, Maini CL, Fuso L, Giordano A, Carbonin PU, Galli G. Effects of aging on mucociliary clearance. Compr Gerontol A 1989; 3:65–68.

206. Goodman RM, Yergin BM, Landa JF, Golinvaux MH, Sackner MA. Relationship of smoking history and pulmonary function tests to tracheal mucous velocity in nonsmokers, young smokers, ex-smokers and patients with chronic bronchitis. Am Rev Respir Dis 1978; 117:205–214.

207. Antonini JM, Roberts JR, Clarke RW, Yang HM, Barger MW, Ma JY, Weissman DN. Effect of age on respiratory defense mechanisms: pulmonary

bacterial clearance in Fischer 344 rats after intratracheal instillation of *Listeria* monocytogenes. Chest 2001; 120(1):240–249.

208. Coonrod JD, Jarrells MC, Bridges RB. Impaired pulmonary clearance of pneumococci in neonatal rats. Pediatr Res. 1987; 22(6):736–742.

209. Pigorini F, Maini CL, Pau F, Giosue S. The influence of age on the pulmonary clearance of 99Tcm-DTPA radioaerosol. Nucl Med Commun 1988; 9(12):965–971.

210. Braga FJ, Manco JC, Souza JF, Ferrioli E, De Andrade J, Iazigi N. Age-related reduction in 99mTc-DTPA alveolar-capillary clearance in normal humans. Nucl Med Commun 1996; 17(11):971–974.

211. Tankersley CG, Shank JA, Flanders SE, Soutiere SE, Rabold R, Mitzner W, Wagner EM. Changes in lung permeability and lung mechanics accompany homeostatic instability in senescent mice. J Appl Physiol 2003; 95(4):1681–1687.

212. Wolff RK, Dolovich MB, Obminski G, Newhouse MT. Effects of exercise and eucapnic hyperventilation on bronchial clearance in man. J Appl Physiol 1977; 43:46–50.

213. Sweeney TD, Tryka AF, Brain JD. Effect of exercise on redistribution and clearance of inhaled particles from hamster lungs. J Appl Physiol 1990; 68(3):967–972.

214. John J, Wollmer P, Dahlbäck M, Luts A, Jonson B. Tidal volume and alveolar clearance of insoluble particles. J Appl Physiol 1994; 76:584–588.

215. Valberg PA, Wolff RK, Mauderly JL. Redistribution of retained particles: effect of hyperpnea. Am Rev Respir Dis 1985; 131:273–280.

216. Su SH, Chen HI, Jen CJ. Severe exercise enhances phagocytosis by murine bronchoalveolar macrophages. J Leukoc Biol 2001; 69(1):75–80.

217. Raidal SL, Love DN, Bailey GD, Rose RJ. The effect of high intensity exercise on the functional capacity of equine pulmonary alveolar macrophages and BAL-derived lymphocytes. Res Vet Sci 2000; 68(3):249–253.

218. Lorino AM, Meignan M, Bouissou P, Atlan G. Effects of sustained exercise on pulmonary clearance of aerosolized 99mTc-DTPA. J Appl Physiol 1989; 67:2055–2059.

219. Meignan M, Rosso J, Leveau J, Katz A, Cinotti L, Madelaine G, Galle P. Exercise increases the lung clearance of inhaled Technetium-99m DTPA. J Nucl Med 1986; 27:274–280.

220. Majima Y, Sakakura Y, Matsubara T, Murai S, Miyoshi Y. Mucociliary clearance in chronic sinusitis: related human nasal clearance and in vitro bullfrog palate clearance. Biorheology 1983; 20:251–262.

221. Stanley PJ, Wilson R, Greenstone MA, Mackay IS, Cole PJ. Abnormal nasal mucociliary clearance in patients with rhinitis and its relationship to concomitant chest disease. Br J Dis Chest 1985; 79:77–82.

222. Rutland J, Cole PJ. Nasal mucociliary clearance and ciliary beat frequency in cystic fibrosis compared with sinusitis and bronchiectasis. Thorax 1981; 36:654–658.

223. Camner P, Mossberg B, Philipson K. Tracheobronchial clearance and chronic obstructive lung disease. Scand J Resp Dis 1973; 54:272–281.

224. Vastag E, Matthys H, Zsamboki G, Kohler D. Mucociliary clearance in smokers. Eur J Respir Dis 1986; 68:107–113.

225. Santa Cruz R, Landa J, Hirsch J. Tracheal mucous velocity in normal man and patients with obstructive lung disease. Am Rev Respir Dis 1974; 109:458–463.

226. Smaldone GC, Foster WM, O'Riordan TG, Messina MS, Langenback EG, Perry RJ. Regional impairment of mucociliary clearance in chronic obstructive pulmonary disease. Chest 1993; 103:1390–1396.

227. Smaldone GC, Itoh H, Swift DL, Wagner HN. Effect of flow-limiting segments and cough on particle deposition and mucociliary clearance in the lung. Am Rev Respir Dis 1979; 120:747–758.

228. Bateman JRM, Pavia D, Sheahan NF, Agnew JE, Clarke SW. Impaired tracheobronchial clearance in patients with mild stable asthma. Thorax 1983; 38:463–467.

229. Ilowite JS, Bennett WD, Sheetz MS, Groth ML, Nierman DM. Permeability of the bronchial mucosa to Tc99m-DTPA in asthma. Am Rev Respir Dis 1989; 139:1139–1143.

230. O'Riordan TG, Zwang J, Smaldone GC. Mucociliary clearance in adult asthma. Am Rev Respir Dis 1992; 146:598–603.

231. Messina MS, O'Riordan TG, Smaldone GC. Changes in mucociliary clearance during acute exacerbations of asthma. Am Rev Respir Dis 1991; 143:993–997.

232. Camner P, Jarstrand C, Philipson K. Tracheobronchial clearance in patients with influenza. Am Rev Respir Dis 1973; 108:131–135.

233. Puchelle E, Zahm JM, Girard F, Bertrand A, Polu JM, Aug F, Sadoul P. Mucociliary transport in vivo and in vitro: relations to sputum properties in chronic bronchitis. Eur J Respir Dis 1980; 61:254–264.

234. Groth ML, Macri K, Foster WM. Cough and mucociliary transport of airway particulate in chronic obstructive lung disease. Ann Occup Hyg 1997; 41(suppl):515–521.

235. Noone PG, Bennett WD, Regnis JA, Zeman KL, Carson JL, King M, Boucher RC, Knowles MR. Effect of aerosolized uridine-5'-triphosphate on airway clearance with cough in patients with primary ciliary dyskinesia. Am J Respir Crit Care Med 1999; 160:144–149.

236. Bohning DE, Atkins HL, Cohn SH. Long term clearance in man: normal and impaired. Ann Occup Hyg 1982; 26(suppl):259–271.

237. Moller W, Barth W, Kohlhaufl M, Haussinger K, Stahlhofen W, Heyder J. Human alveolar long-term clearance of ferromagnetic iron oxide microparticles in healthy and diseased subjects. Exp Lung Res 2001; 27(7): 547–568.

238. Damon EG, Mokler BV, Jones RK. Influence of elastase-induced emphysema and the inhalation of an irritant aerosol on deposition and retention of an inhaled insoluble aerosol in Fischer-344 rats. Toxicol Appl Pharmacol 1983; 67:322–330.

239. Hahn FF, Hobbs CH. The effect of enzyme-induced pulmonary emphysema in Syrian hamsters on the deposition and long-term retention of inhaled particles. Arch Environ Health 1979; 34:203–211.

240. Creasia DA, Nettesheim P, Hammons AS. Impairment of deep lung clearance by influenza virus infection. Arch Environ Health 1973; 26:197–201.

241. Lundgren DL, Hahn FF, Crain CR, Sanchez A. Effect of influenza virus on the pulmonary retention of inhaled Ce-144 and subsequent survival of mice. Health Phys 1978; 34:557–567.

242. Slauson DO, Lay JC, Castleman WL, Neilsen NR. Acute inflammatory lung injury retards pulmonary particle clearance. Inflammation 1989; 13:185–199.

243. Slauson DO, Lay JC, Castleman WL, Neilsen NR. Alveolar macrophage phagocytic kinetics following pulmonary parainfluenza-3 virus infection. J Leukocyte Biol 1987; 41:412–420.

244. Alexis N, Soukup J, Becker S. Association between airways hyperreactivity and bronchial macrophage dysfunction in individuals with mild asthma. Am J Physiol Lung Cell Mol Physiol 2001; 280:L369–L375.

245. Godard P, Chaintreuil J, Damon M, Coupe M, Flandre O, de Paulet AC, Michel FB. Functional assessment of alveolar macrophages: comparison of cells from asthmatics and normal subjects. J Allergy Clin Immunol 1982; 70:88–93.

246. Madl A, Wilson DW, Segall HJ, Pinkerton KE. Alteration in lung particle translocation, macrophage function, and microfilament arrangement in monocrotaline-treated rats. Tox and Appl Pharmacol 1998; 153:28–38.

247. Adamson IYR, Prieditis H. Silica deposition in the lung during epithelial injury potentiates fibrosis and increases particle translocation to lymph nodes. Exp Lung Res 1998; 24:293–306.

248. Laitinen LA, Heino M, Laitinen A, Kava T, Haahtela T. Damage of the airway epithelium and bronchial reactivity in patients with asthma. Am Rev Respir Dis 1985; 131:599–606.

249. Foster WM, Wagner EM. Bronchial edema alters Tc99m-DTPA clearance from the airway surface in sheep. J Appl Physiol 2001; 91:2567–2573.

250. Jones JG, Minty BD, Lawler P, Hulands G, Crawley JC, Veall N. Increased alveolar epithelial permeability in cigarette smokers. Lancet 1980; 121(8159):66–68.

251. Minty BD, Jordan C, Jones JG. Rapid improvement in abnormal pulmonary epithelial permeability after stopping cigarettes. Br Med J 1981; 282:1183.

252. Huchon GJ, Russell JA, Barritault LG, Lipavsky AJA, Murray JF. Chronic air-flow limitation does not increase respiratory epithelial permeability assessed by aerosolized solute, but smoking does. Am Rev Respir Dis 1984; 130:457–460.

253. Braude S, Nolop KB, Hughes JMB, Barnes PJ, Royston D. Comparison of lung vascular and epithelial permeability indices in the adult respiratory distress syndrome. Am Rev Respir Dis 1986; 133:1002–1005.

254. Lin CC, Chang CT, Li TC, Kao A. Objective evidence of impairment of alveolar integrity in patients with non-insulin-dependent diabetes mellitus using radionuclide inhalation lung scan. Lung 2002; 180(3):181–186.

255. Zanobetti A, Schwartz J. Cardiovascular damage by airborne particles: are diabetics more susceptible? Epidemiology 2002; 13(5):588–592.

256. Schlesinger RB. The interaction of inhaled toxicants with respiratory tract clearance mechanisms. Crit Rev Toxicol 1990; 20:257–286.

257. Wolfe RK. Effects of airborne pollutants on mucociliary clearance. Environ Health Perspect 1986; 66:223–237.

258. Albert RE, Berger J, Sanborn K, Lippmann M. Effects of cigarette smoke components on bronchial clearance in the donkey. Arch Environ Health 1974; 29:96–101.

259. Lippmann M, Albert RE, Yeates DB, Berger JM, Foster WM, Bohning DE. Factors affecting tracheobronchial mucociliary transport. In: Walton WH, McGovern B, eds. Inhaled Particles IV: Proceedings of an International Symposium, Part 1. Edinburgh, UK, Oxford, UK: Pergamon Press, Ltd, 1977:305–319.

260. Foster WM, Costa DL, Langenback EG. Ozone exposure alters tracheobronchial mucociliary function in humans. J Appl Physiol 1987; 63:996–1002.

261. Gerrity TR, Bennett WD, Kehrl H, DeWitt PJ. Mucociliary clearance of inhaled particles measured at 2 hr after ozone exposure in humans. J Appl Physiol 1993; 74:2984–2989.

262. Kenoyer JL, Phalen RF, Davis JR. Particle clearance from the respiratory tract as a test of toxicity: effect of ozone on short and long term clearance. Exp Lung Res 1981; 2:111–120.

263. Churg A, Brauer M, Keeling B. Ozone enhances the uptake of mineral particles by tracheobronchial epithelial cells in organ culture. Am J Respir Crit Care Med 1996; 153:1230–1233.

264. Hirsch JA, Swenson E, Wanner A. Tracheal mucous velocity in beagles after long-term exposure to 1 ppm SO_2. Arch Environ Health 1975; 30:249–253.

265. Giordano AM, Morrow PE. Chronic low-level nitrogen dioxide exposure and mucociliary clearance. Arch Environ Health 1972; 25:443.

266. Schlesinger RB. Comparative irritant potency of inhaled sulfate aerosols—effects on bronchial mucociliary clearance. Environ Res 1984; 34:268–279.

267. Leikauf G, Yeates DB, Wales KA, Spektor D, Albert RE, Lippmann M. Effects of sulfuric acid aerosol on respiratory mechanic and mucociliary particle clearance in healthy nonsmoking adults. Am Ind Hyg Assoc J 1981; 42:273–282.

268. Schlesinger RB, Groczynski JE, Dennison J, Richard L, Kinney PL, Bosland MC. Long-term intermittent exposure to sulfuric acid aerosol, ozone, and their combination: alterations in tracheobronchial mucociliary clearance and epithelial secretory cells. Exp Lung Res 1992; 18:505–534.

269. Abraham WM, Sielczak MW, Delehunt JC, Marchette B, Wanner A. Impairment of tracheal mucociliary clearance but not ciliary beat frequency by a combination of low level ozone and sulfur dioxide in sheep. Eur J Respir Dis 1986; 68:114–120.

270. Saldiva PH, King M, Delmonte VL, Macchione M, Parada MA, Daliberto ML, Sakae RS, Criado PM, Silveira PL, Zin WA, et al. Respiratory alterations due to urban air pollution: an experimental study in rats. Environ Res 1992; 57:19–33.

271. Ferin J, Leach LJ. The effects of selected air pollutants on clearance of titanic oxide particles from the lungs of rats. In: Walton WH, McGovern B, eds. Inhaled particles IV: Proceedings of an International Symposium, Part 1: Edinburgh, UK, Oxford, UK: Pergamon Press, Ltd, 1977:333–341.

272. Gardner DE. Alterations in macrophage functions by environmental chemicals. Environ Health Perspect 1984; 55:343–358.

273. Cohen D, Arai SF, Brain JD. Smoking impairs long-term dust clearance from the lung. Science 1979; 204:514–517.
274. Demarest GB, Hudson LD, Altman LC. Impaired alveolar macrophage chemotaxis in patients with acute smoke inhalation. Am Rev Respir Dis 1979; 119:279–286.
275. Holt PG, Keast D. Environmentally induced changes in immunological function. Acute and chronic effects of inhalation of tobacco smoke and other atmospheric contaminants in man and experimental animals. Bacteriol Rev 1977; 41:205–216.
276. Kehrl HR, Vincent LM, Kowalsky RJ, Horstman DH, O'Neil JJ, McCartney WH, Bromberg PA. Ozone exposure increases respiratory epithelial permeability in humans. Am Rev Respir Dis 1987; 135:1124–1128.
277. Foster WM, Stetkiewicz PT. Regional clearance of solute from the respiratory epithelia: 18–20 hr postexposure to ozone. J Appl Physiol 1996; 81(3): 1143–1149.
278. Bhalla DK, Mannix RC, Kleinman MT, Crocker TT. Relative permeability of nasal, tracheal, and bronchoalveolar mucosa to macromolecules in rats exposed to ozone. J Toxicol Environ Health 1986; 17:269–283.
279. Cohen MD, Zelikoff JT, Chen LC, Schlesinger RB. Pulmonary retention and distribution of inhaled chromium: effects of particle solubility and coexposure to ozone. Inhal Tox 1997; 9:843–865.

3

Bioavailability of Particle-Associated Air Pollutants and Relationship to Cardiopulmonary Injury

URMILA P. KODAVANTI and WILLIAM P. WATKINSON

Pulmonary Toxicology Branch, Experimental Toxicology Division,
National Health and Environmental Effects Research Laboratory, ORD,
U.S. Environmental Protection Agency, Research Triangle Park,
North Carolina, U.S.A.

I. Introduction

Over the past decade, numerous epidemiological studies have shown consistent associations between increases in the levels of ambient particulate matter (PM) and increases in human morbidity and mortality (1–7). Furthermore, the evidence suggests that both the cardiovascular and pulmonary systems may be primary targets of these toxic agents. However, despite intensive research efforts, neither the specific constituents of PM responsible for these effects nor their mechanisms of action are well understood.

This article has been reviewed by the National Health and Environmental Effects Research Laboratory, U.S. Environmental Protection Agency, and approved for publication. Approval does not signify that the contents necessarily reflect the views and the policies of the Agency nor does mention of trade names or commercial products does constitute endorsement or recommendation for use.

Although ambient particles arise from a variety of sources and processes and cover a wide range of sizes and compositional materials, respirable particles clearly present the greatest health concern. The larger particles are mostly derived from crustal materials, but the smaller particles are linked to combustion processes. These highly respirable particles are formed through the agglomeration and binding of a variety of microscopic fumes and condensates to core entities. The resultant particles, generally in the nanometer to micrometer size range, may consist of both organic and inorganic species on surfaces while their cores are often composed of carbon or silicate. In general, these particles are dynamic and undergo continual modifications due to changes in atmospheric temperature, humidity, and pressure, as well as exposure to oxidant gases and sunlight (8). When particles come in contact with the liquid media of airway and alveolar lining fluids composed of various aqueous, protein, and lipid substances, or with cells, the soluble and loosely-bound material may dissociate from the core and be released, whereas surface-bound components may react or otherwise interact with airway fluid and cells. Chemical interactions involving the released material, as well as the remaining particle core, with airway and alveolar lining fluids and macrophages ultimately determine their fate and biological action.

Many studies suggest that the toxicity of PM is a function of both its specific constituents and the availability of these constituents to interact with biological systems. This chapter will focus on the leachable and solid components of PM with reactive or nonreactive surfaces, which come in contact with cells or cellular components (airway and alveolar lining fluids), their association with the induction of pulmonary and/or cardiac injuries, and the primary mechanisms by which these effects may be mediated. The specific topics covered include: (1) the determinants of bioavailability, with emphasis on the physical and chemical characteristics of PM and the evidence for translocation of PM or its constituents to remote organs; (2) the bioavailability of PM constituents and the mechanisms of lung injury; (3) the cardiovascular impact, i.e., the roles of endothelial activation, oxidative stress, microvascular thrombosis, and vascular injury in the induction of cardiac impairment; and (4) the impact of pre-existing cardiopulmonary diseases on individual susceptibility and the subsequent manifestation of PM-related injury.

II. Regional Composition of PM and Associated Health Outcomes

The composition and characteristics of both anthropogenic and natural source PM vary markedly from region to region and from source to source (Tables 1–4), and differences in constituents and their respective bioavailabilities may greatly influence the toxicity of PM (9–11). In general, PM

Table 1 Bulk Chemical Composition (%) of Ambient Air PM from Various International Cities

Element	Eastern U.S.A. (<2.5 μm)	Western U.S.A. (<2.5 μm)	Leeds, U.K. (<2.5 μm)	Birmingham, U.K. (<10 μm)	Brisbane, Australia (<2.5 μm)	Sapporo, Japan (<10 μm)	Lahore, Pakistan (TSP)	Hong Kong (TSP)	Antwerp, Belgium (0.2–15 μm)
EC	3.9	14.7	—	18.0	19.3	13.9	2.9	—	—
OC	14.9	27.8	—	20.0	—	14.2	13.1	—	—
TC	18.8	15.7	50.0	38.0	—	28.1	16	57.1	21.3
Organic	20.9	38.9	—	—	27.0	—	—	—	—
Nitrate	1.1	24.0	6.6	6.0	2.6	4.2	16.0	2.8	—
Sulfate	34.1	4.6	26.1	17.0	5.0	16.4	2.1	14.4	18.9
Ammonium	13.0	6.7	9.9	6.0	10.0	2.9	3.0	3.3	—
Chloride	—	—	1.8	2.0	9.7	2.2	—	2.3	3.2
Crustal	—	—	—	—	6.1	—	—	—	—
Minerals	4.3	36.3	5.6	—	—	9.7	16.4	6.1	30.0
Other	22.8	0.0	0.0	31.0	20.3	36.5	61.3	14.0	26.6

Source: From Ref. 9. EC=Elemental carbon, OC=Organic carbon, TC=Total carbon, TSP=Total suspended particles.

Table 2   Elemental Composition of Total Suspended Ambient Air PM from Various Cities Within the United States (ng/m^3)

Element	Boston, MA	Phoenix, AZ	Los Angeles, CA	Chicago, IL	Houston, TX	St. Louis, MO
Aluminum	3,458	2,670	847	269	1,216	1,412
Silicates	6,904	7,440	2,162	831	3,200	4,928
Barium	—	10	127	< 130	139	54
Lead	462	60	251	32	589	877
Nickel	34	10	5	< 1.8	8	9
Vanadium	28	—	9	< 13	< 45	6
Iron	1,733	1,470	2,192	432	766	1,493
Zinc	100	90	293	90	142	175
Copper	58	40	178	17	46	43
Titanium	154	140	165	19	36	587
Manganese	30	50	63	13	35	71

Source: From Ref. 9.

from the eastern United States contains high levels of industrial source-derived sulfate, whereas PM from the western portions of the country has high levels of nitrate, mostly from agricultural and automotive sources (12–15) (Table 1). Significant quantities of zinc, iron, vanadium, and nickel are found in PM collected from areas dominated by oil and coal burning power plants (16–18) (Table 2), whereas PM collected from the vicinity of the Baltimore Turnpike (Baltimore, MD: a mid-Atlantic region of the United States) contains organics on a carbonaceous core and is mostly a product of vehicle emissions (19) (Table 3). In more rural areas, such as Arizona, PM is dominated by the presence of silicates from crustal materials (20). It is widely believed that research aimed at identification of the causative constituents of PM and the mechanisms of action that result in pathological manifestations will facilitate future predictions relating to the types of pollutants and likely health outcomes. Such source-apportionment studies may be crucial to understand the toxic effects of PM and to developing the strategies to control air pollution emissions.

Unfortunately, epidemiological studies have provided only limited information on the role of causative constituents in the development of observed health effects. Furthermore, the PM epidemiological literature demonstrates that, despite large variations in the components of PM at different locations (Table 3), there is a remarkable consistency in health outcomes. This consistency may be explained by the following rationale: (1) most ambient air PM for which positive epidemiological data are available has components that are toxic; (2) the endpoints most frequently measured by epidemiological studies are cardiorespiratory deaths and morbidity, common outcomes of a variety of component-specific mechanisms; and

Table 3 Chemical Composition of Collected Bulk Ambient PM Samples from Selected Sources

Element	NIST[a] Standard: 1648 St. Louis, MO (298)[b]	NIST Standard: Washington DC (298)[b]	NIST Standard: Düsseldorf, Germany (298)[b]	Ambient PM: Baltimore, MD (19)[c]	Ambient PM: Bag-house, Ottawa, Canada (299)[d]
Sulfate (µg/mg)	143	93.5	137.3	—	45
Carbon (%)	—	—	—	—	
Aluminum (µg/mg)	—	—	—	3.8	9.8
Barium (µg/mg)	—	—	—	0.3	0.3
Lead (µg/mg)	—	—	—	0.23	6.7
Nickel (µg/mg)	0.11	0.02	0.24	0.1	0.07
Vanadium (µg/mg)	0.11	0.2	0.18	0.1	0.09
Iron (µg/mg)	8.91	6.6	9.7	21.6	14.9
Zinc (µg/mg)	3.56	1.5	3.7	1.1	10.4
Copper (µg/mg)	0.37	0.14	0.42	1.4	0.85
Cobalt (µg/mg)	—	—	—	0.0	0.005
Manganese (µg/mg)	—	—	—	1.2	0.48
Endotoxin, (EU/mg)[e]	—	—	—	< 1.0	—

[a]National Institute of Technology Standards.
[b]Metals analyzed in 1 M hydrochloric acid extract of particulate sample.
[c]Collected using high-volume cyclone collector and metal content represent total metal content.
[d]Concentrated nitric acid extracts were analyzed for elemental content.
[e]Endotoxin was measured semi-quantitatively using a limulus amebocyte lysate agglutination assay kit (19).

(3) many components of PM generate reactive oxygen species during their interactions with bioactive molecules, resulting in common secondary mechanisms leading to cardiopulmonary impairment, despite the diversity of the initial mediators. Thus, there is a clear need to conduct both epidemiological and toxicological studies aimed at identifying

Table 4 Water-Leachable Elemental, and Organic Composition of Combustion Source PM of Different Origins

Element	Oil combustion: within boiler, precipitator (Ref. 21)	Oil combustion: fugitive emission in 1970s (Ref. 74)	Oil combustion: within boiler, precipitator (Ref. 217)	Oil combustion: fugitive emission in 1990s (Ref. 140)	Coal combustion: SRM 1633 (Ref. 19)
Sulfate (μg/mg)	267.3	530.6	212.7	107.0	—
Carbon (%)	17.3	1.2	4.6	18.8	—
Aluminum (μg/mg)	—	—	0.23	—	150.5
Barium (μg/mg)	BD	—	—	BD	0.71
Lead (μg/mg)	BD	—	0.04	BD	0.07
Nickel (μg/mg)	14.2	26.3	6.9	3.0	0.01
Vanadium (μg/mg)	20.6	32.8	1.3	0.1	0.29
Iron (μg/mg)	4.7	15.7	0.02	2.5	77.8
Zinc (μg/mg)	6.4	0.08	11.5	14.5	0.21
Copper (μg/mg)	0.7	0.18	0.23	0.1	0.11
Cobalt (μg/mg)	BD	—	—	BD	0.05
Manganese (μg/mg)	0.2	—	—	0.4	0.13
Endotoxin	—	2.5 pg/mg	0.08 EU/mg	0.57 EU/mg	—

Note: The level of water-leachable content of individual metals varies with the type of combustion fly ash. BD, below detectable levels. The empty cells with dashes indicate data not available.

component-specific mechanisms, rather than merely documenting end-biological responses, in order to gain a more complete understanding of how ambient PM may cause injury to the lung, heart, systemic vasculature, and other organs.

III. Composition and Characteristics of PM Determine Bioavailability

Before producing an effect, the particle or its components must interact with biological tissues; the extent or ease of this interaction is directly related to the *bioavailability* of the particle and its constituents (both soluble and insoluble). Bioavailability is determined by the physical and chemical characteristics of the particle, as well as the degree to which the constituents are bound to the particle core. Similarly, these characteristics determine the ease with which a particle or its constituents may translocate to a remote tissue or organ after deposition within the lung. The components that remain unexposed to biological material are not considered bioavailable. Thus, as defined in this chapter, the term bioavailable refers to any PM components, soluble or insoluble, reactive or nonreactive, which come into contact with biological fluid.

Much of the information on the component-specific effects of PM comes from recently conducted in vitro and in vivo toxicological studies using surrogates of different compositions, such as residual oil fly ashes (21–24), synthetic particles coated with materials (25,26), individual metals (27–30), diesel (31–35), carbon, printex, titanium of different sizes (26,36,37), and ambient PM from different sources (17,38–41). Although past PM research has focused primarily on pulmonary effects, recently, more consideration has been given to the study of the cardiovascular effects of PM. The recognition of the significant cardiovascular impact of PM has also prompted interest in particle translocation mechanisms. Thus, in order to elicit a cardiac response, pulmonary-delivered PM must induce a systemic response or toxic components of the PM must migrate to the heart to produce a direct effect. Therefore, before discussing studies on the mechanisms of pulmonary and cardiac effects, it is imperative to understand the kinetics of the delivery of bioavailable PM and/or its constituents to both pulmonary and extrapulmonary sites. On the basis of chemical composition, PM components can be found in the following fractions: (1) water soluble, (2) water insoluble fine core with reactive surface, (3) water insoluble fine core with non-reactive surface, (4) protein and lipid soluble organic, (5) ultrafine reactive particles, and (6) ultrafine nonreactive particles. A hypothetical framework based on information gathered from recent studies of PM translocation and health effects (42–45), and pulmonary drug transport mechanisms (46), outlining how different PM components may reach

Particulate Matter Causative Constituents and Size Interactions with Cells

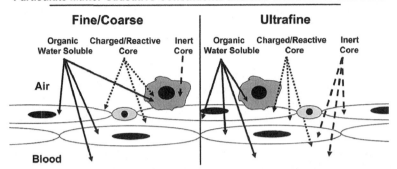

Figure 1 Schematic of PM and PM component interactions with lung cells and translocation to the circulation. Cell layers at the air phase represent alveolar epithelial cells and at the blood phase represent endothelial cells of pulmonary capillary walls. The arrow indicates potential sites of PM component translocation.

different cells, enter the circulation and be transported to other organ systems, is given in Fig. 1. As the particles land on the alveolar lining fluid, soluble components can be released and translocated while particle cores of 0.1–10 μm are likely to be phagocytosed. The ultrafine particles are less likely to be phagocytosed but may readily enter macrophages, pulmonary epithelial and endothelial cells, the interstitial space, and the circulation. The biological interactions of these components, often separating into different fractions, may determine the pulmonary and cardiovascular effects of these PM species.

A. Soluble Elemental Constituents

Soluble components of PM represent the most bioavailable fraction of constituents (Table 4). They are readily leached from the particle surface and, given their physical and chemical characteristics, they are also amenable to other modes of transport. Thus, these constituents, when toxic, may play a key role in the induction of adverse health effects, both at the site of their deposition in the lung, as well as at remote tissues and organ systems. When inhaled, particles encounter the mucus and liquid lining that covers airway and alveolar surfaces; water- and lipid-soluble PM components likely leach off and are absorbed by epithelial cells, macrophages, and ultimately, the systemic circulation. Some of the soluble PM components, such as the metals, can carry a charge (47,48) and bind to proteins of the surfactant or on the cell surface. The mechanisms of their translocation can vary depending on the chemical properties of differentially soluble components; such as metals (49–53) or organics (54,55). Water-soluble, lipid- and protein-soluble, and low molecular weight PM components may migrate to the circulation and then to other target organs. Experimental studies show that PM-associated metals may be translocated to the circulation and other extrapulmonary organs following pulmonary exposure (56–58).

Although there is evidence for transport of drug molecules via pulmonary delivery mechanisms involving drug aerosols—often bound to a carrier protein or encapsulated in liposomes—the current level of understanding of how components of ambient particles are transported to and through the circulation is still in its infancy. Further studies of these drug delivery mechanisms should help scientists conceptualize how different components of PM may be transported to the circulation and other organ systems.

Nasal uptake of particulate metals and their transport to the brain have also been considered to be important factors in the generation of extrapulmonary effects of PM. Indeed, absorption of manganese and its transport to the olfactory bulbs have been postulated in manganese-induced neurotoxicity (59,60). However, recent studies have shown that inhaled iron is neither taken up by nasal neurons nor transported to the brain (61). Little is known about PM neurotoxicity and clearly, more research is needed to investigate the potential roles of PM components in neuronal effects. Although developmental and neurotoxic effects of PM have been speculated, there is meager experimental evidence for such effects at the present time, and the mechanisms of component-specific effects, as well as the potential for components to traverse through capillary barriers of the brain and placenta, are less well understood.

B. Organic Constituents

Organic species can constitute a large portion of motor vehicle exhaust particles and are considered among the most significant causative constituents of ambient PM (62). The organic fraction of diesel exhaust is composed of a complex mixture of carbonaceous particles, potentially carcinogenic polycyclic aromatic hydrocarbons (PAHs), and nitrated PAHs (35,63). Polycyclic aromatic hydrocarbons are often condensed on ultrafine soot particles. Although the impact of diesel exhaust on pulmonary host defense mechanisms has been widely studied for many years (64–68), recent evidence suggests a potential cardiovascular risk as well (69).

Using labeled PAHs readsorbed to soot of diesel origin, Gerde et al. (54) have recently reported that a large fraction of the soot-adsorbed PAHs translocates to the circulation within minutes following inhalation. A more tightly-bound fraction may remain on the particles and translocate to the lymph nodes where further dissolution may occur. Although these authors have demonstrated the translocation of unmetabolized organic PAHs, it is not clear whether the reported endothelial effects of PAHs are due to the metabolites or their parent compounds or, if bioactivation does occur, whether it takes place in the liver or at the endothelial surface. Parent compounds and DNA adducts of PAHs have been detected in the blood in humans exposed to fine ambient PM (10,34), suggesting that extrapulmonary targets are critical in the induction and expression of health effects. Although chronic inhalation exposures have been conducted to investigate the carcinogenic effects of diesel exhaust (70–72), research on its potential cardiovascular effects is insufficient. In addition at this time, there is no evidence linking inhaled diesel exhaust or its constituents to adverse effects in the brain or reproductive organs.

C. Particle Surface Characteristics and Reactivity

The surface and chemical properties of PM undergo continuous transformations in the atmosphere due to changes in temperature and humidity, interactions with gaseous components, and photochemical reactions. Once particles impact the surface of the airway lining fluid, highly soluble components are released and the less soluble remnant particles are likely phagocytosed or cleared via mucociliary action. The more acidic environment of the phagolysosome may leach yet more material. Although it appears that these soluble bioavailable constituents are responsible for many of the adverse effects seen following exposure to PM (21,24,29,73–75), recent evidence demonstrates that the insoluble fraction may also play an independent role in observed toxic responses (39,76). For example, it is known that the surface chemistry of the particle can affect its opsonization and/or phagocytosis and the subsequent activation and release of mediators from phagocytes and epithelial cells (42,43,50,77–79). A number of studies have investigated the influence of surface chemical properties on the biological responses of cells, both in vitro and in vivo. However, no information is available on whether there are specific differences in surface chemistries and biological actions associated with the insoluble core of PM obtained from different sources. The metabolic rate of benzo-[a]-pyrene adsorbed onto the carbonaceous core of diesel soot was carefully studied by Gerde et al. (54), who demonstrated that although most of the fraction was rapidly translocated into the circulation, a small percentage of benzo-[a]-pyrene remained attached to the particles for months. As with the water-soluble components, organic constituents bound to the particle surface may be released into the alveolar lining fluid. The surfactant material contains high concentrations of lipids and proteins, which may facilitate release of organic constituents in the airway/alveolar lining fluid. These constituents can then be taken up by airway and alveolar cells. More information on this subject can be found in an excellent review on particle deposition in Chapter 2 of this book.

The role of particle surface reactivity in the pathogenic response to PM is complex and dependent upon a number of factors (42,80,81). For example, the relationship between surface reactivity and pathogenicity is not readily predictable from the knowledge of the chemical composition of the bulk sample because the particle surface can have several reactive sites with differing chemical compositions. Furthermore, the reactivity is not linear but depends upon surface area and the chemical composition of the surrounding airway lining. The effects of insoluble particles may persist for long periods of time because of particle retention in the various lung compartments. In his detailed review, Fubini (42) proposed four major points to consider: (a) poorly coordinated atoms and ions on the particle surface constitute local centers of more pronounced reactivity and, therefore, no generalization about biological effect can be made using mass; (b) while in the lung or in the atmosphere, the surface properties age from more reactive to less reactive over time; (c) chemical treatments may affect the particle surface without modifying the core; for example, acid washing can remove surface ions and modify the surface chemistry of silica, thus modifying its toxicity (82,83); and (d) temperature modifications may also affect the particle surface properties. In the lung, the surface properties of the particle may modulate scavenger receptor-mediated alveolar macrophage function, including apoptosis (84).

There has been significant research on the role of sequestration of iron on the surface of asbestos fibers and silica, and on the potential oxidant production (85,86). Studies have shown that particle-bound iron may catalyze Fenton-like reactions in the presence of antioxidants and oxygen. Additional studies report that ferruginous bodies are formed in vivo around asbestos fibers; these bodies represent endogenous iron deposits in the form of iron oxyhydroxides mixed with organic materials. The significance of this process is not known, but it is thought to be an adaptive response whereby foreign material is encapsulated or otherwise isolated from the tissues of its biological host. A number of specific proteins that control iron uptake in the gastrointestinal tract are also present in the lung where they serve to facilitate iron transport to epithelial cells and sequester it as catalytically inactive ferritin. Ferritin is subsequently transported to the reticuloendothelial system for clearance (87). Because of the presence of active sequestration mechanisms, inhaled bioavailable iron may not cause oxidative lung injury unless the sequestration mechanisms are saturated because of high exposure concentrations. However, this does not eliminate the possibility of interactions of iron with other metals, which might modify their toxicities.

Recently, zeta potential—the electrical potential that exists across the interface of all solids and liquids—has been implicated in the biological activity of ambient and combustion source PM. Suspensions of a variety of combustion and ambient PM demonstrated differential surface charges (zeta potential), as measured by microelectrophoresis. Significant positive correlations between PM zeta potential and the release of inflammatory

mediators from human bronchial airway epithelial cells suggest the importance of surface charge in eliciting a biological response (48). However,
because zeta potential can also be generated by soluble components, such
as metals, it is not clear whether this response is due to surface-bound
metals or ionic solutes in the media. It remains to be investigated how
ambient-derived particles, which differ in their core structure, physico-
chemistry, and surface-bound materials, may impact cells and pulmonary
structures with similar zeta potential-mediated mechanisms.

One approach to better investigate the relationship between the surface reactivity and the biological action of PM would be to physicochemically characterize the surfaces of the insoluble remnants of a variety of
particles obtained from different ambient sources. After characterization,
these insoluble fractions can be employed in in vitro and in vivo toxicological studies. Berg et al. (50) correlated various types of dusts composed of
different elemental mixtures and demonstrated that hydrogen peroxide
release from exposed bovine alveolar macrophages was metal dependent.
Further, Schluter et al. (51) compared the production of reactive oxygen
species in bovine alveolar macrophages incubated with metal salts such
as metal oxides, sulfates, and metal-coated silica particles. A number of
redox active metals were chosen. Interestingly, these studies demonstrated
that the coating of silica particles with different metal oxides did not alter
the potency of the particles to produce reactive oxygen intermediates,
whereas exposure of macrophages to metal salts by themselves produced
a metal-dependant oxidative burst. The response to metal-coated carbonaceous particles is unknown; however, investigating these effects will be
essential in identifying chemical processes that lead to the formation of
more toxic particles.

D. Particle Size and Reactivity

Particle size influences bioavailability in a number of ways. Most importantly, the physical size of a particle determines whether or not the particle
is respirable. The particles of greatest health concern range in diameter from
$\sim$10 μm to $\sim$10 nm. These particles are generally grouped into three modes:
coarse (10.0–2.5 μm); fine (2.5–0.1 μm); and ultrafine (<100 nm); with the
final size being determined, in large part, by the respective generation process. Particles also differ by shape, porosity, and composition, which in turn,
may influence the type of material (e.g., organic, acid) that can condense
onto the particle matrix (11). This diversity in physicochemical attributes
not only influences the level and extent of particle deposition in the pulmonary tree, but also affects the dissolution of constituents in the airways, and
the subsequent biological action on lung cells or remote tissues (88).

Phagocytosis of particles by macrophages is likely to facilitate release
of soluble components within phagolysosomes because of their acidic

content (54,89). The solubilized material may then activate these cells or exert other effects (90–92). Particle-laden macrophages are also known to be retained within the alveolar spaces for long periods of time (93) and, depending on the dissolution kinetics of the bioactive materials, may have long-lasting effects.

Ultrafine particles, on the other hand, are phagocytosed much less efficiently, but may be taken up by endocytosis or pinocytosis into epithelial cells to be translocated to the systemic circulation (44,94–96). Translocation of ultrafines has been primarily studied using a variety of synthetic particles. Depending upon the chemical nature of these particles, differential degrees of translocation have been reported. Recent evidence demonstrates that ultrafine carbon particles may be translocated to the liver—and to a lesser extent to the brain—following whole-body exposure (94). Translocation of polystyrene nanoparticles to the liver after their absorption through the gut has also been reported (97). Both routes of exposure involve absorption of particles through the epithelium to the blood. Interestingly, there is evidence for the preferential translocation and accumulation of particles within the liver (94–96), raising questions as to whether the liver may be a target organ or merely a site for particle storage/metabolism. Additional studies have detected fluorescent microspheres in the brain following pulmonary exposure (98). It is very likely that the rate of transport of ultrafine particles depends upon their chemical composition and their binding affinity to biomolecules. Clearly, ongoing research on the biological fate of insoluble particles of different sizes will provide needed mechanistic data on ultrafine composition and transport.

Another emerging concept regarding ultrafine particle translocation involves the affinity of these particles to bind to proteins. It has been hypothesized that proteins may act as selective transporters to enable ultrafines to enter the circulation, and this area of research is under active investigation (46). The evidence that ultrafine carbon particles accumulate in the liver after pulmonary exposure suggests a carrier-mediated transport, possibly involving membrane proteins (94). Furthermore, it has long been known that metals, such as zinc, iron, copper, and cadmium, which appear to be the important constituents of urban PM atmospheres, can readily bind to proteins (99). A related area of research is currently examining the capability of some proteins to selectively transport chemicals and ultrafines from the pulmonary epithelium to the circulation. The information gained from these studies may yield clues regarding the transport of ultrafine particles and soluble components to extrapulmonary organs such as the heart, the liver, and the brain. To gain further insights into the mechanisms of transport and cell injury due to nanoparticles, readers are encouraged to read Chapter 9 in this book on Nanoparticles and Mechanisms of Injury.

IV. Bioavailability of PM and Links to Pulmonary Injury

It is clear that the lung encounters particles that have survived their passage through nasal airways. Those particles scrubbed out by the nasal epithelium may induce effects in that compartment, but the lung remains the primary target for reported PM health effects. The specific mechanisms of particle-induced injuries depend on the bioavailable PM components, their physical properties, and their interaction with the microenvironment where these particles deposit. This section will focus on PM effects in the lung and bioavailable component-specific mechanisms.

Although attempts have been made to associate anthropogenic components to adverse health effects since the great air pollution episodes of Donora, Pennsylvania in 1932 (100) and London in 1954 (101,102), the past decade has seen extensive efforts expended to determine the component-specific effects of PM on pulmonary cells. Metals, given their anthropogenic origins, ubiquitous presence in ambient PM, and established toxicity, have been hypothesized to be a primary causative constituent group, and thus, a great deal of work has been carried out to elucidate the role of metals in PM-induced health effects. More recently, research on organic PM constituents and ultrafines has gained attention, based on the reactivity of these components, their capacity to cause oxidative stress, and their potential vascular and extrapulmonary bioavailability.

A. Particulate-Associated Metals and Lung Injury

In the early 1980s, Hatch and colleagues (53,103) proposed that bioavailable or water-soluble metals contribute to the adverse biological effects of ambient particles. Using oil combustion particles collected from the stacks of electric power plants burning no. 6 residual oil, as well as particles collected from ambient air, these researchers showed that: (a) fine fugitive emissions escaping into the air contained large quantities of metals; (b) these metals were soluble in water; and (c) the pulmonary toxicity of these particles in mice was primarily dependent on the presence of soluble metals (53,103). Follow-up studies conducted in the mid-1990s by Ghio and colleagues (104–107) using the same and additional residual oil fly ashes, along with ambient PM samples, provided further evidence that lung injury in exposed animals was best correlated with total metal content. Subsequently, using one of the previous fly ash samples known to contain high concentrations of elemental metals, Dreher et al. (74) demonstrated that water-soluble metals present in this fly ash were responsible for most of the acute pulmonary injury, and furthermore, that the washed particles caused no significant lung damage in rats. Taking this one step further, Dreher et al. (74) and Kodavanti et al. (27) reported that iron, vanadium, and nickel, the three predominant metals present in this fugitive oil combustion ash, accounted for most of the lung injury, and that nickel appeared to be the most potent of these metals in inducing injury in vivo. Kodavanti et al. (27) also reported metal-specific temporal differences in the ability of these different metals to induce pulmonary injury. In contrast, in vitro studies using both rat and human bronchial epithelial cells reported that vanadium was the most toxic among these three metals while nickel caused little, if any, effects on these cells (105,108).

These differences in the results of in vivo and in vitro studies prompted further investigations using a variety of oil fly ashes of different metal compositions. A follow-up study conducted by Kodavanti et al. (21) using 10 surrogate combustion PM samples of varied metals in differing quantities indicated that PM-associated vanadium was primarily responsible for acute neutrophilic inflammation, whereas alveolar space vascular damage was most correlated with nickel (Fig. 2). Further,

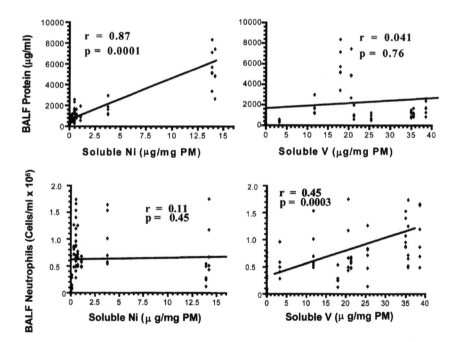

Figure 2 Association of metal content of combustion PM and pulmonary inflammatory response. Residual oil combustion particulate samples were collected from various locations within an oil burning power plant and were physicochemically characterized. Male Sprague–Dawley rats were intratracheally exposed to 10 particulate samples of differing elemental composition. Pulmonary injury and inflammation, determined at 24-hr postexposure, were correlated with water-soluble vanadium and nickel content of PM using multiple regression analyses (21). Note that protein leakage is significantly correlated with nickel content of PM, whereas neutrophilic inflammation is significantly correlated with vanadium content. (From Ref. 21.)

vanadium has been shown to inhibit tyrosine phosphatase activity, which results in the accumulation of phosphotyrosine and the subsequent activation of signaling pathways in mediating its inflammatory effects in the airways (109,110). Nickel, on the other hand, has been reported to directly interact with VCAM-1 and E-selectin, which are cell surface adhesion molecules (111). Thus, the injuries induced by vanadium and nickel are likely to be cell-type specific. Vanadium and nickel are primarily encountered in oil combustion-derived PM and thus can be detected in the vicinity of power plants burning residual oil (58,112). However, all ambient air samples may not contain these metals in significant quantities or in high proportions. A fly ash studied by Gavett et al. (113) contained a high concentration of zinc and another studied by Ghio and Quigley (114) contained primarily iron: the lung injuries caused by these samples were attributable to their bioavailable zinc and iron, respectively. Hence, a variety of metals may be toxic when inhaled with PM.

Numerous in vitro and in vivo studies have been conducted since the mid-1990s in different laboratories using either individual metals or fly ash as PM surrogates (Table 4), and the results of these studies have generally supported a role for bioavailable metals as potential causative components of PM-induced pulmonary injury. These studies are summarized in a recent review by Ghio et al. (24). Toxicological studies done with fly ash samples at high concentrations are often criticized as irrelevant to real ambient situations, as environmental exposures occur at relatively low concentrations and with more compositionally-complex PM. However, this body of work has provided strong evidence implicating metals as causative constituents, as well as insight into the source-specific compositional influence on health outcomes.

The role of metals has also been investigated in both clinical and animal studies using ambient PM samples obtained from locations where epidemiological evidence has demonstrated adverse health outcomes. These studies establish coherence between epidemiological and toxicological findings and link causality to specific constituents (73,115–117). A number of studies have used factorial analysis to demonstrate component-specific pulmonary effects of concentrated ambient particles in humans and animals and have shown associations between metals and injury profiles (17,73).

Although a variety of metals may coexist on the particle surface (Tables 2 and 3), it is likely that these metals may interact in a competitive or antagonistic manner. Metal–metal interactions can also take place in the alveolar lining fluid and affect Fenton-like chemical reactions, as well as at the cell surface where competition can occur in binding to surface receptors and other proteins. A few in vitro and in vivo studies have reported such interactions and have shown metal-specific antagonistic or additive effects. Exposures to combinations of nickel and cobalt or nickel and chromium have been shown to induce greater lung injury than exposure to an equivalent quantity of either metal alone (118,119). Dreher et al. (74) suggested residual oil fly ash-induced injury might result from the interactions of metals, and Kodavanti et al. (27) reported that nickel-induced lung pathology and cytokine gene expression were less severe when nickel was present with other metals such as iron and vanadium. Currently, the mechanisms of these interactions are not known with regard to PM-induced health effects.

Some of the earlier studies prompted by occupational exposures investigated the effects of inhaled metals in animals and in vitro redox activity in the induction of cellular toxicity (30,37,50–54). Metals, in the presence of oxygen and ascorbate, can facilitate a Fenton-like reaction and generate reactive oxygen species. As alveolar lining fluid is rich in ascorbate and other reducing agents, these reducing agents act as cofactors for the metal–oxygen interactions and produce reactive oxygen species (24,43,120). The ensuing chemical chain reaction continues to generate reactive oxygen species until there is a deficiency of a critical reactant in the lining fluid. This has been proposed to occur within the milieu of the alveolar surface (121–123). Metals have different redox potentials and, based on their redox properties, can cause different levels of oxidant production and different types of cell injuries. The redox potentials of metals have been studied with respect to their relationship to the mechanism of the macrophage oxidative burst (49–52). Because of the high reactivity of free radical species, the half-life of these unstable reactants is short and the potential for damage is most likely at the site of their production. Thus, the reactive oxygen species can signal the cell to induce an inflammatory response. Intracellularly-produced free radicals are known to induce phosphorylation of kinases, metabolism by phosphatases, and subsequent signal transduction (124).

The mechanisms by which metals interact depend upon the type of metal, its capacity to bind to macromolecules or cell surface receptors, and the cell type encountered by the metal ion. The field of metal toxicology has been well studied for many years, as many metals, such as iron, zinc, copper, and selenium, are essential for protein structures and functions.

Iron is one of the major elemental constituents of ambient PM. Biologically, it is at the core of the hemoglobin complex and it is essential for oxygen transport. It is also complexed with a variety of other proteins and, in its free form, is effectively taken up by tissues via iron sequestration mechanisms (99,125,126). Lung cells and alveolar lining fluid are rich in transferrin and lactoferrin, both important iron-binding proteins, whose primary function is iron sequestration (127). Given the abundance of these iron-binding proteins, the toxic effects of inhaled iron are only manifested if the sequestration mechanisms are impaired or overwhelmed. Thus, iron exposure is generally associated with minimal pulmonary injury if the exposures involve relatively low concentrations. However, when iron exposures occur at high concentrations, the extent of pulmonary injury can be remarkable. In addition, there is evidence that iron can be mobilized by endogenous substances such as citrate which may contribute to local toxicity (128). Iron can interact with other metals to increase or decrease their toxicity. Interactions of iron with metals have been shown to decrease the toxicity of metals, such as nickel and vanadium, in vivo (28,74).

Vanadium is a common component of fossil fuel burning, especially residual oils (129). In addition, vanadium has been shown to have insulin mimetic properties (130) and can function as a potent inhibitor of phosphotyrosine phosphatases (131). It is not clear whether the effect of this metal is due to a direct action or to vanadium-induced oxidative stress, but inactivation of phosphatases leads to activation of tyrosine kinases, which in turn regulate the PI3-kinase and ras/MAP kinase signaling pathways (132). Vanadium exposure to rat airway epithelial cells has been shown to cause oxidative stress (133). Vanadium has also been shown to induce activation of STAT-1 and P38 MAPK in lung myofibroblasts, a process inhibited by the epidermal growth factor (EGF) receptor inhibitor AG1478, suggesting that EGF receptor signaling activates STAT-1 and NF-$\kappa\beta$ signaling pathways (134). Activation of these transcription factors by vanadium has been shown to generate inflammatory responses in the lung following transcriptional activation of proinflammatory genes (135).

Metals can induce cell signaling by interacting with receptors. For example, zinc, another abundant metal of ambient PM (9), is redox inactive and yet can induce EGF receptor signaling by direct activation of the EGF receptor tyrosine kinase, with activation of downstream kinases MEK1/2 and ERK1/2, and subsequent translocation of NF-$\kappa\beta$ (136). Activation of EGF signaling has also been shown to occur with other metals such as arsenic (136). This activation and nuclear DNA binding increase the promoter activities of genes that regulate the inflammatory response (137). Similarly, at high concentrations, zinc fume exposures are known to cause metal fume fever and acute pulmonary toxicity (138,139). At high intratracheal instillation doses, zinc sulfate causes acute pulmonary inflammation (140). However, when the exposure occurs through inhalation at lower concentrations, the inflammatory response is not manifested, suggesting that smaller quantities of zinc may be captured by binding proteins in pulmonary cells without eliciting a toxic response (140). Induction of metallothionein and zinc binding to this protein are the likely mechanisms of zinc sequestration. Exposure to zinc has been shown to induce metallothionein in the liver and the heart upon uptake into the body (141,142). Similarly, zinc readily binds to proteins: more than 1000 proteins are known to bind zinc, and are considered catalytically important components for protein functioning (143,144).

Copper is another biologically essential metal, frequently found in ambient PM; however, unlike zinc, it is redox active (9,145,146). Although the sequestration of essential metals through metallothionein binding can reduce their potential toxicity, pulmonary exposure to copper has been shown to cause substantial pulmonary inflammation (75). In vitro exposures of bronchial epithelial cells to copper or to ambient particle extracts containing copper are known to cause activation of NF-$\kappa\beta$ and secretion of the proinflammatory cytokine IL-8 (75,108). It is not clear whether this copper-associated effect is mediated by its interaction with the cell surface receptor or via formation of reactive oxygen species. However, its effect on IL-8 production can be diminished by incubation of the cells with antioxidants, suggesting the involvement of oxidative stress (75).

Another significant elemental component of ambient PM is silica, generally found in the form of silicates derived primarily from crustal materials (147,148). Because of the limited solubility of silicates, they are more likely to have local pulmonary effects when exposures occur at high concentrations. However, solubilization in protein- and lipid-rich alveolar lining fluid may occur more readily, and thus, extension of its effects to extrapulmonary organs has been suggested. Recently, pulmonary and vascular effects of concentrated ambient particles have been shown to be associated with the levels of silica in the PM (148), although it is not clear if the silicates detected in PM the sample were bioavailable or simply were surrogates for other toxicants. Silicates are often complex and differ from free silica that is highly reactive and pathogenic due to free surface electrons (149,150).

In addition to iron, vanadium, zinc, and copper, other metals often detected in significant quantities in ambient PM include aluminum, arsenic, lead, manganese, cobalt, and nickel (9,15–19) (Table 2). Although individually, these metals have been well studied with respect to their biological actions, their relative contributions to ambient PM-induced health effects are unclear. Studies involving source-specific composition and correlations with specific health outcomes will be important in clarifying the role of bioavailable metals in ambient PM health effects and in developing emission control strategies.

B. Particle-Associated Organics and Lung Injury

Although organic constituents of ambient PM may originate from numerous sources, it has been estimated that two-thirds of the primary PM organic mass is derived from diesel and motor vehicle emissions in areas of high vehicular traffic (71). Diesel particulates contain a variety of organic species, including PAHs and pyrenes (151,152), which are likely bioactive. Many of the surface constituents of diesel exhaust particles are likely bioavailable at the airway and alveolar surfaces, as well as at extrapulmonary sites (54). Diesel exhausts have been studied for potential health hazards for decades in animal bioassays focusing on cancer and chronic pulmonary effects, and the majority of these studies have found positive correlations associated with particle overload (70,153–155). More recently, research interest has focused on the role of diesel exhaust PM in the exacerbation of allergic airway diseases, including asthma (64–68,155). It has been shown in many experimental models of asthma that diesel exposure can enhance the allergic response caused by allergen stimulation and act as an adjuvant (156,157). Diesel exhausts have also been widely studied with respect to their DNA binding properties. DNA adduct formation has been considered the primary mechanism of carcinogenic effects of diesel, and these effects have been detected in vitro, in animal models, and in humans (158–160).

In recent years, interest in the potential health hazards associated with diesel and gasoline emissions has been rekindled on the basis of the potential role of organic constituents of ambient PM in the induction of adverse health effects, primarily involving the pulmonary and cardiovascular systems (68,161,162). The mechanisms of action of diesel constituents have been studied in a variety of in vitro cell cultures and in vivo allergic animal models and, depending on the type of cells/animals and the type of diesel exhausts studied, clear differences in the mechanisms have been shown (157,163). For example, in a mouse model of dust mite antigen-induced allergenicity, it has been shown that eotaxin and IL-5 are induced after diesel enhancement of the allergic response (157). However, eotaxin was not induced in the A549 cell line following exposure to components of diesel exhaust (163). These differences in mechanism of injury may relate to the type of constituents, the exposure protocol, and/or the specific biological system studied.

The most extensively studied area involves induction of oxidative stress in vivo and in vitro in the lung and DNA adduct formation (160,164). This oxidative stress, likely induced by bioactive PAHs, may play a major role in diesel exhaust-induced chronic pulmonary inflammation, enhancement of allergenicity, and cancer (165). Currently, studies related to diesel constituent-specific effects use different diesel sources with varied combustion protocols that complicate interpretations of many mechanistic studies. As the emissions are better defined in terms of their constituents, the role of organic PM constituents should become clearer.

C. Particle-Associated Biological Components and Lung Injury

Bacterial, fungal, and other plant- and animal-derived biological components containing endotoxins (LPS; lipopolysaccharides) may adhere to particles or may exist as a separate entity (166). A detailed account of the role of biological contaminants of ambient PM can be found in Chapter 10 of this book on biological air pollutants. Although these components are readily bioavailable to pulmonary epithelial cells and alveolar macrophages regardless of the nature of their transport state, the observed biological effects can vary with the type of protein. For example, if LPS is adherent to the particle with other constituent materials such as organics or metals, the effect of LPS may modulate or be modulated by other PM components. The adjuvant effects of diesel-exhaust particles on LPS-induced inflammation have been well documented (167–169). The results of studies related to the role of LPS in PM-induced pulmonary responses are likely to vary depending upon the exposure protocol (e.g., whether LPS is given prior to, simultaneously, or post-PM exposure) (170,171). The mechanism by which LPS induces a pulmonary inflammatory response involves Toll-like receptor 4-mediated cell signaling, NF-$\kappa\beta$ activation, and induction of proinflammatory chemokines such as IL-8/MIP-2 (172–174). It has been shown that PM can induce the same chemokines, but apparently by a mechanism independent of Toll-4 receptor activation (172). How these mechanisms interlink to explain some of these interactions is yet to be determined.

The adjuvant effect of PM has been suggested in bacterial endotoxin-induced inflammation. However, the specific signaling mechanisms involved are likely dependent upon the PM components and the level of endotoxin activity. The role of ambient PM-associated LPS has been studied using alveolar macrophages from both animals and humans (39,76,175). The role of Toll-like receptors has also been suggested, but it is not clear how the PM components may modify these signaling events. Finally, it has been shown that LPS-neutralizing antibody reverses the effectiveness of coarse PM in inducing macrophage responses. This suggests that LPS may be a significant causative component of a select ambient PM.

D. Ultrafine Particles and Pulmonary Injury

It is difficult to distinguish between the roles of the fine vs. the ultrafine fractions of ambient PM, as ultrafine particles are continuously generated while simultaneously agglomerating into the fine PM size distribution (11). Although the health effects of ultrafines have been studied for several years using synthetic materials (36,37,176–178), interest in ambient ultrafines has recently increased (45) due to new epidemiological evidence (179,180) of their impact and toxicological evidence suggesting potential particle translocation through the circulation to other organs such as the brain, the liver, and the heart (5,44,45,178). Animal toxicological studies undertaken to address causality of ultrafine PM are emerging but thus far have not been able to attribute the effects on a mass basis in relation to either fine or coarse particles. The toxicity of ultrafines, based on mass, has generally been shown to be greater than that of fines (181); however, there are not enough data to confirm the relative roles of surface area and particle number in this outcome. It is likely that some ultrafines have reactive surfaces, whereas others may not. Likewise, some ultrafines can carry organic constituents, whereas others may carry transition metals. Using size-fractionated synthetic carbon particles, it has been shown that synthetic ultrafines induce greater toxicity than synthetic fines made of the same material. However, this relationship cannot be established using size-fractionated ambient PM, suggesting that, in addition to size, composition plays a critical role in toxicity (41,182). Using synthetic ultrafines of the same size but composed of different materials, Dick et al. (41) have shown that in vitro and in vivo oxidative stress, proinflammatory gene expression, and DNA damage are modulated by compositional differences in the ultrafines. However, ultrafine particles of a given composition with low-solubility materials are more inflammogenic in the rat lung than fine respirable particles made from the same material (181), when compared on a mass basis. The additional evidence supporting the importance of the composition of ultrafines comes from a study reporting stimulation of granulocyte macrophage colony-stimulating factor via a mitogen-activated protein kinase pathway in human bronchial epithelial cells following exposure to New York City ultrafines. The effect was attributed to their composition, as this effect was not evident with similar-sized carbon particles (38).

A variety of synthetic ultrafines have been employed in vitro using different cell types and in vivo using different animal species to determine the mechanisms of action. However, it is not clear which types of synthetic ultrafines may be more toxic or what mechanisms are involved in mediating their toxicity to cells. A number of studies have demonstrated the induction of oxidative stress with synthetic and ambient ultrafines (181). Ultrafine carbon particles can cause inflammation via processes independent of the release of transition metals, as no transition metals are present in carbon particles (183–185). The property that drives the greater inflammogenicity of ultrafines is unknown but may relate to the particle surface area and oxidative stress (186). Increases in intracellular $Ca(++)$ may underlie the cellular effects of ultrafines, although the mechanism whereby ultrafines produce this effect, is not understood (187).

Oxidative stress and mitochondrial DNA damage have been reported with exposures to ambient ultrafines from Los Angeles, CA, U.S.A. (184). By damaging cytoskeleton structures, ultrafine particles can impair the ability of macrophages to phagocytize and clear other particles (188). In alveolar epithelial cell lines, ultrafine ambient PM induced proliferative responses via activation of proto-oncogene expression (189). These and other emerging studies (190–193) may provide the mechanistic insight to link the relative roles of size, composition, and surface area in ultrafine-induced pulmonary and extrapulmonary health effects. On the basis of the available literature on ultrafines, it can be postulated that particle size and composition are important interdependent factors that may play significant roles in the observed toxic outcomes.

E. Oxidative Stress and Cell Signaling in PM-Induced Pulmonary Injury

Although metal mass concentrations in ambient air may be lower than the concentrations of other components, the ready bioavailability and the reactivity of metals may contribute significantly to adverse health outcomes. Metals can bind to proteins and regulate their functions, their ability to generate reactive oxygen species, and their systemic translocation. The PM-induced oxidative stress has been attributed to the presence of metals and/or organics (17,24,31,33,133,194) and ultrafines (184). The role of oxidative stress has been studied extensively both in vitro and in vivo (in rats) with metal-rich residual oil fly ash PM samples, as well as with PM samples of ambient origin (24,133,184,194). Residual oil fly ash exposures at high intratracheal doses in rats caused increased electron spin resonance signals in the alveolar lining fluid (195). Recently, a rapid increase in the steady state concentrations of reactive oxygen species, as measured by in vivo chemiluminescence, has been reported in the lungs of rats inhaling either combustion source or concentrated ambient particles (196). These authors also demonstrated an increase in the water content of the lung and in the activities of superoxide dismutase and catalase, consistent with oxidative processes. These rather striking changes were not triggered by inert carbon black aerosols suggesting that soluble and toxic components, such as metals, may play a critical role in eliciting pulmonary oxidative stress. In other studies, a transgenic mouse overexpressing superoxide dismutase, an antioxidant enzyme, demonstrated less pulmonary injury and inflammation following oil fly ash exposure (197), supporting the involvement of oxidative stress. Furthermore, the injury caused by the same fly ash was diminished in rats by their pretreatment with dimethylthiourea (194). Finally, numerous in vitro studies have shown that treatment of cells with antioxidants can diminish toxicity caused by a variety of metal-containing particles and individual metals (52,75,83,104,105,108,133,194). All these studies support the concept that metal-induced injury to the lung involves oxidative stress and cell signaling, and they also support a potential role for redox-active metal induction of Fenton-like reactions in the alveolar lining fluid.

Although many earlier toxicological studies have focused on the carcinogenic effects of diesel exhaust particles, the role of these particles in the induction of oxidative stress was not investigated until recently. Oxidative stress has now been demonstrated in a number of studies involving exposure of macrophages to diesel exhaust particles and extracts (31,33). Mitochondrial oxidative stress and apoptosis were also attributable to the extracts of diesel exhausts (198). Further, Kumagai et al. (199,200) have reported that organics of diesel exhausts cause oxidation of protein sulfhydryls and their bioactivation is involved in DNA damage. Quinones present in PM can directly catalyze reactive oxygen species formation and cause oxidative damage to cells (201). Polycyclic aromatic hydrocarbons present in diesel exhaust can indirectly induce oxidative stress through their bioactivation by cytochrome P450, epoxide hydrolase, and dihydrodiol dehydrogenase, leading to the generation of quinones (165). Pro-oxidative effects of diesel extracts have been shown in bronchial epithelial cells and macrophages (202). Interestingly, oxidative stress has also been reported in macrophages and epithelial cells following exposure to ambient ultra-fines (203,204). These authors attributed the oxidative stress and mito-chondrial damage to the process of redox cycling of organic chemicals within ultrafine ambient particles. One likely source of ultrafines in ambi-ent particles is diesel exhaust, as these particles are of nanometer size range when generated.

Intracellular signaling is critical in manifesting the response of a cell or an organism to a toxic insult (Fig. 3). A variety of signaling mechan-isms have been studied to determine how different causative components of PM may cause adverse pulmonary and cardiovascular effects. Metals such as vanadium, zinc, and arsenic have been well studied and are known to activate/inhibit protein phosphatases/kinases, leading to phospho-rylation of the EGF receptor and other proteins which, in turn, induce MAP kinase and NF-$\kappa\beta$ signaling cascades, and subsequent transcription of proinflammatory genes (131,132). Similarly, bacterial components of ambient air cause inflammatory responses via stimulation of Toll-like receptors and downstream signaling involving MAP kinases and the NF-$\kappa\beta$ pathway (39,76,172–175). These may directly or indirectly culmi-nate in oxidative stress augmented by organics, PAHs or diesel, and ultra-fines to stimulate NF-$\kappa\beta$, AP-1, STAT, and JAK pathways. In addition, the antioxidant response element can be induced by components mediat-ing oxidative stress, which further activate gene transcriptions involved in compensatory antioxidant mechanisms. Thus, we have just begun to unravel the role of oxidative stress and the molecular mechanisms of the cell signaling involved in the pathogenesis of ambient PM-induced pulmonary diseases in animals and humans. The availability of high-throughput screening for phosphoproteins (phosphatases and kinases), families of transcription factors, and gene expression, along with protein expression profiling, will provide insight into the mechanisms of the complex bionetworking of responses. Studies have also begun to invest-igate the roles of single nucleotide polymorphisms, which modify gene transcriptional machinery and translational events. These factors subsequently cause variations in individual susceptibilities to given envir-onmental exposures (205–207). Added to this are DNA binding proteins, which provide yet another control on gene transcription, and post-transcriptional protein modifications, which might modulate responses to air pollutants.

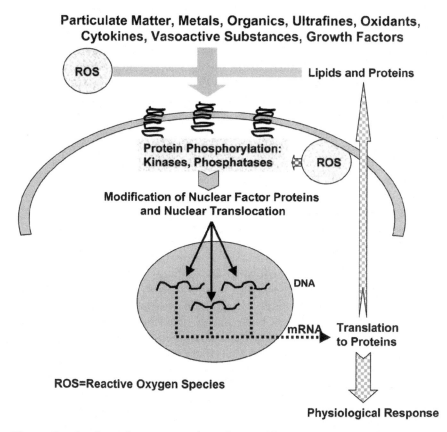

Figure 3 A schematic representation of potential cell signaling events, which can be induced in the lung or in the heart following the PM exposure. A comprehensive analysis of phosphoproteins, nuclear factor translocation, and gene expression can provide mechanistic information on the biological network of signaling and cross-talk between signaling pathways in PM-induced cell injury.

F. Host Susceptibility and Lung Injury

Epidemiological associations indicating greater morbidity and mortality in individuals with pre-existing diseases have stimulated research on the impact of susceptibility to PM health effects. Groups with chronic obstructive pulmonary diseases (COPD), asthma/allergic airway diseases, pneumonia, and other infectious diseases have been shown to have stronger associations with increased adverse effects following exposure to PM than healthy individuals (1–7). In order to understand how pre-existing pulmonary disease may exacerbate PM-induced health effects and how this susceptibility can be considered in the risk assessment process, toxicologists have employed transgenic and pharmaceutically-induced animal models of human diseases in PM health effect studies (205,208). The PM health effects have been studied extensively in rodent models of allergic airway diseases. However, there are relatively fewer studies using models of chronic pulmonary disease, such as COPD, fibrosis, and pulmonary hypertension. There are a number of possible reasons for this discrepancy: (1) the health concern for exacerbated PM effects in COPD patients was only recently recognized; (2) the skepticism in using animal models which poorly mimic human disease; (3) the complexity and variability of disease phenotype; and (4) the lack of consistent data to demonstrating exacerbation of PM effects.

Mechanisms underlying susceptibility are likely to reflect the pathological expression of disease/host physiology and may be mediated via differences in gene/protein expression (e.g., single nucleotide polymorphisms or dysregulation of transcription) (205–207,209). Animal models of various diseases can provide mechanistic evidence on the susceptibility variation following air pollution/PM exposures and perhaps shed light on common host features that contribute to risk.

The reported studies on PM health effects using animal models have provided mixed results. It has been shown that PM effects may be either exacerbated or decreased due to the presence of experimental bronchitis or emphysema, respectively, and that these differences in susceptibility may relate to differences in the bioavailability of PM and its distribution in the diseased lung (210,211). Studies done with a bronchitic rat model have shown exacerbated inflammatory responses to concentrated ambient PM from Boston, MA, U.S.A. (17) and Research Triangle Park, NC, U.S.A. (18). However, a rat model with coexisting bronchitis and emphysema did not demonstrate increased toxicity or inflammation when exposed to combustion-derived PM (208). A rat model of monocrotaline-induced vasculitis has been shown to demonstrate exacerbated pulmonary injury and mortality following exposures to combustion-derived PM and its metal constituents (28,212). The mechanisms are unclear but may relate to underlying endothelial damage caused by monocrotaline. The same model demonstrated an enhanced toxicity when exposed to concentrated ambient PM in Boston (213) but not when exposed to concentrated New York City PM (214). Clearly, the mechanisms underlying the variabilities in susceptibility are poorly understood at this time.

Genetic models with unigenic or polygenic disease phenotypes may be critical to understanding the gene–environmental interactions responsible for variations in susceptibility to PM-induced injury. A rat strain exhibiting naturally-occurring systemic hypertension (the Wistar–Kyoto-derived spontaneously hypertensive rat) that likely involves polygenic traits as in humans, has been shown to be susceptible to combustion-derived PM health effects (23) and airway diseases caused by exposure to tobacco smoke and sulfur dioxide (215,216). Although many phenotypic and genetic differences exist between this disease model and its healthy control strain (Wistar-Kyoto rat), the mechanisms and genetic make-up that governs its susceptibility are not fully understood. However, it has recently been demonstrated that the lungs and hearts of spontaneously hypertensive rats express higher baseline levels of many inflammatory cytokines (209), Toll-like receptors, and activated nuclear factors (217). It has also been demonstrated that this rat strain is more susceptible to increased blood coagulability, which may predispose these animals to exacerbated cardiovascular effects of PM (23). A number of mouse strains demonstrating variable susceptibility to ozone have also been shown to be differentially susceptible to PM, due to their genetic make-up (205–207). It has been shown that increased susceptibility of a mouse strain to hyperoxia is associated with a mutation in NRF-2, which regulates phase II metabolism enzyme genes, including the one regulating glutathione homeostasis (218). This study provides a genetic basis for susceptibility differences in an oxidative stress-mediated toxic response. Similarly, differences in the responsiveness to LPS, but not to PM, have been associated with a mutation in Toll-like receptors, which mediates LPS-induced inflammatory responses in the lung (219). It would be interesting to investigate whether analogous polymorphisms exist in humans susceptible to pulmonary diseases and PM-induced lung injury.

Our understanding of susceptibility differences can only be enhanced by using a variety of transgenic and animal disease models, in conjunction with epidemiological evaluations of susceptibility differences in human populations. This complicated biological discipline is being slowly but increasingly addressed in relation to environmental exposures, as we enter an era of biotechnology evolution. The issues remain as to how this will be integrated into the human risk assessment arena.

V. Bioavailability of PM and Links to Cardiovascular Effects

A number of epidemiological studies have demonstrated positive associations between levels of air pollution and risk factors for cardiovascular diseases, reporting increases in plasma viscosity (220), plasma fibrinogen (221), circulating band cells (222), C-reactive protein (223), systemic inflammation (222), and oxidative stress (224) as indices of pollution-induced effects. Both panel and clinical studies have investigated functional cardiophysiological impairments in humans after air pollution episodes and following occupational exposures to fuel oil ash; increases in pulse rate, blood pressure, and arrhythmias, along with decreases in heart rate variability, have been reported (112,225–228). Further, clinical studies have shown that concentrated ambient particles can increase acute phase reactants, such as plasma fibrinogen (229), and induce vasoconstriction in the brachial artery (230), a possible marker for coronary artery constriction. Animal toxicological studies, designed to verify the epidemiological findings showing increases in risk factors of cardiovascular disease following PM exposure, have largely supported the notion that air pollution exposure can cause cardiovascular toxicity. These associations have provided some insight into how air pollution may promote cardiac toxicity via systemic impairment; however, the mechanisms have not yet been identified.

A. Cardiopulmonary Interactions

Positive associations linking cardiovascular mortality and morbidity and increased particulate air pollution have also stimulated interest in the physiologic interactions between the cardiac and pulmonary systems. Given that the lung is the portal of entry for air pollutants, it is intriguing that the heart can sometimes be the primary target for the adverse effects produced by these agents. Although the intimate anatomical and physiological relationships between the heart and the lung have been appreciated for a number of years, the cross-linking of toxicological responses is only now being investigated. For example, environmental exposures and chronic pulmonary diseases have been associated with right heart impairments (231–234). As the entire cardiac output passes through the low-pressure pulmonary capillaries for oxygenation and removal of carbon dioxide, any PM-induced increase in pulmonary vasculature resistance can impede blood flow and result in increased right ventricular pressure. Sustained extrapressure in the right ventricle will lead to hypertrophy of the right ventricle, a condition known as cor pulmonale (235). Air pollution-induced changes in right and left ventricular function may not be detectable at lower degrees of pulmonary injury; however, generalized vascular effects may result. Another potentially relevant cardiopulmonary interaction may occur as a consequence of changes in carbon dioxide and oxygen exchange occurring in the pulmonary vasculature. Vascular chemoreceptors can sense blood gas changes (236) that are likely to occur during pulmonary injury; activation of these receptors can shift the balance between sympathetic and parasympathetic tone and thereby alter cardiac output. Other functional cardiopulmonary interactions may also occur through neurohumoral and vagal-mediated changes in respiration, cardiac conductance, and vascular resistance (237–239). Additionally, pulmonary injury can stimulate the release of mediators that may impair blood coagulation, fibrinolysis, and clearance of vasoactive substances such as endothelin. Finally, the capillary network can facilitate the uptake of toxic air pollutants, which may travel to and directly impact the heart before their clearance through the liver and kidney. These integral physiological events make the pulmonary and cardiovascular systems inseparable and make epidemiological associations between pulmonary air pollution exposure and cardiac morbidity/mortality likely.

B. Mechanisms of PM-Induced Cardiovascular Effects

Attempts to more fully evaluate the proposed mechanisms of cardiovascular injury following exposure to PM have been generally unsuccessful for a number of reasons. First, there are no appropriate animal models sensitive enough to exhibit frank cardiac toxicity following exposure to environmentally relevant concentrations of PM. Second, clinically useful plasma markers of cardiac injury are currently unable to detect subtle inflammatory and degenerative changes in the heart. Although histological evaluation of cardiac tissue—using a variety of staining techniques—remains the most accurate method of detecting subtle cardiac toxicity, these techniques are not routinely employed in air pollution studies and may not yield quantifiable changes with acute exposures at ambient levels. Finally, environmental PM contains diverse causative constituents. Therefore, without sufficient knowledge of constituent-specific effects on cardiac tissue, it is difficult to identify appropriate PM samples that can be used to study cardiovascular effects.

Three primary pathophysiological mechanisms have been proposed to account for the observed PM-induced cardiovascular effects (240–242) (Fig. 4). According to the first proposed mechanism, it is likely that toxic PM and/or its constituents deposit in the lung and cause a localized inflammatory response. Mediators and products of the inflammatory response may then enter the systemic circulation and thereby adversely affect the systemic vasculature, as well as other remote tissues or organ systems, including the heart. This pulmonary injury/inflammation-induced systemic activation can increase microvascular thrombogenic activity, expression of endothelial adhesion molecules, endothelial activation, oxidative stress, and inflammation leading to subsequent cardiac events. The second mechanistic hypothesis involves stimulation of vagal reflexes generated by sensory C-fibers on the respiratory epithelium. These reflexes, in turn, may alter the ratio of sympathetic/parasympathetic activation and can lead to profound changes in vascular tone, as well as decrements in cardiac performance and rhythmicity. More details on neurologically-mediated cardiovascular responses to PM can be found in Chapter 6 of this book. The third proposed mechanism involves the concept that metallic substances bound to PM are water soluble and therefore readily translocated to the systemic circulation. Thus, these soluble metals may pass freely into the pulmonary circulation and migrate to the heart where they may induce cardiac injury by direct interactions with myocardial tissues and cells.

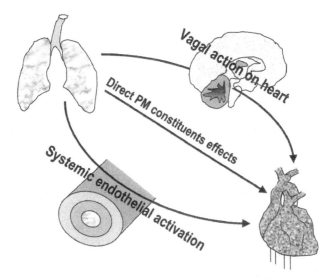

Figure 4   Potential mechanisms of PM-induced cardiac effects. Three primary mechanisms have been proposed for cardiac impairments induced by pulmonary exposure to PM: (1) pulmonary injury/inflammation causes systemic responses (activation of blood coagulation cascade, release of vasoactive substances, release of cytokines in the circulation, release of immature polymorphonuclear cells from bone marrow, and direct endothelial activation), which cause changes in the heart; (2) neuronal-mediated alteration in cardiac parasympathetic and sympathetic tone; and (3) soluble and bioavailable components migrate to the heart and cause direct effects on cardiac cells.

1. Systemic Vascular Response to PM Exposure

Systemic endothelial activation can result in a variety of biological phenomena (Fig. 5). For example, PM-induced pulmonary inflammation may activate endothelial cells in the lung, stimulate the blood coagulation cascade, and inhibit clot degradation (Fig. 6) (243,244). Fibrinogen, an important component of the coagulation cascade, is involved in the final stage of clot formation where it is converted to fibrin to form the clot (245,246). Hence, the concentration of fibrinogen in the plasma is often used as an index of the degree of activation of the coagulation response. Furthermore, fibrinogen is considered to be one of the critical risk factors for cardiovascular disease, as it has long been known that humans and animals with hypertension and cardiovascular disease have higher levels of plasma fibrinogen (247–249). Although the relationship between this plasma marker and PM exposure was initially examined in epidemiological studies, a number of other studies have since evaluated the roles of blood coagulation and clot retention in metal- and PM-induced pulmonary injuries. Increases in plasma fibrinogen levels following exposures to particles have been noted

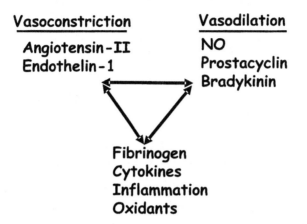

Figure 5 A schematic representation of interactions between released vasoactive substances and cytokines, oxidants, and mediators of blood coagulation following endothelial activation and inflammation in the vasculature. Note that endothelial responses can be triggered by activation of endothelial cells via cytokines, circulating vasoactive substances, oxidants, and circulating proteins involved in the blood coagulation cascade.

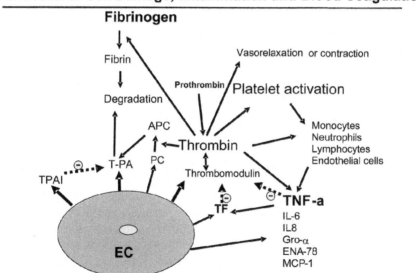

Figure 6 Blood coagulation and clot degradation events that are likely to be altered following PM-induced pulmonary injury. EC, endothelial cells; APC, activated protein C; TPAI, tissue-plasminogen activator inhibitor; T-PA, tissue-plasminogen activator; PC, protein C, TF, tissue factor.

in animal studies, as well as in clinical studies following combustion and real-time ambient particle exposures (23,28,229,250). Microvascular clot formation in the pulmonary capillary bed has also been postulated to be important in the cardiopulmonary response.

A number of metals that are components of ambient PM have been studied with respect to their cardiac and vascular effects. Exposure to nickel, a major constituent of combustion particles, promotes activation of plasminogen activator inhibitor-1 (PAI-1), along with the formation of tissue plasminogen activator (tPA) and plasminogen complex, ultimately leading to the prolongation of clot retention in the lung (251). Inflammatory mediators released by pulmonary cells following particle exposure can also increase clot retention. Many studies have shown that a variety of PM and PM-metallic constituents increase the levels of inflammatory cytokines in the lung (137,182,209). It has recently been reported that zinc exposure can cause an increase in tissue factor mRNA expression in the heart, likely via a systemic increase in blood coagulation (252). Ambient particulates may stimulate endothelial release of vasoactive substances, such as endothelin and bradykinin, that may trigger systemic activation and alterations in cardiac function and cellular biochemistry (253).

PM-induced extrapulmonary vascular thrombosis has been studied in rabbits and hamsters following pulmonary exposure to fine and ultrafine PM. A number of these studies have been conducted by Nemmar and colleagues (193,254,255). Their unique approach involved combining intravenous injection of Rose Bengal dye with exposure to UV radiation to stimulate thrombi formation in the femoral artery. Animals were then intratracheally exposed to PM, and platelet aggregation and thrombi formation were quantitated using computer-assisted tomography. These studies have provided critical information regarding the pathways by which PM may cause increases in thrombi formation away from the lung. Using a variety of PM with both soluble and insoluble constituents, these authors have further demonstrated that exposures to ultrafine carbon particles and soluble metals—but not coarse carbon particles—may promote thrombi formation (253). These studies suggest a potential role for circulating PM constituents in systemic thrombi formation and also argue for a role for local pulmonary inflammation in mediating systemic events. However, many questions remain regarding the thrombi-producing ability of insoluble PM, which is more likely to be retained within the lung, as well as the effects of combined exposures to locally-acting pulmonary irritants, such as ozone or LPS, and PM containing bioavailable metals.

The induction of systemic inflammation by pulmonary phagocyte-mediator release has been examined in a number of different human and animal studies (32,40,222,256,257), and these studies support a role for bone marrow stimulation in the production of PM-associated cardiovascular effects. It has been shown that the initial recruitment of inflammatory cells following exposure to PM causes activation of macrophages and the release of mediators that remotely stimulate the bone marrow (222,258). In response, the bone marrow releases polymorphonuclear cells into the circulation. A persistent increase in the presence of these band cells has been noted in Singapore residents following nearby forest fires and biomass burning (259), as well as in rabbits repeatedly exposed by intratracheal instillation to ambient PM (258). These cells are phenotypically and functionally unique and have an enhanced capacity to cause tissue damage. Studies by van Eeden et al. (260) have shown that these cells are stiffer and less mobile than normal polymorphonuclear cells and that they contain more myeloperoxidases and exhibit higher expression of surface adhesion molecules, such as L-selectin. These authors further postulated that, because of these characteristics, these newly-released polymorphonuclear cells could be more readily activated in the lung endothelium by locally-released cytokines. Studies conducted by this same group of investigators (40) demonstrated that the systemic inflammation caused by repeated PM exposures in rabbits was associated with a progression of atherosclerotic plaque formation in both coronary and abdominal arteries. They demonstrated that the volume fraction of atherosclerotic lesions in coronary arteries was significantly greater after repeated exposure to PM in plaque-prone Watanabe rabbits, and that this effect was significantly correlated with the number of particles phagocytosed by macrophages. This sequence of events has been proposed to play a role in PM-induced systemic inflammation (222) and cigarette smoke-induced emphysema (261,262). However, at this time, the role of this inflammatory response in PM-induced cardiac pathology, rhythm changes, and chronic cardiovascular diseases is still unclear. Furthermore, it is not clear if systemic inflammation can be induced as a result of bone marrow stimulation following pulmonary injury mediated by gaseous air pollutants, such as ozone. Although increased inflammatory mediators such as IL-6 and TNF-α have been detected in patients with cardiovascular disease and are considered important risk factors (263), to date there is no consistent evidence that demonstrates increases in these mediators in response to PM exposure in humans or in animals.

2. Neuronal Mechanisms

The second mechanism proposed to explain the observed cardiovascular effects following inhalation of PM involves the neuronal mediation of physiological responses in the heart. Numerous studies have demonstrated that inhaled pollutants stimulate airway sensory receptors that reflexively induce changes in cardiovascular tone and electrocardiogram traces (264). The heterogeneous distribution of sensory receptors along the nasal passages, tracheobronchial tree, and alveoli accounts for the variety of reported responses. Thus, different receptor types sense different stimuli, e.g., rapidly-adapting receptors sense touch and irritants (265), whereas neuroepithelial bodies sense hypoxia (266). C-fibers also respond to irritant stimuli (267) and have been implicated in PM-induced neurogenic inflammation (268). Rapidly-adapting receptors and C-fiber receptors in the alveolar wall are very sensitive to irritants and pollutants and reflexively cause pronounced bradycardia and hypotension (264,269,270). In other studies, human bronchial airway epithelial cells were pretreated with capsazepine and amiloride, antagonists to vanilloid and acid-sensitive receptors, respectively, and subsequently exposed to PM of different origins. These studies demonstrated significant reductions in the release of IL-6, suggesting their potential role in neurogenic inflammation (271,272). Peptides, such as substance P and neurokinins, are released from sensory C-fibers that penetrate between airway epithelial cells following irritant exposures. Substance P causes vasodilatation, plasma exudation, and mucus secretion, whereas neurokinin A causes bronchoconstriction and enhanced cholinergic reflexes (273,274). The anatomic and physiological properties of afferent neurons have been shown to change following irritation and inflammation in the airways (275,276). These studies demonstrate cardiorespiratory interactions, mediated through vagal and spinal ganglion neurons, that lead to changes in cardiac conductance. However, it is still not well understood if these physiological reflexes have any pathological manifestations. Thus, although remarkable correlations have been reported between exposure to PM and cardiophysiological impairments in epidemiological and animal toxicological studies, the pathobiologic links are less well understood.

3. Potential Role of Soluble Components in Cardiac Injury Caused by PM

The ready bioavailability of the soluble constituents of PM and their capacity for transport to the heart provides an additional potential mechanism whereby inhaled pollutants may promote cardiac injury. These causative constituents are mostly metals, soluble organics, and ultrafine particles. Thus, inhaled PM-associated constituents may be taken up by the pulmonary capillary bed and delivered to the left side of the heart prior to their processing or trapping in the liver or other tissues. Metals may bind to reactive plasma proteins and then circulate into the coronary bed before their filtration or storage as metal–metallothionein complexes in the hepatic tissue. Importantly, the concentration of soluble PM components traversing the pulmonary capillary bed, entering the heart via the pulmonary vein, and perfusing the myocardium via the coronary circulation can be substantially higher than the concentrations seen following the subsequent dilution within the systemic circulation. Soluble components may also be circulated to the brain before they are cycled through the liver where they are subject to filtration or storage. These potential mechanisms are not fully understood and represent an area for future investigation.

There have been a few occupational toxicological studies which demonstrated cardiovascular impairments with exposure to metals, and many of these elemental components have been detected at high concentrations in ambient PM. For example, cadmium has been linked to increased cardiovascular toxicity, especially at lower, more environmentally-relevant concentrations (277,278). Although cadmium has been detected in some ambient particles, it is also a prominent elemental component of cigarette smoke (279), and smoking has long been linked to increased cardiovascular morbidity and mortality (280,281). The argument can be made that at higher concentration acute exposures (e.g., smoking), the toxicity to the lung may overwhelm the cardiovascular effects of this metal. However, the impact on the heart in chronic exposure scenarios may be substantial. Exposure to cobalt, which also has been detected in ambient PM, has been linked to cardiomyopathy (282). Mortality in aluminum smelter workers has been ascribed to circulatory complications, suggesting a potential role of this metal in cardiovascular disorders (283). Exposure to copper has been linked to increases in the risk factors for coronary diseases (284), whereas exposure to silica has been epidemiologically associated with an increased incidence of autoimmune vasculitis in humans (285). Higher mortality from cardiovascular diseases has been specifically noted among ferroalloy plant workers (286). Importantly, all of these elemental components, e.g., cadmium, cobalt, aluminum, copper, silica, and iron have been detected in significant concentrations in most ambient PM (9,15,19). Because epidemiological studies specifically suggest a greater risk of morbidity and mortality due to cardiovascular diseases following exposure to ambient PM, experimental studies linking each component to specific cardiovascular health effects will provide a better mechanistic understanding of PM and cardiopulmonary interactions.

Although most PM animal studies have been focused on cardiophysiological impairments, a few recent studies have utilized other approaches. As in the case with the lung, a rapid increase in the steady state concentrations of reactive oxygen species has also been found in the hearts of rats inhaling combustion source and concentrated ambient particles (196). The reported changes include an increase in the water content of the heart, along with increases in the activities of superoxide dismutase and catalase. These rather striking changes were attributable to soluble metals, as inert carbon black aerosols did not elicit cardiac toxicity. Although in vitro studies have demonstrated changes in redox sensitive cell signaling and an increased production of inflammatory cytokines, in vivo chemiluminescence techniques have not been extensively employed in PM studies. It remains to be determined if such changes induce any pathological manifestations in the heart, especially following exposures to low levels of particles.

A recent episodic inhalation study of combustion source PM (287) retrospectively analyzed cardiac histopathology in three rat strains that had undergone both shorter/acute and long-term exposures. The PM sample selected for this study contained a large amount of bioavailable zinc and minimal quantities of nickel, vanadium, and iron, distinguishing it from other extensively studied residual oil fly ashes that contained much higher levels of these transition metals (27–29,74). Furthermore, the elemental and organic compositions of this combustion PM were similar to those of ambient PM obtained from selected urban locations (9,29,288,289). This study provided causative evidence of cardiac injury in Wistar–Kyoto rats following episodic, long-term inhalation of PM with the suggestion of a potential role for zinc (Fig. 7). Myocardial injury was characterized predominantly by degenerating cardiomyocytes, active inflammatory foci, and

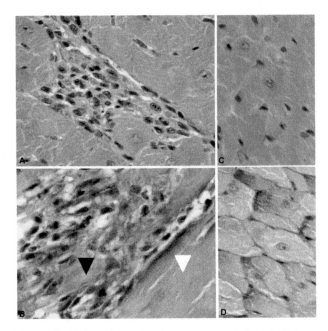

Figure 7 Myocardial injury following long-term episodic inhalation exposures to fugitive oil combustion PM in the rat. Rats were exposed to fugitive combustion oil fly ash by nose-only inhalation, $10\,mg/m^3$, 6 hr/day; 1 day/week for 16 consecutive weeks, and cardiac histology was performed using hematoxylin–eosin and PAS staining. Note significant focal myocardial degeneration and inflammation (A and B). Normal myocardium is shown in C and D. In B, the black arrow indicates degenerating myocyte, whereas the white arrow indicates intact striated myocyte. (From Ref. 287.)

accumulation of collagen in the ventricles and interventricular septum. Furthermore, injury was apparent at exposure concentrations that resulted in minimal pulmonary toxicity.

A potential role for bioavailable organic constituents, especially PAHs, in cardiovascular injury is also likely; for example, these constituents have been known to cause atherogenic stimulation that lead to proliferation of vascular smooth muscle cells (290,291). Diesel soot particles contain a variety of PAHs and can contribute significantly to the mass of ambient PM, especially in heavy motor vehicle traffic areas (19,34,292). These particles have been shown to have mutagenic and carcinogenic potentials in a variety of organ systems. Some of these organic components are readily taken up by epithelial and endothelial cells (54), and thus, these cells may be the target sites for inhaled bioactive organic constituents. Extensive research by Ramos and colleagues (293–295) has examined the underlying mechanisms responsible for the vascular atherogenic effects caused by exposure to benzo-[a]-pyrene and methylcholanthrene in animals. Their studies have further demonstrated that both in vivo and in vitro oxidative metabolites of benzo-[a]-pyrene cause activation of antioxidant/electrophile response element nuclear binding and c-Ha-ras transactivation in vascular smooth muscle cells, leading to proliferative responses (295). Although the effects of bioactive PAHs on vascular smooth muscles cells have been studied extensively, similar studies have not been conducted using diesel exhaust or ambient particles in vivo. The efforts to study the potential atherogenic effects of particles may be limited by the availability of appropriate animal models. As described earlier, to date only one study has demonstrated the progression of atherosclerotic lesions in rabbits following repeated intratracheal instillations of ambient particles at high concentrations (40). Although these authors did not postulate that the observed coronary vascular effects were caused by organic constituents of PM, they did demonstrate systemic inflammation and the appearance of band cells in the activation of endothelial surface-bearing atherosclerosis plaque. Thus, while progress has been made, much remains to be done in order to understand the role of individual constituents in stimulating cardiovascular responses, and many more mechanistic studies will be required to fully understand the potential constituent-specific mechanisms.

4. Host Susceptibility to Cardiovascular Effects of PM

As discussed earlier with respect to pulmonary disease models, our understanding of the impact of acute or chronic myocardial and vascular disease on susceptibility to adverse PM-associated cardiovascular effects is limited. Only a few PM health studies have employed animal models exhibiting experimental and genetic cardiac disease. PM has been shown to exacerbate ischemia-related myocardial dysfunction in surgically-induced rat (296) and dog (148) models of myocardial infarction. The incidence of myocardial effects has been statistically correlated with bioavailable components of ambient PM. Studies using a rat polygenic model of cardiovascular disease demonstrated greater fibrinogen change relative to healthy rats and demonstrated the suppression of the ST-segment area of the ECG, following the exposure to inhaled combustion particles (23,209). Hypertensive rats have also been used for identifying cardiovascular risk factors and immediate cardiovascular effects of PM (297). Rats with acute myocardial infarction have been exposed to combustion source (253) and concentrated ambient particles to identify biological indicators demonstrating exacerbated cardiovascular effects of PM (296). Rats with monocrotaline-induced pulmonary vasculitis demonstrated increased mortality, along with increased arrhythmias and decreased heart rate, following a bolus exposure to combustion-derived PM and its bioavailable metal constituents (28). These studies, which imply causality and demonstrate differences in susceptibility, were not designed to probe the underlying mechanisms. Greater integration of a variety of experimental and genetic models with improved molecular and genetic characterization will be crucial in the identification of PM cardiovascular effects among diverse human populations with cardiopulmonary diseases.

VI. Summary

The PM health effects may be largely driven by the individual PM constituents and their respective bioavailabilities at pulmonary and extrapulmonary sites. The bioavailability of PM components can be affected by host factors, such as the presence of disease, and more importantly, by the solubility and the reactivity of the components in biological fluids, the size of the inhaled particles, and the physicochemical properties of the PM. Although soluble and insoluble components can be bioavailable at the site of their deposition in the airways and on alveolar epithelial surfaces, some components such as leachable metals, organics, and ultrafine PM can be transported to extrapulmonary sites. Endothelial surfaces of the vasculature may be greatly affected by these components. Nonsoluble components are phagocytosed by alveolar macrophages and, depending on their structure and chemical properties, may cause the macrophages to be activated. Local pulmonary inflammation is also likely to stimulate the systemic vasculature, as inflammation can trigger blood coagulation and vasoconstriction. Although the mechanisms of PM health effects can vary depending on the composition of the PM, they likely involve oxidative stress and component-specific signaling cascades that govern phenotype expression of toxicity via gene expression. Although in vitro approaches using a variety of cells of cardiopulmonary origin can provide a mechanistic understanding of component-specific biological effects, the inherent integration of the cardiac and pulmonary systems necessitates the use of acute and chronic in vivo approaches to understand the complex and interactive biological network affecting the physiology of cardiopulmonary diseases.

Acknowledgments

The authors thank Drs. Daniel L. Costa, Linda S. Birnbaum, Janice A. Dye, and Jane Gallagher of the US EPA and W. Mike Foster of the Duke University Medical Center, Durham, NC, for their critical reviews of the manuscript. The authors also thank Dr. Peter S. Gilmour, for his help in the preparation of the manuscript and Ms. Preeti P. Kodavanti, for her help in conducting a computerized literature search.

References

1. Dockery DW. Epidemiologic evidence of cardiovascular effects of particulate air pollution. Environ Health Perspect 2001; 109(suppl 4):483–486.
2. Morris RD. Airborne particulates and hospital admissions for cardiovascular disease: a quantitative review of the evidence. Environ Health Perspect 2001; 109(suppl 4):495–500.
3. Pope CA III. Epidemiology of fine particulate air pollution and human health: biologic mechanisms and who's at risk? Environ Health Perspect 2000; 108(suppl 4):713–723.
4. Schwartz J. Air pollution and blood markers of cardiovascular risk. Environ Health Perspect 2001; 109(suppl 3):405–409.
5. Ibald-Mulli A, Wichmann HE, Kreyling W, Peters A. Epidemiological evidence on health effects of ultrafine particles. J Aerosol Med 2002; 15(2): 189–201.
6. Leikauf GD. Hazardous air pollutants and asthma. Environ Health Perspect 2002; 110(suppl 4):505–526.
7. Bell ML, Samet JM, Dominici F. Time-series studies of particulate matter. Annu Rev Public Health 2004; 25:247–280.
8. Derwent RG. Atmospheric chemistry. In: Holgate ST, Samet JM, Koren HS, Maynard RL, eds. Air Pollution and Health. London: Academic Press, 1999.
9. Harrison RM, Yin J. Particulate matter in the atmosphere: which particle properties are important for its effects on health? Sci Total Environ 2000; 249(1–3):85–101.
10. Levy JI, Houseman EA, Spengler JD, Loh P, Ryan L. Fine particulate matter and polycyclic aromatic hydrocarbon concentration patterns in Roxbury, Massachusetts: a community-based GIS analysis. Environ Health Perspect 2001; 109(4):341–347.
11. Xiong C, Friedlander SK. Morphological properties of atmospheric aerosol aggregates. Proc Natl Acad Sci USA 2001; 98(21):11851–11856.

12. Motallebi N, Taylor CA Jr, Croes BE. Particulate matter in California: part 2—Spatial, temporal, and compositional patterns of PM2.5, PM10–2.5, and PM10. J Air Waste Manag Assoc 2003; 53(12):1517–1530.
13. Green LC, Armstrong SR. Particulate matter in ambient air and mortality: toxicologic perspectives. Regul Toxicol Pharmacol 2003; 38(3):326–335.
14. Mysliwiec MJ, Kleeman MJ. Source apportionment of secondary airborne particulate matter in a polluted atmosphere. Environ Sci Technol 2002; 36(24):5376–5384.
15. Smith KR, Kim S, Recendez JJ, Teague SV, Menache MG, Grubbs DE, Sioutas C, Pinkerton, KE. Airborne particles of the California Central Valley alter the lungs of healthy adult rats. Environ Health Perspect 2003; 111(7): 902–908; discussion A408–A409.
16. Goldsmith CA, Ning Y, Qin G, Imrich A, Lawrence J, Murthy GG, Catalano PJ, Kobzik L. Combined air pollution particle and ozone exposure increases airway responsiveness in mice. Inhal Toxicol 2002; 14(4):325–347.
17. Saldiva PH, Clarke RW, Coull BA, Stearns RC, Lawrence J, Murthy GG, Diaz E, Koutrakis P, Suh H, Tsuda A, Godleski JJ. Lung inflammation induced by concentrated ambient air particles is related to particle composition. Am J Respir Crit Care Med 2002; 165(12):1610–1617.
18. Kodavanti UP, Mebane R, Ledbetter A, Krantz T, McGee J, Jackson MC, Walsh L, Hilliard H, Chen BY, Richards J, Costa DL. Variable pulmonary responses from exposure to concentrated ambient air particles in a rat model of bronchitis. Toxicol Sci 2000; 54(2):441–451.
19. Walters DM, Breysse PN, Wills-Karp M. Ambient urban Baltimore particulate-induced airway hyperresponsiveness and inflammation in mice. Am J Respir Crit Care Med 2001; 164(8 Pt 1):1438–1443.
20. Smith RL, Spitzner D, Kim Y, Fuentes M. Threshold dependence of mortality effects for fine and coarse particles in Phoenix, Arizona. J Air Waste Manag Assoc 2000; 50(8):1367–1379.
21. Kodavanti UP, Hauser R, Christiani DC, Meng ZH, McGee J, Ledbetter A, Richards J, Costa DL. Pulmonary responses to oil fly ash particles in the rat differ by virtue of their specific soluble metals. Toxicol Sci 1998; 43(2):204–212.
22. Watkinson WP, Campen MJ, Costa DL. Cardiac arrhythmia induction after exposure to residual oil fly ash particles in a rodent model of pulmonary hypertension. Toxicol Sci 1998; 41(2):209–216.
23. Kodavanti UP, Schladweiler MC, Ledbetter AD, Hauser R, Christiani DC, McGee J, Richards JR, Costa DL. Temporal association between pulmonary and systemic effects of particulate matter in healthy and cardiovascular compromised rats. J Toxicol Environ Health A 2002; 65(20):1545–1569.
24. Ghio AJ, Silbajoris R, Carson JL, Samet JM. Biologic effects of oil fly ash. Environ Health Perspect 2002; 110(suppl 1):89–94.
25. Driscoll KE, Lindenschmidt RC, Maurer JK, Perkins L, Perkins M, Higgins J. Pulmonary response to inhaled silica or titanium dioxide. Toxicol Appl Pharmacol 1991; 111(2):201–210.
26. Drumm K, Oettinger R, Smolarski R, Bay M, Kienast K. In vitro study of human alveolar macrophages inflammatory mediator transcriptions and

releases induced by soot FR 101, Printex 90, titandioxide and Chrysotile B. Eur J Med Res 1998; 3(9):432–438.

27. Kodavanti UP, Jaskot RH, Costa DL, Dreher KL. Pulmonary proinflammatory gene expression induction following acute exposure to residual oil fly ash: roles of particle-associated metals. Inhal Toxicol 1997; 9:679–701.

28. Campen MJ, Nolan JP, Schladweiler MC, Kodavanti UP, Costa DL, Watkinson WP. Cardiac and thermoregulatory effects of instilled particulate matter-associated transition metals in healthy and cardiopulmonary-compromised rats. J Toxicol Environ Health A 2002; 65(20):1615–1631.

29. Adamson IY, Prieditis H, Hedgecock C, Vincent R. Zinc is the toxic factor in the lung response to an atmospheric particulate sample. Toxicol Appl Pharmacol 2000; 166(2):111–119.

30. Hirano S, Shimada T, Osugi J, Kodama N, Suzuki KT. Pulmonary clearance and inflammatory potency of intratracheally instilled or acutely inhaled nickel sulfate in rats. Arch Toxicol 1994; 68(9):548–554.

31. Hiura TS, Kaszubowski MP, Li N, Nel AE. Chemicals in diesel exhaust particles generate reactive oxygen radicals and induce apoptosis in macrophages. J Immunol 1999; 163(10):5582–5591.

32. Salvi S, Blomberg A, Rudell B, Kelly F, Sandstrom T, Holgate ST, Frew A. Acute inflammatory responses in the airways and peripheral blood after short-term exposure to diesel exhaust in healthy human volunteers. Am J Respir Crit Care Med 1999; 159(3):702–709.

33. Hashimoto S, Gon Y, Takeshita I, Matsumoto K, Jibiki I, Takizawa H, Kudoh S, Horie T. Diesel exhaust particles activate p38 MAP kinase to produce interleukin 8 and RANTES by human bronchial epithelial cells and N-acetylcysteine attenuates p38 MAP kinase activation. Am J Respir Crit Care Med 2000; 161(1):280–285.

34. Pandya RJ, Solomon G, Kinner A, Balmes JR. Diesel exhaust and asthma: hypotheses and molecular mechanisms of action. Environ Health Perspect 2002; 110(suppl 1):103–112.

35. Singh P, DeMarini, DM, Dick CAJ, Tabor DG, Ryan JV, Linak WP, Kobayashi T, Gilmour MI. Sample characterization of automobile and forklift diesel exhaust particles and comparative pulmonary toxicity in mice. Environ Health Perspect. 2004; 112(8):814–819.

36. Warheit DB, Laurence BR, Reed KL, Roach DH, Reynolds GA, Webb TR. Comparative pulmonary toxicity assessment of single-wall carbon nanotubes in rats. Toxicol Sci 2004; 77(1):117–125.

37. Zhang Q, Kusaka Y, Zhu X, Sato K, Mo Y, Kluz T, Donaldson K. Comparative toxicity of standard nickel and ultrafine nickel in lung after intratracheal instillation. J Occup Health 2003; 45(1):23–30.

38. Reibman J, Hsu Y, Chen LC, Kumar A, Su WC, Choy W, Talbot A, Gordon T. Size fractions of ambient particulate matter induce granulocyte macrophage colony-stimulating factor in human bronchial epithelial cells by mitogen-activated protein kinase pathways. Am J Respir Cell Mol Biol 2002; 27(4): 455–462.

39. Imrich A, Ning Y, Kobzik L. Insoluble components of concentrated air particles mediate alveolar macrophage responses in vitro. Toxicol Appl Pharmacol 2000; 167(2):140–150.

40. Suwa T, Hogg JC, Quinlan KB, Ohgami A, Vincent R, van Eeden SF. Particulate air pollution induces progression of atherosclerosis. J Am Coll Cardiol 2002; 39(6):935–942.

41. Dick CA, Singh P, Daniels M, Evansky P, Becker S, Gilmour MI. Murine pulmonary inflammatory responses following instillation of size-fractionated ambient particulate matter. J Toxicol Environ Health A 2003; 66(23): 2193–2207.

42. Fubini B. Surface reactivity in the pathogenic response to particulates. Environ Health Perspect 1997; 105(suppl 5):1013–1020.

43. Guthrie GD Jr. Mineral properties and their contributions to particle toxicity. Environ Health Perspect 1997; 105S(suppl 5):1003–1011.

44. Nemmar A, Vanbilloen H, Hoylaerts MF, Hoet PH, Verbruggen A, Nemery B. Passage of intratracheally instilled ultrafine particles from the lung into the systemic circulation in hamster. Am J Respir Crit Care Med 2001; 164(9): 1665–1668.

45. Oberdorster G, Utell MJ. Ultrafine particles in the urban air: to the respiratory tract—and beyond? Environ Health Perspect 2002; 110(8):A440–A441.

46. Hermans C, Bernard A. Lung epithelium-specific proteins: characteristics and potential applications as markers. Am J Respir Crit Care Med 1999; 159(2):646–678.

47. Abbracchio MP, Heck JD, Costa M. The phagocytosis and transforming activity of crystalline metal sulfide particles are related to their negative surface charge. Carcinogenesis 1982; 3(2):175–180.

48. Veronesi B, Haar C, Lee L, Oortgiesen M. The surface charge of visible particulate matter predicts biological activation in human bronchial epithelial cells. Toxicol Appl Pharmacol 2002; 178(3):144–154.

49. Kuhn DC, Demers LM. Influence of mineral dust surface chemistry on eicosanoid production by the alveolar macrophage. J Toxicol Environ Health 1992; 35(1):39–50.

50. Berg I, Schluter T, Gercken G. Increase of bovine alveolar macrophage superoxide anion and hydrogen peroxide release by dusts of different origin. J Toxicol Environ Health 1993; 39(3):341–354.

51. Schluter T, Berg I, Dorger M, Gercken G. Effect of heavy metal ions on the release of reactive oxygen intermediates by bovine alveolar macrophages. Toxicology 1995; 98(1–3):47–55.

52. Tian L, Lawrence DA. Metal-induced modulation of nitric oxide production in vitro by murine macrophages: lead, nickel, and cobalt utilize different mechanisms. Toxicol Appl Pharmacol 1996; 141(2):540–547.

53. Hatch GE, Boykin E, Graham JA, Lewtas J, Pott F, Loud K, Mumford JL. Inhalable particles and pulmonary host defense: in vivo and in vitro effects of ambient air and combustion particles. Environ Res 1985; 36(1):67–80.

54. Gerde P, Muggenburg BA, Lundborg M, Dahl AR. The rapid alveolar absorption of diesel soot-adsorbed benzo[a]pyrene: bioavailability, metabo-

lism and dosimetry of an inhaled particle-borne carcinogen. Carcinogenesis 2001; 22(5):741–749.

55. Binkova B, Cerna M, Pastorkova A, Jelinek R, Benes I, Novak J, Sram RJ. Biological activities of organic compounds adsorbed onto ambient air particles: comparison between the cities of Teplice and Prague during the summer and winter seasons 2000–2001. Mutat Res 2003; 525(1–2):43–59.

56. Rhoads K, Sanders CL. Lung clearance, translocation, and acute toxicity of arsenic, beryllium, cadmium, cobalt, lead, selenium, vanadium, and ytterbium oxides following deposition in rat lung. Environ Res 1985; 36(2):359–378.

57. Takenaka S, Karg E, Roth C, Schulz H, Ziesenis A, Heinzmann U, Schramel P, Heyder J. Pulmonary and systemic distribution of inhaled ultrafine silver particles in rats. Environ Health Perspect 2001; 109(suppl 4):547–551.

58. Kim JY, Hauser R, Wand MP, Herrick RF, Houk RS, Aeschliman DB, Woodin MA, Christiani DC. Association of expired nitric oxide with urinary metal concentrations in boilermakers exposed to residual oil fly ash. Am J Ind Med 2003; 44(5):458–466.

59. Tjalve H, Henriksson J. Uptake of metals in the brain via olfactory pathways. Neurotoxicology 1999; 20(2–3):181–195.

60. Dorman DC, Brenneman KA, McElveen AM, Lynch SE, Roberts KC, Wong BA. Olfactory transport: a direct route of delivery of inhaled manganese phosphate to the rat brain. J Toxicol Environ Health A 2002; 65(20): 1493–1511.

61. Rao DB, Wong BA, McManus BE, McElveen AM, James AR, Dorman DC. Inhaled iron, unlike manganese, is not transported to the rat brain via the olfactory pathway. Toxicol Appl Pharmacol 2003; 193(1):116–126.

62. Earth Watch, Global Environmental Monitoring. Urban air pollution in megacities of the world. Chapter 2. In: Understanding Urban Air Pollution Problems. Blackwell on behalf of the World Health Organization and United Nations Environment Programme.

63. Manchester-Neesvig JB, Schauer JJ, Cass GR. The distribution of particle-phase organic compounds in the atmosphere and their use for source apportionment during the Southern California Children's Health Study. J Air Waste Manag Assoc 2003; 53(9):1065–1079.

64. Diaz-Sanchez D, Dotson AR, Takenaka H, Saxon A. Diesel exhaust particles induce local IgE production in vivo and alter the pattern of IgE messenger RNA isoforms. J Clin Invest 1994; 94(4):1417–1425.

65. van Zijverden M, van der Pijl A, Bol M, van Pinxteren FA, de Haar C, Penninks H, van Loveren H, Pieters R. Diesel exhaust, carbon black, and silica particles display distinct Th1/Th2 modulating activity. Toxicol Appl Pharmacol 2000; 168(2):131–139.

66. Diaz-Sanchez D, Proietti L, Polosa R. Diesel fumes and the rising prevalence of atopy: an urban legend? Curr Allergy Asthma Rep 2003; 3(2):146–152.

67. Yang HM, Butterworth L, Munson AE, Meade BJ. Respiratory exposure to diesel exhaust particles decreases the spleen IgM response to a T cell-dependent antigen in female B6C3F1 mice. Toxicol Sci 2003; 71(2): 207–216.

68. Siegel PD, Saxena RK, Saxena QB, Ma JK, Ma JY, Yin XJ, Castranova V, Al-Humadi N, Lewis DM. Effect of diesel exhaust particulate (DEP) on immune responses: contributions of particulate versus organic soluble components. J Toxicol Environ Health A 2004; 67(3):221–231.

69. Campen MJ, McDonald JD, Gigliotti AP, Seilkop SK, Reed MD, Benson JM. Cardiovascular effects of inhaled diesel exhaust in spontaneously hypertensive rats. Cardiovasc Toxicol 2003; 3(4):353–361.

70. Boffetta P, Jourenkova N, Gustavsson P. Cancer risk from occupational and environmental exposure to polycyclic aromatic hydrocarbons. Cancer Causes Control 1997; 8(3):444–472.

71. Kagawa J. Health effects of diesel exhaust emissions—a mixture of air pollutants of worldwide concern. Toxicology 2002; 181–182:349–353.

72. Schins RP. Mechanisms of genotoxicity of particles and fibers. Inhal Toxicol 2002; 14(1):57–78.

73. Huang YC, Ghio AJ, Stonehuerner J, McGee J, Carter JD, Grambow SC, Devlin RB. The role of soluble components in ambient fine particle-induced changes in human lungs and blood. Inhal Toxicol 2003; 15(4):327–342.

74. Dreher KL, Jaskot RH, Lehmann JR, Richards JH, McGee JK, Ghio AJ, Costa DL. Soluble transition metals mediate residual oil fly ash induced acute lung injury. J Toxicol Environ Health 1997; 50(3):285–305.

75. Kennedy T, Ghio AJ, Reed W, Samet J, Zagorski J, Quay J, Carter J, Dailey L, Hoidal JR, Devlin RB. Copper-dependent inflammation and nuclear factor-kappaB activation by particulate air pollution. Am J Respir Cell Mol Biol 1998; 19(3):366–378.

76. Soukup JM, Becker S. Human alveolar macrophage responses to air pollution particulates are associated with insoluble components of coarse material, including particulate endotoxin. Toxicol Appl Pharmacol 2001; 171(1): 20–26.

77. Goldsmith CA, Frevert C, Imrich A, Sioutas C, Kobzik L. Alveolar macrophage interaction with air pollution particulates. Environ Health Perspect 1997; 105(suppl 5):1191–1195.

78. Catelas I, Huk OL, Petit A, Zukor DJ, Marchand R, Yahia L. Flow cytometric analysis of macrophage response to ceramic and polyethylene particles: effects of size, concentration, and composition. J Biomed Mater Res 1998; 41(4):600–607.

79. Dorger M, Krombach F. Interaction of alveolar macrophages with inhaled mineral particulates. J Aerosol Med 2000; 13(4):369–380.

80. Fenoglio I, Prandi L, Tomatis M, Fubini B. Free radical generation in the toxicity of inhaled mineral particles: the role of iron speciation at the surface of asbestos and silica. Redox Rep 2001; 6(4):235–241.

81. Fubini B, Fenoglio I, Elias Z, Poirot O. Variability of biological responses to silicas: effect of origin, crystallinity, and state of surface on generation of reactive oxygen species and morphological transformation of mammalian cells. J Environ Pathol Toxicol Oncol 2001; 20(suppl 1):95–108.

82. Donaldson K, Stone V, Duffin R, Clouter A, Schins R, Borm P. The quartz hazard: effects of surface and matrix on inflammogenic activity. J Environ Pathol Toxicol Oncol 2001; 20(suppl 1):109–118.

83. Schins RP, Duffin R, Hohr D, Knaapen AM, Shi T, Weishaupt C, Stone V, Donaldson K, Borm PJ. Surface modification of quartz inhibits toxicity, particle uptake, and oxidative DNA damage in human lung epithelial cells. Chem Res Toxicol 2002; 15(9):1166–1173.

84. Obot CJ, Morandi MT, Beebe TP, Hamilton RF, Holian A. Surface components of airborne particulate matter induce macrophage apoptosis through scavenger receptors. Toxicol Appl Pharmacol 2002; 184(2):98–106.

85. Shen Z, Bosbach D, Hochella MF Jr, Bish DL, Williams MG Jr, Dodson RF, Aust AE. Using in vitro iron deposition on asbestos to model asbestos bodies formed in human lung. Chem Res Toxicol 2000; 13(9):913–921.

86. Fenoglio I, Fonsato S, Fubini B. Reaction of cysteine and glutathione (GSH) at the freshly fractured quartz surface: a possible role in silica-related diseases? Free Radic Biol Med 2003; 35(7):752–762.

87. Turi JL, Yang F, Garrick MD, Piantadosi CA, Ghio AJ. The iron cycle and oxidative stress in the lung. Free Radic Biol Med 2004; 36(7):850–857.

88. Foster WM. Deposition and clearance of inhaled particles. In: Holgate ST, Samet JM, Koren, HS, Maynard RL, eds. Air Pollution and Health. London: Academic Press, 1999.

89. Geiser M. Morphological aspects of particle uptake by lung phagocytes. Microsc Res Tech 2002; 57(6):512–522.

90. Lehnert BE. Pulmonary and thoracic macrophage subpopulations and clearance of particles from the lung. Environ Health Perspect 1992; 97:17–46.

91. Palecanda A, Kobzik L. Receptors for unopsonized particles: the role of alveolar macrophage scavenger receptors. Curr Mol Med 2001; 1(5):589–595.

92. Becker S, Soukup JM, Sioutas C, Cassee FR. Response of human alveolar macrophages to ultrafine, fine, and coarse urban air pollution particles. Exp Lung Res 2003; 29(1):29–44.

93. Oberdorster G. Toxicokinetics and effects of fibrous and nonfibrous particles. Inhal Toxicol 2002; 14(1):29–56.

94. Oberdorster G, Sharp Z, Atudorei V, Elder A, Gelein R, Lunts A, Kreyling W, Cox C. Extrapulmonary translocation of ultrafine carbon particles following whole-body inhalation exposure of rats. J Toxicol Environ Health A 2002; 65(20):1531–1543.

95. Kreyling WG, Semmler M, Erbe F, Mayer P, Takenaka S, Schulz H, Oberdorster G, Ziesenis A. Translocation of ultrafine insoluble iridium particles from lung epithelium to extrapulmonary organs is size dependent but very low. J Toxicol Environ Health A 2002; 65(20):1513–1530.

96. Khandoga A, Stampfl A, Takenaka S, Schulz H, Radykewicz R, Kreyling W, Krombach F. Ultrafine particles exert prothrombotic but not inflammatory effects on the hepatic microcirculation in healthy mice in vivo. Circulation 2004; 109(10):1320–1325.

97. Florence AT, Hillery AM, Hussain N, Jani PU. Factors affecting the oral uptake and translocation of polystyrene nanoparticles: histological and analytical evidence. J Drug Target 1995; 3(1):65–70.

98. Oberdorster G. Translocation of inhaled ultrafine particles to the brain. Inhal Toxicol. 2004; 16(6–7):437–445.

99. Garrick MD, Dolan KG, Horbinski C, Ghio AJ, Higgins D, Porubcin M, Moore G, Hainsworth LN, Umbreit JN, Conrad ME, Feng L, Lis A, Roth JA, Singleton S, Garrick LM. DMT1: a mammalian transporter for multiple metals. Biometals 2003; 16(1):41–54.

100. Nemery B, Hoet PH, Nemmar A. The Meuse Valley fog of 1930: an air pollution disaster. Lancet 2001; 357(9257):704–708.

101. Logan WP. Mortality in the London fog incident, 1952. Lancet 1953; 1(7):336–338.

102. Anderson HR. Health effects of air pollution episodes. In: Holgate ST, Samet JM, Koren HS, Maynard RL, eds. Air Pollution and Health. London: Academic Press, 1999.

103. Hatch GE, Gardner DE, Menzel DB. Stimulation of oxidant production in alveolar macrophages by pollutant and latex particles. Environ Res 1980; 23(1):121–136.

104. Ghio AJ, Stonehuerner J, Dailey LA, Carter JD. Metals associated with both the water-soluble and insoluble fractions of an ambient air pollution particle catalyze an oxidative stress. Inhal Toxicol 1999; 11(1):37–49.

105. Carter JD, Ghio AJ, Samet JM, Devlin RB. Cytokine production by human airway epithelial cells after exposure to an air pollution particle is metal-dependent. Toxicol Appl Pharmacol 1997; 146(2):180–188.

106. Ghio AJ, Carter JD, Richards JH, Brighton LE, Lay JC, Devlin RB. Disruption of normal iron homeostasis after bronchial instillation of an iron-containing particle. Am J Physiol 1998; 274(3 Pt 1):L396–L403.

107. Ghio AJ, Richards JH, Dittrich KL, Samet JM. Metal storage and transport proteins increase after exposure of the rat lung to an air pollution particle. Toxicol Pathol 1998; 26(3):388–394.

108. Samet JM, Graves LM, Quay J, Dailey LA, Devlin RB, Ghio AJ, Wu W, Bromberg PA, Reed W. Activation of MAPKs in human bronchial epithelial cells exposed to metals. Am J Physiol 1998; 275(3 Pt 1): L551–L558.

109. Samet JM, Stonehuerner J, Reed W, Devlin RB, Dailey LA, Kennedy TP, Bromberg PA, Ghio AJ. Disruption of protein tyrosine phosphate homeostasis in bronchial epithelial cells exposed to oil fly ash. Am J Physiol 1997; 272(3 Pt 1):L426–L432.

110. Wang YZ, Bonner JC. Mechanism of extracellular signal-regulated kinase (ERK)-1 and ERK-2 activation by vanadium pentoxide in rat pulmonary myofibroblasts. Am J Respir Cell Mol Biol 2000; 22(5):590–596.

111. Goebeler M, Roth J, Brocker EB, Sorg C, Schulze-Osthoff K. Activation of nuclear factor-kappaB and gene expression in human endothelial cells by the common haptens nickel and cobalt. J Immunol 1995; 155(5): 2459–2467.

112. Magari SR, Schwartz J, Williams PL, Hauser R, Smith TJ, Christiani DC. The association of particulate air metal concentrations with heart rate variability. Environ Health Perspect 2002; 110(9):875–880.

113. Gavett SH, Madison SL, Dreher KL, Winsett DW, McGee JK, Costa DL. Metal and sulfate composition of residual oil fly ash determines airway hyper-reactivity and lung injury in rats. Environ Res 1997; 72(2):162–172.

114. Ghio AJ, Quigley DR. Complexation of iron by humic-like substances in lung tissue: role in coal workers' pneumoconiosis. Am J Physiol 1994; 267(2 Pt 1):L173–L179.

115. Ghio AJ, Devlin RB. Inflammatory lung injury after bronchial instillation of air pollution particles. Am J Respir Crit Care Med 2001; 164(4):704–708.

116. Pagan I, Costa DL, McGee JK, Richards JH, Dye JA. Metals mimic airway epithelial injury induced by in vitro exposure to Utah Valley ambient particulate matter extracts. J Toxicol Environ Health A 2003; 66(12):1087–1112.

117. Gavett SH, Haykal-Coates N, Copeland LB, Heinrich J, Gilmour MI. Metal composition of ambient PM2.5 influences severity of allergic airways disease in mice. Environ Health Perspect 2003; 111(12):1471–1477.

118. Johansson A, Curstedt T, Jarstrand C, Camner P. Alveolar macrophages and lung lesions after combined exposure to nickel, cobalt, and trivalent chromium. Environ Health Perspect 1992; 97:215–219.

119. Johansson A, Curstedt T, Robertson B, Camner P. Lung lesions after experimental combined exposure to nickel and trivalent chromium. Environ Res 1989; 50(1):103–119.

120. Rojanasakul Y, Wang L, Hoffman AH, Shi X, Dalal NS, Banks DE, Ma JK. Mechanisms of hydroxyl free radical-induced cellular injury and calcium overloading in alveolar macrophages. Am J Respir Cell Mol Biol 1993; 8(4):377–383.

121. Madden MC, Thomas MJ, Ghio AJ. Acetaldehyde (CH_3CHO) production in rodent lung after exposure to metal-rich particles. Free Radic Biol Med 1999; 26(11–12):1569–1577.

122. Mouithys-Mickalad A, Mathy-Hartert M, Du G, Sluse F, Deby C, Lamy M, Deby-Dupont G. Oxygen consumption and electron spin resonance studies of free radical production by alveolar cells exposed to anoxia: inhibiting effects of the antibiotic ceftazidime. Redox Rep 2002; 7(2):85–94.

123. Ding M, Shi X, Castranova V, Vallyathan V. Predisposing factors in occupational lung cancer: inorganic minerals and chromium. J Environ Pathol Toxicol Oncol 2000; 19(1–2):129–138.

124. Barchowsky A, O'Hara KA. Metal-induced cell signaling and gene activation in lung diseases. Free Radic Biol Med 2003; 34(9):1130–1135.

125. Ball BR, Smith KR, Veranth JM, Aust AE. Bioavailability of iron from coal fly ash: mechanisms of mobilization and of biological effects. Inhal Toxicol 2000; 12(suppl 4):209–225.

126. Gutteridge JM, Quinlan GJ, Evans TW. The iron paradox of heart and lungs and its implications for acute lung injury. Free Radic Res 2001; 34(5): 439–443.

127. Ghio AJ, Carter JD, Richards JH, Richer LD, Grissom CK, Elstad MR. Iron and iron-related proteins in the lower respiratory tract of patients with acute respiratory distress syndrome. Crit Care Med 2003; 31(2):395–400.

128. Aust AE, Ball JC, Hu AA, Lighty JS, Smith KR, Straccia AM, Veranth JM, Young WC. Particle characteristics responsible for effects on human lung epithelial cells. Res Rep Health Eff Inst 2002; 110:1–65.

129. Kim JY, Hauser R, Wand MP, Herrick RF, Amarasiriwardena CJ, Christiani DC. The association of expired nitric oxide with occupational particulate metal exposure. Environ Res 2003; 93(2):158–166.

130. Morinville A, Maysinger D, Shaver A. From Vanadis to Atropos: vanadium compounds as pharmacological tools in cell death signalling. Trends Pharmacol Sci 1998; 19(11):452–460.

131. Samet JM, Silbajoris R, Wu W, Graves LM. Tyrosine phosphatases as targets in metal-induced signaling in human airway epithelial cells. Am J Respir Cell Mol Biol 1999; 21(3):357–364.

132. Theberge JF, Mehdi MZ, Pandey SK, Srivastava AK. Prolongation of insulin-induced activation of mitogen-activated protein kinases ERK 1/2 and phosphatidylinositol 3-kinase by vanadyl sulfate, a protein tyrosine phosphatase inhibitor. Arch Biochem Biophys 2003; 420(1):9–17.

133. Dye JA, Adler KB, Richards JH, Dreher KL. Role of soluble metals in oil fly ash-induced airway epithelial injury and cytokine gene expression. Am J Physiol 1999; 277:L498–L510.

134. Wang YZ, Ingram JL, Walters DM, Rice AB, Santos JH, Van Houten B, Bonner JC. Vanadium-induced STAT-1 activation in lung myofibroblasts requires H_2O_2 and P38 MAP kinase. Free Radic Biol Med 2003; 35(8): 845–855.

135. Wang L, Medan D, Mercer R, Overmiller D, Leornard S, Castranova V, Shi X, Ding M, Huang C, Rojanasakul Y. Vanadium-induced apoptosis and pulmonary inflammation in mice: role of reactive oxygen species. J Cell Physiol 2003; 195(1):99–107.

136. Wu W, Jaspers I, Zhang W, Graves LM, Samet JM. Role of Ras in metal-induced EGF receptor signaling and NF-kappaB activation in human airway epithelial cells. Am J Physiol Lung Cell Mol Physiol 2002; 282(5): L1040–L1048.

137. Samet JM, Silbajoris R, Huang T, Jaspers I. Transcription factor activation following exposure of an intact lung preparation to metallic particulate matter. Environ Health Perspect 2002; 110(10):985–990.

138. Gordon T, Chen LC, Fine JM, Schlesinger RB, Su WY, Kimmel TA, Amdur MO. Pulmonary effects of inhaled zinc oxide in human subjects, guinea pigs, rats, and rabbits. Am Ind Hyg Assoc J 1992; 53(8):503–509.

139. Fine JM, Gordon T, Chen LC, Kinney P, Falcone G, Sparer J, Beckett WS. Characterization of clinical tolerance to inhaled zinc oxide in naive subjects and sheet metal workers. J Occup Environ Med 2000; 42(11): 1085–1091.

140. Kodavanti UP, Schladweiler MC, Ledbetter AD, Hauser R, Christiani DC, Samet JM, McGee J, Richards JH, Costa DL. Pulmonary and systemic effects of zinc-containing emission particles in three rat strains: multiple exposure scenarios. Toxicol Sci 2002; 70(1):73–85.

141. Ye B, Maret W, Vallee BL. Zinc metallothionein imported into liver mitochondria modulates respiration. Proc Natl Acad Sci USA 2001; 98(5): 2317–2322.

142. Ali MM, Frei E, Straub J, Breuer A, Wiessler M. Induction of metallothionein by zinc protects from daunorubicin toxicity in rats. Toxicology 2002; 179(1–2):85–93.
143. Finney LA, O'Halloran TV. Transition metal speciation in the cell: insights from the chemistry of metal ion receptors. Science 2003; 300(5621):931–936.
144. Kambe T, Yamaguchi-Iwai Y, Sasaki R, Nagao M. Overview of mammalian zinc transporters. Cell Mol Life Sci 2004; 61(1):49–68.
145. Kim JH, Cho H, Ryu SE, Choi MU. Effects of metal ions on the activity of protein tyrosine phosphatase VHR: highly potent and reversible oxidative inactivation by Cu^{2+} ion. Arch Biochem Biophys 2000; 382(1):72–80.
146. Li Y, Seacat A, Kuppusamy P, Zweier JL, Yager JD, Trush MA. Copper redox-dependent activation of 2-tert-butyl(1,4)hydroquinone: formation of reactive oxygen species and induction of oxidative DNA damage in isolated DNA and cultured rat hepatocytes. Mutat Res 2002; 518(2):123–133.
147. Muhle H, Mangelsdorf I. Inhalation toxicity of mineral particles: critical appraisal of endpoints and study design. Toxicol Lett 2003; 140–141: 223–228.
148. Wellenius GA, Coull BA, Godleski JJ, Koutrakis P, Okabe K, Savage ST, Lawrence JE, Murthy GG, Verrier RL. Inhalation of concentrated ambient air particles exacerbates myocardial ischemia in conscious dogs. Environ Health Perspect 2003; 111(4):402–408.
149. Cohen R, Velho V. Update on respiratory disease from coal mine and silica dust. Clin Chest Med 2002; 23(4):811–826.
150. Hnizdo E, Vallyathan V. Chronic obstructive pulmonary disease due to occupational exposure to silica dust: a review of epidemiological and pathological evidence. Occup Environ Med 2003; 60(4):237–243.
151. Fernandes MB, Brooks P. Characterization of carbonaceous combustion residues: II. Nonpolar organic compounds. Chemosphere 2003; 53(5):447–458.
152. Tobias HJ, Beving DE, Ziemann PJ, Sakurai H, Zuk M, McMurry PH, Zarling D, Waytulonis R, Kittelson DB. Chemical analysis of diesel engine nanoparticles using a nano-DMA/thermal desorption particle beam mass spectrometer. Environ Sci Technol 2001; 35(11):2233–2243.
153. Stayner L, Dankovic D, Smith R, Steenland K. Predicted lung cancer risk among miners exposed to diesel exhaust particles. Am J Ind Med 1998; 34(3):207–219.
154. Valberg PA, Watson AY. Analysis of diesel-exhaust unit-risk estimates derived from animal bioassays. Regul Toxicol Pharmacol 1996; 24(1 Pt 1):30–44.
155. Stenfors N, Nordenhall C, Salvi SS, et al. Different airway inflammatory responses in asthmatic and healthy humans exposed to diesel. Eur Respir J 2004; 23(1):82–86.
156. Steerenberg PA, Withagen CE, Dormans JA, van Dalen WJ, van Loveren H, Casee FR. Adjuvant activity of various diesel exhaust and ambient particles in two allergic models. J Toxicol Environ Health A 2003; 66(15):1421–1439.
157. Ichinose T, Takano H, Sadakane K, Yanagisawa R, Yoshikawa T, Sagai M, Shibamoto T. Mouse strain differences in eosinophilic airway inflammation caused by intratracheal instillation of mite allergen and diesel exhaust particles. J Appl Toxicol 2004; 24(1):69–76.

158. Yang K, Airoldi L, Pastorelli R, Restano J, Guanci M, Hemminki K. Aromatic DNA adducts in lymphocytes of humans working at high and low traffic density areas. Chem Biol Interact 1996; 101(2):127–136.

159. Pohjola SK, Lappi M, Honkanen M, Rantanen L, Savela K. DNA binding of polycyclic aromatic hydrocarbons in a human bronchial epithelial cell line treated with diesel and gasoline particulate extracts and benzo[a]pyrene. Mutagenesis 2003; 18(5):429–438.

160. Risom L, Dybdahl M, Bornholdt J, Vogel U, Wallin H, Moller P, Loft S. Oxidative DNA damage and defence gene expression in the mouse lung after short-term exposure to diesel exhaust particles by inhalation. Carcinogenesis 2003; 24(11):1847–1852.

161. Nemmar A, Hoet PH, Dinsdale D, Vermylen J, Hoylaerts MF, Nemery B. Diesel exhaust particles in lung acutely enhance experimental peripheral thrombosis. Circulation 2003; 107(8):1202–1208.

162. Hirano S, Furuyama A, Koike E, Kobayashi T. Oxidative-stress potency of organic extracts of diesel exhaust and urban fine particles in rat heart microvessel endothelial cells. Toxicology 2003; 187(2–3):161–170.

163. Bommel H, Haake M, Luft P, Horejs-Hoeck J, Hein H, Bartels J, Schauer C, Poschl U, Kracht M, Duschl A. The diesel exhaust component pyrene induces expression of IL-8 but not of eotaxin. Int Immunopharmacol 2003; 3(10–11):1371–1379.

164. Mudway IS, Stenfors N, Duggan ST, Roxborough H, Zielinski H, Marklund SL, Blomberg A, Frew AJ, Sandstrom T, Kelly FJ. An in vitro and in vivo investigation of the effects of diesel exhaust on human airway lining fluid antioxidants. Arch Biochem Biophys 2004; 423(1):200–212.

165. Ma JY, Ma JK. The dual effect of the particulate and organic components of diesel exhaust particles on the alteration of pulmonary immune/inflammatory responses and metabolic enzymes. J Environ Sci Health Part C Environ Carcinog Ecotoxicol Rev 2002; 20(2):117–147.

166. Monn C, Koren HS. Bioaerosols in ambient air particulates: a review and research needs. Rev Environ Health 1999; 14(2):79–89.

167. Long CM, Suh HH, Kobzik L, Catalano PJ, Ning YY, Koutrakis P. A pilot investigation of the relative toxicity of indoor and outdoor fine particles: in vitro effects of endotoxin and other particulate properties. Environ Health Perspect 2001; 109(10):1019–1026.

168. Takano H, Yanagisawa R, Ichinose T, Sadakane K, Yoshino S, Yoshikawa T, Morita M. Diesel exhaust particles enhance lung injury related to bacterial endotoxin through expression of proinflammatory cytokines, chemokines, and intercellular adhesion molecule-1. Am J Respir Crit Care Med 2002; 165(9):1329–1335.

169. Rylander R. Endotoxin in the environment—exposure and effects. J Endotoxin Res 2002; 8(4):241–252.

170. Imrich A, Ning YY, Koziel H, Coull B, Kobzik L. Lipopolysaccharide priming amplifies lung macrophage tumor necrosis factor production in response to air particles. Toxicol Appl Pharmacol 1999; 159(2):117–124.

171. Amakawa K, Terashima T, Matsuzaki T, Matsumaru A, Sagai M, Yamaguchi K. Suppressive effects of diesel exhaust particles on cytokine release from human and murine alveolar macrophages. Exp Lung Res 2003; 29(3):149–164.

172. Hollingsworth IJ, Cook DN, Brass DM, Walker JK, Morgan DL, Foster WM, Schwartz DA. The role of toll-like receptor 4 in environmental airway injury in mice. Am J Respir Crit Care Med. 2004; 170(2):126–132.

173. Becker S, Fenton MJ, Soukup JM. Involvement of microbial components and toll-like receptors 2 and 4 in cytokine responses to air pollution particles. Am J Respir Cell Mol Biol 2002; 27(5):611–618.

174. Gilmour PS, Rahman I, Hayashi S, Hogg JC, Donaldson K, MacNee W. Adenoviral E1A primes alveolar epithelial cells to PM(10)-induced transcription of interleukin-8. Am J Physiol Lung Cell Mol Physiol 2001; 281(3): L598–L606.

175. Monn C, Becker S. Cytotoxicity and induction of proinflammatory cytokines from human monocytes exposed to fine (PM2.5) and coarse particles (PM10–2.5) in outdoor and indoor air. Toxicol Appl Pharmacol 1999; 155(3):245–252.

176. Oberdorster G, Ferin J, Gelein R, Soderholm SC, Finkelstein J. Role of the alveolar macrophage in lung injury: studies with ultrafine particles. Environ Health Perspect 1992; 97:193–199.

177. Oberdorster G, Finkelstein J, Ferin J, Godleski J, Chang LY, Gelein R, Johnston C, Crapo JD. Ultrafine particles as a potential environmental health hazard. Studies with model particles. Chest 1996; 109(suppl 3): 68S–69S.

178. Oberdorster G. Pulmonary effects of inhaled ultrafine particles. Int Arch Occup Environ Health 2001; 74(1):1–8.

179. Wichmann HE, Spix C, Tuch T, Wolke G, Peters A, Heinrich J, Kreyling WG, Heyder J. Daily mortality and fine and ultrafine particles in Erfurt, Germany part I: role of particle number and particle mass. Res Rep Health Eff Inst 2000; 98:5–86.

180. de Hartog JJ, Hoek G, Peters A, Timonen K, Ibald-Mulli A, Brunekreef B, Heinrich J, Tiittanen P, van Wijnen JH, Kreyling W, Kulmala M, Pekkanen J. Effects of fine and ultrafine particles on cardiorespiratory symptoms in elderly subjects with coronary heart disease: the ULTRA study. Am J Epidemiol 2003; 157(7):613–623.

181. Brown DM, Wilson MR, MacNee W, Stone V, Donaldson K. Size-dependent proinflammatory effects of ultrafine polystyrene particles: a role for surface area and oxidative stress in the enhanced activity of ultrafines. Toxicol Appl Pharmacol 2001; 175(3):191–199.

182. Dick CA, Brown DM, Donaldson K, Stone V. The role of free radicals in the toxic and inflammatory effects of four different ultrafine particle types. Inhal Toxicol 2003; 15(1):39–52.

183. Brown DM, Donaldson K, Borm PJ, Schins RP, Dehnhardt M, Gilmour P, Jimenez LA, Stone V. Calcium and ROS-mediated activation of transcription factors and TNF-α cytokine gene expression in macrophages exposed to ultrafine particles. Am J Physiol Lung Cell Mol Physiol 2004; 286(2):L344–L353.

184. Li N, Sioutas C, Cho A, Schmitz D, Misra C, Sempf J, Wang M, Oberley T, Froines J, Nel A. Ultrafine particulate pollutants induce oxidative stress and mitochondrial damage. Environ Health Perspect 2003; 111(4):455–460.

185. Brown DM, Stone V, Findlay P, MacNee W, Donaldson K. Increased inflammation and intracellular calcium caused by ultrafine carbon black is independent of transition metals or other soluble components. Occup Environ Med 2000; 57(10):685–691.

186. MacNee W, Donaldson K. Mechanism of lung injury caused by PM10 and ultrafine particles with special reference to COPD. Eur Respir J Suppl 2003; 40:47s–51s.

187. Stone V, Tuinman M, Vamvakopoulos JE, Shaw J, Brown D, Petterson S, Faux SP, Borm P, MacNee W, Michaelangeli F, Donaldson K. Increased calcium influx in a monocytic cell line on exposure to ultrafine carbon black. Eur Respir J 2000; 15(2):297–303.

188. Moller W, Hofer T, Ziesenis A, Karg E, Heyder J. Ultrafine particles cause cytoskeletal dysfunctions in macrophages. Toxicol Appl Pharmacol 2002; 182(3):197–207.

189. Timblin CR, Shukla A, Berlanger I, BeruBe KA, Churg A, Mossman BT. Ultrafine airborne particles cause increases in protooncogene expression and proliferation in alveolar epithelial cells. Toxicol Appl Pharmacol 2002; 179(2):98–104.

190. Wilson MR, Lightbody JH, Donaldson K, Sales J, Stone V. Interactions between ultrafine particles and transition metals in vivo and in vitro. Toxicol Appl Pharmacol 2002; 184(3):172–179.

191. Gallagher J, Sams R II, Inmon J, Gelein R, Elder A, Oberdorster G, Prahalad AK. Formation of 8-oxo-7,8-dihydro-2'-deoxyguanosine in rat lung DNA following subchronic inhalation of carbon black. Toxicol Appl Pharmacol 2003; 190(3):224–231.

192. Gilmour PS, Ziesenis A, Morrison ER, Vickers MA, Drost EM, Ford I, Karg E, Mossa C, Schroeppel A, Ferron GA, Heyder J, Greaves M, MacNee W, Donaldson K. Pulmonary and systemic effects of short-term inhalation exposure to ultrafine carbon black particles. Toxicol Appl Pharmacol 2004; 195(1):35–44.

193. Hamoir J, Nemmar A, Halloy D, Wirth D, Vincke G, Vanderplasschen A, Nemery B, Gustin P. Effect of polystyrene particles on lung microvascular permeability in isolated perfused rabbit lungs: role of size and surface properties. Toxicol Appl Pharmacol 2003; 190(3):278–285.

194. Dye JA, Adler KB, Richards JH, Dreher KL. Epithelial injury induced by exposure to residual oil fly-ash particles: role of reactive oxygen species? Am J Respir Cell Mol Biol 1997; 17(5):625–633.

195. Kadiiska MB, Mason RP, Dreher KL, Costa DL, Ghio AJ. In vivo evidence of free radical formation in the rat lung after exposure to an emission source air pollution particle. Chem Res Toxicol 1997; 10(10):1104–1108.

196. Gurgueira SA, Lawrence J, Coull B, Murthy GG, Gonzalez-Flecha B. Rapid increases in the steady-state concentration of reactive oxygen species in the lungs and heart after particulate air pollution inhalation. Environ Health Perspect 2002; 110(8):749–755.

197. Ghio AJ, Suliman HB, Carter JD, Abushamaa AM, Folz RJ. Overexpression of extracellular superoxide dismutase decreases lung injury after exposure to oil fly ash. Am J Physiol Lung Cell Mol Physiol 2002; 283(1): L211–L218.

198. Hiura TS, Li N, Kaplan R, Horwitz M, Seagrave JC, Nel AE. The role of a mitochondrial pathway in the induction of apoptosis by chemicals extracted from diesel exhaust particles. J Immunol 2000; 165(5):2703–2711.

199. Kumagai Y, Arimoto T, Shinyashiki M, Shimojo N, Nakai Y, Yoshikawa T, Sagai M. Generation of reactive oxygen species during interaction of diesel exhaust particle components with NADPH-cytochrome P450 reductase and involvement of the bioactivation in the DNA damage. Free Radic Biol Med 1997; 22(3):479–487.

200. Kumagai Y, Koide S, Taguchi K, Endo A, Nakai Y, Yoshikawa T, Shimojo N. Oxidation of proximal protein sulfhydryls by phenanthraquinone, a component of diesel exhaust particles. Chem Res Toxicol 2002; 15(4): 483–489.

201. Penning TM, Burczynski ME, Hung CF, McCoull KD, Palackal NT, Tsuruda LS. Dihydrodiol dehydrogenases and polycyclic aromatic hydrocarbon activation: generation of reactive and redox active o-quinones. Chem Res Toxicol 1999; 12(1):1–18.

202. Li N, Wang M, Oberley TD, Sempf JM, Nel AE. Comparison of the pro-oxidative and proinflammatory effects of organic diesel exhaust particle chemicals in bronchial epithelial cells and macrophages. J Immunol 2002; 169(8):4531–4541.

203. Li N, Kim S, Wang M, Froines J, Sioutas C, Nel A. Use of a stratified oxidative stress model to study the biological effects of ambient concentrated and diesel exhaust particulate matter. Inhal Toxicol 2002; 14(5):459–486.

204. Li N, Hao M, Phalen RF, Hinds WC, Nel AE. Particulate air pollutants and asthma. A paradigm for the role of oxidative stress in PM-induced adverse health effects. Clin Immunol 2003; 109(3):250–265.

205. Ohtsuka Y, Brunson KJ, Jedlicka AE, Mitzner W, Clarke RW, Zhang LY, Eleff SM, Kleeberger SR. Genetic linkage analysis of susceptibility to particle exposure in mice. Am J Respir Cell Mol Biol 2000; 22(5):574–581.

206. Zhang Q, Kleeberger SR, Reddy SP. DEP-induced fra-1 expression correlates with a distinct activation of AP-1-dependent gene transcription in the lung. Am J Physiol Lung Cell Mol Physiol 2004; 286(2):L427–L436.

207. Kleeberger SR. Genetic aspects of susceptibility to air pollution. Eur Respir J Suppl 2003; 40:52s–56s.

208. Kodavanti UP, Costa DL. Rodent models of susceptibility: what is their place in inhalation toxicology? Respir Physiol 2001; 128(1):57–70.

209. Kodavanti UP, Schladweiler MC, Ledbetter AD, Watkinson WP, Campen MJ, Winsett DW, Richards JR, Crissman KM, Hatch GE, Costa DL. The spontaneously hypertensive rat as a model of human cardiovascular disease: evidence of exacerbated cardiopulmonary injury and oxidative stress from inhaled emission particulate matter. Toxicol Appl Pharmacol 2000; 164(3): 250–263.

210. Sweeney TD, Brain JD, Leavitt SA, Godleski JJ. Emphysema alters the deposition pattern of inhaled particles in hamsters. Am J Pathol 1987; 128(1): 19–28.

211. Sweeney TD, Skornik WA, Brain JD, Hatch V, Godleski JJ. Chronic bronchitis alters the pattern of aerosol deposition in the lung. Am J Respir Crit Care Med 1995; 151(2 Pt 1):482–488.

212. Kodavanti UP, Jackson MC, Ledbetter AD, Richards JR, Gardner SY, Watkinson WP, Campen MJ, Costa DL. Lung injury from intratracheal and inhalation exposures to residual oil fly ash in a rat model of monocrotaline-induced pulmonary hypertension. J Toxicol Environ Health A 1999; 57(8):543–563.

213. Killingsworth CR, Shore SA, Alessandrini F, Dey RD, Paulauskis JD. Rat alveolar macrophages express preprotachykinin gene-I mRNA-encoding tachykinins. Am J Physiol 1997; 273(5 Pt 1):L1073–L1081.

214. Gordon T, Nadziejko C, Schlesinger R, Chen LC. Pulmonary and cardiovascular effects of acute exposure to concentrated ambient particulate matter in rats. Toxicol Lett 1998; 96–97:285–288.

215. Smith KR, Uyeminami DL, Kodavanti UP, Crapo JD, Chang LY, Pinkerton KE. Inhibition of tobacco smoke-induced lung inflammation by a catalytic antioxidant. Free Radic Biol Med 2002; 33(8):1106–1114.

216. Schladweiler MC, Ledbetter AD, Pinkerton KE, Smith KR, Gilmour PS, Evansky PA, Costa DL, Watkinson WP, Nolan JP, Kodavanti UP. Experimental induction of chronic pulmonary disease in genetically susceptible rat model. Am J Respir Crit Care Med 2003; 167:A76.

217. Gilmour PS, Schladweiler MC, Richards JH, Ledbetter AD, Kodavanti, UP. Hypertensive Rats are Susceptible to TLR4-mediated signalling following exposure to combustion source particulate matter (PM). Inhal Toxicol 2004; 16(suppl 1):5–18.

218. Cho HY, Jedlicka AE, Reddy SP, Kensler TW, Yamamoto M, Zhang LY, Kleeberger SR. Role of NRF2 in protection against hyperoxic lung injury in mice. Am J Respir Cell Mol Biol 2002; 26(2):175–182.

219. Schwartz DA. Inhaled endotoxin, a risk for airway disease in some people. Respir Physiol 2001; 128(1):47–55.

220. Peters A, Doring A, Wichmann HE, Koenig W. Increased plasma viscosity during an air pollution episode: a link to mortality? Lancet 1997; 349(9065):1582–1587.

221. Pekkanen J, Brunner EJ, Anderson HR, Tiittanen P, Atkinson RW. Daily concentrations of air pollution and plasma fibrinogen in London. Occup Environ Med 2000; 57(12):818–822.

222. van Eeden SF, Hogg JC. Systemic inflammatory response induced by particulate matter air pollution: the importance of bone-marrow stimulation. J Toxicol Environ Health A 2002; 65(20):1597–1613.

223. Peters A, Frohlich M, Doring A, Immervoll T, Wichmann HE, Hutchinson WL, Pepys MB, Koenig W. Particulate air pollution is associated with an acute phase response in men; results from the MONICA-Augsburg Study. Eur Heart J 2001; 22(14):1198–1204.

224. Sorensen M, Daneshvar B, Hansen M, et al. Personal PM2.5 exposure and markers of oxidative stress in blood. Environ Health Perspect 2003; 111(2): 161–166.

225. Gold DR, Litonjua A, Schwartz J, Lovett E, Larson A, Nearing B, Allen G, Verrier M, Cherry R, Verrier R. Ambient pollution and heart rate variability. Circulation 2000; 101(11):1267–1273.

226. Devlin RB, Ghio AJ, Kehrl H, Sanders G, Cascio W. Elderly humans exposed to concentrated air pollution particles have decreased heart rate variability. Eur Respir J Suppl 2003; 40:76s–80s.

227. Brauer M, Ebelt ST, Fisher TV, Brumm J, Petkau AJ, Vedal S. Exposure of chronic obstructive pulmonary disease patients to particles: respiratory and cardiovascular health effects. J Expo Anal Environ Epidemiol 2001; 11(6): 490–500.

228. Holguin F, Tellez-Rojo MM, Hernandez M, Cortez M, Chow JC, Watson JG, Mannino D, Romieu I. Air pollution and heart rate variability among the elderly in Mexico City. Epidemiology 2003; 14(5):521–527.

229. Ghio AJ, Kim C, Devlin RB. Concentrated ambient air particles induce mild pulmonary inflammation in healthy human volunteers. Am J Respir Crit Care Med 2000; 162(3 Pt 1):981–988.

230. Brook RD, Brook JR, Urch B, Vincent R, Rajagopalan S, Silverman F. Inhalation of fine particulate air pollution and ozone causes acute arterial vasoconstriction in healthy adults. Circulation 2002; 105(13):1534–1536.

231. Wang XL, Raveendran M, Wang J. Genetic influence on cigarette-induced cardiovascular disease. Prog Cardiovasc Dis 2003; 45(5):361–382.

232. Angerer P, Nowak D. Working in permanent hypoxia for fire protection-impact on health. Int Arch Occup Environ Health 2003; 76(2):87–102.

233. Gong H Jr, Wong R, Sarma RJ, Linn WS, Sullivan ED, Shamoo DA, Anderson KR, Prasad SB. Cardiovascular effects of ozone exposure in human volunteers. Am J Respir Crit Care Med 1998; 158(2):538–546.

234. Pekdemir H, Camsari A, Akkus MN, Cicek D, Tuncer C, Yildirim Z. Impaired cardiac autonomic functions in patients with environmental asbestos exposure: a study of time domain heart rate variability. J Electrocardiol 2003; 36(3):195–203.

235. Rigolin VH, Robiolio PA, Wilson JS, Harrison JK, Bashore TM. The forgotten chamber: the importance of the right ventricle. Cathet Cardiovasc Diagn 1995; 35(1):18–28.

236. Spyer KM, Thomas T. Sensing arterial CO_2 levels: a role for medullary P2X receptors. J Auton Nerv Syst 2000; 81(1–3):228–235.

237. Yasuma F, Hayano J. Respiratory sinus arrhythmia: why does the heartbeat synchronize with respiratory rhythm? Chest 2004; 125(2):683–690.

238. Lee LY, Pisarri TE. Afferent properties and reflex functions of bronchopulmonary C-fibers. Respir Physiol 2001; 125(1–2):47–65.

239. Murata K, Araki S. Assessment of autonomic neurotoxicity in occupational and environmental health as determined by ECG R–R interval variability: a review. Am J Ind Med 1996; 30(2):155–163.

240. Donaldson K, Stone V, Seaton A, MacNee W. Ambient particle inhalation and the cardiovascular system: potential mechanisms. Environ Health Perspect 2001; 109(suppl 4):523–527.

241. Anderson HR, Atkinson RW, Bremner SA, Marston L. Particulate air pollution and hospital admissions for cardiorespiratory diseases: are the elderly at greater risk? Eur Respir J Suppl 2003; 40:39s–46s.

242. Brook RD, Brook JR, Rajagopalan S. Air pollution: the "Heart" of the problem. Curr Hypertens Rep 2003; 5(1):32–39.

243. Welty-Wolf KE, Carraway MS, Ortel TL, Piantadosi CA. Coagulation and inflammation in acute lung injury. Thromb Haemost 2002; 88(1):17–25.

244. Russell JA. Genetics of coagulation factors in acute lung injury. Crit Care Med 2003; 31(suppl 4):S243–S247.

245. Kurata M, Horii I. Blood coagulation tests in toxicological studies—review of methods and their significance for drug safety assessment. J Toxicol Sci 2004; 29(1):13–32.

246. Pinsky DJ, Liao H, Lawson CA, Yan SF, Chen J, Carmeliet P, Loskutoff DJ, Stern DM. Coordinated induction of plasminogen activator inhibitor-1 (PAI-1) and inhibition of plasminogen activator gene expression by hypoxia promotes pulmonary vascular fibrin deposition. J Clin Invest 1998; 102(5): 919–928.

247. Hughes S. Novel cardiovascular risk factors. J Cardiovasc Nurs 2003; 18(2): 131–138.

248. Magliano DJ, Liew D, Ashton EL, Sundararajan V, McNeil JJ. Novel biomedical risk markers for cardiovascular disease. J Cardiovasc Risk 2003; 10(1): 41–55.

249. Koenig W. Fibrin(ogen) in cardiovascular disease: an update. Thromb Haemost 2003; 89(4):601–609.

250. Gardner SY, Lehmann JR, Costa DL. Oil fly ash-induced elevation of plasma fibrinogen levels in rats. Toxicol Sci 2000; 56(1):175–180.

251. Andrew A, Barchowsky A. Nickel-induced plasminogen activator inhibitor-1 expression inhibits the fibrinolytic activity of human airway epithelial cells. Toxicol Appl Pharmacol 2000; 168(1):50–57.

252. Gilmour PS, Schladweiler MC, Richards JH, Kodavanti UP. Pro-coagulant cardic gene expression in response to pulmonary zinc exposure. Am J Respir Crit Care Med 169(7):A884.

253. Kang YJ, Li Y, Zhou Z, Roberts AM, Cai L, Myers SR, Wang L, Schuchke DA. Elevation of serum endothelins and cardiotoxicity induced by particulate matter (PM2.5) in rats with acute myocardial infarction. Cardiovasc Toxicol 2000; 2:253–261.

254. Nemmar A, Hoylaerts MF, Hoet PH, Dinsdale D, Smith T, Xu H, Vermylen J, Nemery B. Ultrafine particles affect experimental thrombosis in an in vivo hamster model. Am J Respir Crit Care Med 2002; 166(7):998–1004.

255. Nemmar A, Nemery B, Hoet PH, Vermylen J, Hoylaerts MF. Pulmonary inflammation and thrombogenicity caused by diesel particles in hamsters: role of histamine. Am J Respir Crit Care Med 2003; 168(11):1366–1372.

256. van Eeden SF, Tan WC, Suwa T, Mukae H, Terashima T, Fujii T, Qui D, Vincent R, Hogg JC. Cytokines involved in the systemic inflammatory

response induced by exposure to particulate matter air pollutants (PM(10)). Am J Respir Crit Care Med 2001; 164(5):826–830.

257. Mukae H, Vincent R, Quinlan K, English D, Hards J, Hogg JC, van Eeden SF. The effect of repeated exposure to particulate air pollution (PM10) on the bone marrow. Am J Respir Crit Care Med 2001; 163(1):201–209.

258. Fujii T, Hayashi S, Hogg JC, Mukae H, Suwa T, Goto Y, Vincent R, van Eeden SF. Interaction of alveolar macrophages and airway epithelial cells following exposure to particulate matter produces mediators that stimulate the bone marrow. Am J Respir Cell Mol Biol 2002; 27(1):34–41.

259. Tan WC, Qiu D, Liam BL, Ng TP, Lee SH, van Eeden SF, D'Yachkova Y, Hogg JC. The human bone marrow response to acute air pollution caused by forest fires. Am J Respir Crit Care Med 2000; 161(4 Pt 1):1213–1217.

260. van Eeden SF, Hogg JC. The response of human bone marrow to chronic cigarette smoking. Eur Respir J 2000; 15(5):915–921.

261. Hunninghake GW, Crystal RG. Cigarette smoking and lung destruction. Accumulation of neutrophils in the lungs of cigarette smokers. Am Rev Respir Dis 1983; 128(5):833–838.

262. Terashima T, English D, Hogg JC, van Eeden SF. Release of polymorphonuclear leukocytes from the bone marrow by interleukin-8. Blood 1998; 92(3): 1062–1069.

263. Lind L. Circulating markers of inflammation and atherosclerosis. Atherosclerosis 2003; 169(2):203–214.

264. Widdicombe J, Lee LY. Airway reflexes, autonomic function, and cardiovascular responses. Environ Health Perspect 2001; 109(suppl 4):579–584.

265. Ma A, Bravo M, Kappagoda CT. Responses of bronchial C-fiber afferents of the rabbit to changes in lung compliance. Respir Physiol Neurobiol 2003; 138(2–3):155–163.

266. Cutz E, Fu XW, Nurse CA. Ionotropic receptors in pulmonary neuroepithelial bodies (NEB) and their possible role in modulation of hypoxia signalling. Adv Exp Med Biol 2003; 536:155–161.

267. Nowak D. Chemosensory irritation and the lung. Int Arch Occup Environ Health 2002; 75(5):326–331.

268. Veronesi B, Oortgiesen M. Neurogenic inflammation and particulate matter (PM) air pollutants. Neurotoxicology 2001; 22(6):795–810.

269. Lee LY, Widdicombe JG. Modulation of airway sensitivity to inhaled irritants: role of inflammatory mediators. Environ Health Perspect 2001; 109(suppl 4):585–589.

270. Long NC, Abraham J, Kobzik L, Weller EA, Krishna Murthy GG, Shore SA. Respiratory tract inflammation during the induction of chronic bronchitis in rats: role of C-fibres. Eur Respir J 1999; 14(1):46–56.

271. Veronesi B, de Haar C, Roy J, Oortgiesen M. Particulate matter inflammation and receptor sensitivity are target cell specific. Inhal Toxicol 2002; 14(2): 159–183.

272. Veronesi B, Oortgiesen M, Carter JD, Devlin RB. Particulate matter initiates inflammatory cytokine release by activation of capsaicin and acid receptors in a human bronchial epithelial cell line. Toxicol Appl Pharmacol 1999; 154(1):106–115.

273. Barnes PJ. Airway neuropeptides. In: Busse WM, Holgate ST, eds. Asthma and Rhinitis. Boston: Blackwell Scientific Publications; 1995:667–685.
274. Maggi CA. Tachykinin receptors and airway pathophysiology. Eur Respir J 1993; 6(5):735–742.
275. Undem BJ, Kajekar R, Hunter DD, Myers AC. Neural integration and allergic disease. J Allergy Clin Immunol 2000; 106(suppl 5):S213–S220.
276. Carr MJ, Hunter DD, Undem BJ. Neurotrophins and asthma. Curr Opin Pulm Med 2001; 7(1):1–7.
277. Kopp SJ, Perry HM Jr, Perry EF, Erlanger M. Cardiac physiologic and tissue metabolic changes following chronic low-level cadmium and cadmium plus lead ingestion in the rat. Toxicol Appl Pharmacol 1983; 69(1):149–160.
278. Kisling GM, Kopp SJ, Paulson DJ, Hawley PL, Tow JP. Inhibition of rat heart mitochondrial respiration by cadmium chloride. Toxicol Appl Pharmacol 1987; 89(3):295–304.
279. Grasseschi RM, Ramaswamy RB, Levine DJ, Klaassen CD, Wesselius LJ. Cadmium accumulation and detoxification by alveolar macrophages of cigarette smokers. Chest 2003; 124(5):1924–1928.
280. Benowitz NL. Cigarette smoking and cardiovascular disease: pathophysiology and implications for treatment. Prog Cardiovasc Dis 2003; 46(1):91–111.
281. Burke A, Fitzgerald GA. Oxidative stress and smoking-induced vascular injury. Prog Cardiovasc Dis 2003; 46(1):79–90.
282. Seghizzi P, D'Adda F, Borleri D, Barbic F, Mosconi G. Cobalt myocardiopathy. A critical review of literature. Sci Total Environ 1994; 150(1–3):105–109.
283. Ronneberg A. Mortality and cancer morbidity in workers from an aluminium smelter with prebaked carbon anodes—part III: mortality from circulatory and respiratory diseases. Occup Environ Med 1995; 52(4):255–261.
284. Adam B, Aslan S, Bedir A, Alvur M. The interaction between copper and coronary risk indicators. Jpn Heart J 2001; 42(3):281–286.
285. Ebihara I, Kawami M. Mineral dust exposure and systemic diseases. J Environ Pathol Toxicol Oncol 2000; 19(1–2):109–127.
286. Hobbesland A, Kjuus H, Thelle DS. Mortality from cardiovascular diseases and sudden death in ferroalloy plants. Scand J Work Environ Health 1997; 23(5):334–341.
287. Kodavanti UP, Moyer CF, Ledbetter AD, Schladweiler MC, Costa DL, Hauser R, Christiani DC, Nyska A. Inhaled environmental combustion particles cause myocardial injury in the Wistar Kyoto rat. Toxicol Sci 2003; 71(2):237–245.
288. Dye JA, Lehmann JR, McGee JK, Winsett DW, Ledbetter AD, Everitt JI, Ghio AJ, Costa DL. Acute pulmonary toxicity of particulate matter filter extracts in rats: coherence with epidemiologic studies in Utah Valley residents. Environ Health Perspect 2001; 109(suppl 3):395–403.
289. Balachandran S, Meena BR, Khillare PS. Particle size distribution and its elemental composition in the ambient air of Delhi. Environ Int 2000; 26(1–2):49–54.
290. Sadhu DN, Merchant M, Safe SH, Ramos KS. Modulation of protooncogene expression in rat aortic smooth muscle cells by benzo[a]pyrene. Arch Biochem Biophys 1993; 300(1):124–131.

291. Moorthy B, Miller KP, Jiang W, Williams ES, Kondraganti SR, Ramos KS. Role of cytochrome P4501B1 in benzo[a]pyrene bioactivation to DNA-binding metabolites in mouse vascular smooth muscle cells: evidence from 32P-postlabeling for formation of 3-hydroxybenzo[a]pyrene and benzo[a]pyrene-3,6-quinone as major proximate genotoxic intermediates. J Pharmacol Exp Ther 2003; 305(1):394–401.

292. Levy JI, Bennett DH, Melly SJ, Spengler JD. Influence of traffic patterns on particulate matter and polycyclic aromatic hydrocarbon concentrations in Roxbury, Massachusetts. J Expo Anal Environ Epidemiol 2003; 13(5): 364–371.

293. Johnson CD, Balagurunathan Y, Lu KP, Tadesse M, Falahatpisheh MH, Carroll RJ, Dougherty ER, Afshari CA, Ramos KS. Genomic profiles and predictive biological networks in oxidant-induced atherogenesis. Physiol Genomics 2003; 13(3):263–275.

294. Miller KP, Ramos KS. Impact of cellular metabolism on the biological effects of benzo[a]pyrene and related hydrocarbons. Drug Metab Rev 2001; 33(1): 1–35.

295. Miller KP, Chen YH, Hastings VL, Bral CM, Ramos KS. Profiles of antioxidant/electrophile response element (ARE/EpRE) nuclear protein binding and c-Ha-ras transactivation in vascular smooth muscle cells treated with oxidative metabolites of benzo[a]pyrene. Biochem Pharmacol 2000; 60(9):1285–1296.

296. Wellenius GA, Saldiva PH, Batalha JR, Krishna Murthy GG, Coull BA, Verrier RL, Godleski JJ. Electrocardiographic changes during exposure to residual oil fly ash (ROFA) particles in a rat model of myocardial infarction. Toxicol Sci 2002; 66(2):327–335.

297. Nadziejko C, Fang K, Nadziejko E, Narciso SP, Zhong M, Chen LC. Immediate effects of particulate air pollutants on heart rate and respiratory rate in hypertensive rats. Cardiovasc Toxicol 2002; 2:245–252.

298. Costa DL, Dreher KL. Bioavailable transition metals in particulate matter mediate cardiopulmonary injury in healthy and compromised animal models. Environ Health Perspect 1997; 105(suppl 5):1053–1060.

299. Vincent R, Goegan P, Johnson G, Brook JR, Kumarathasan P, Bouthillier LB, Richard T. Regulation of promoter-CAT stress genes in HepG2 cells by suspensions of particles from ambient air. Fundam Appl Toxicol 1997; 39(1): 18–32.

4

Genetic Susceptibility Factors in the Cardiopulmonary Response to Air Pollution

TERRY GORDON

School of Medicine, New York University, Tuxedo,
New York, U.S.A.

I. Introduction

A myriad number of factors influence the cardiopulmonary response to the inhaled particles and gases which we encounter in the ambient environment or in the workplace. This chapter will focus upon the host genetic factors, rather than physiologic or anatomic factors such as age or particle deposition patterns, which can influence the cardiovascular and pulmonary response of human individuals or test animals to air pollutants. The vulnerability of sensitive subpopulations, such as the aged or ill, to air pollutants is covered elsewhere in this book (Chapters 1, 2, 8, and 11).

Since the time when workers carried canaries into mines, health professionals have taken advantage of differences in genetic susceptibility to air pollutants to protect and understand human health. Modern toxicology uses three major approaches in the use of animal genetic models of cardiopulmonary disease to understand the role of susceptibility in human disease. The oldest approach is the identification and use of animals which develop cardiopulmonary disease from spontaneous mutations or functional polymorphisms (e.g., spontaneously hypertensive rats). This use of animals with spontaneous disease is decades old. One newer approach utilizes mice and rats in classic genetic studies using methods which were pioneered by plant geneticists. This classic genetics approach has been used extensively in the field of air pollution by Kleeberger (1) and Leikauf (2). The third approach to studying the role of genetic susceptibility in the cardiopulmonary effects of inhaled particles and gases is the use of genetically modified mice. These genetically modified mouse models include transgenic mice, in which extra or foreign genes are introduced into the mouse genome, and knockout mice, in which a particular gene is removed from the mouse genome. Variations in the extent of the introduction or removal of DNA segments can also be performed. Such genome modifications have been accomplished in the rat but to a far lesser extent than in the mouse.

The following review will explore these three approaches to the examination of individual susceptibility to air pollutants in animal models. Although investigators have used these models, especially the classic mouse genetic approach, for gene discovery, the majority of this chapter will review the use of animal models of cardiopulmonary disease in the context of understanding the mechanisms which underlie the response to inhaled particles and gases.

II. Classic Genetic Models

Scientists have used a variety of research approaches to evaluate the relative contribution of genes and environment to the response of the mammalian lung to inhaled particles and gases. These methodologies have both advantages and disadvantages and, to date, have provided important insight into the genes that predispose adults to inhaled toxicants. A common approach to the identification of susceptibility genes has been on a "gene-by-gene" basis. For example, investigators have hypothesized that certain enzymatic processes, such as the cytochrome P450 system, may predispose individuals to the carcinogenic effects of PAHs present in inhaled cigarette smoke and, they have tested for differences in function and polymorphisms in these genes on a one polymorphism-by-one polymorphism basis. Researchers have also examined the role of polymorphisms in particular genes within individuals with a pulmonary disease, such as asthma, by comparing relevant genomic sequences to that in control populations. While these findings suggest that a particular gene may contribute to the susceptibility to pollutant-induced adverse pulmonary effects, the "gene-by-gene" approach is limited in scope. Unless one has tremendous insight into the role of a particular gene, it is generally inefficient to investigate susceptibility using a "gene-by-gene" or "polymorphism-by-polymorphism" approach. Moreover, in multi-genetic mechanisms, which are frequently the case (e.g., asthma), these studies cannot typically identify the magnitude to which a particular gene contributes to increased host susceptibility. Therefore, to examine the role of genes in the enhanced susceptibility of the mammalian cardiovascular and pulmonary systems to inhaled pollutants on a genome-wide basis, scientists have turned to classic genetic approaches. These methods have been developed primarily by plant geneticists, make no a priori assumption about which gene(s) is involved, and utilize a genome-wide analysis to identify regions of the genome linked to the observed phenotype (i.e., response). Moreover, this genetic approach is forward-looking and starts with a well-defined and quantitative response (a.k.a., phenotype) that moves toward the identification of individual genes that are responsible for or contribute to the observed phenotype. As suggested by Silver (3) and Williams et al. (4), this forward genetics approach is not a fishing expedition but can be directed toward the discovery of genes which are the key controllers in molecular pathways that underlie the cardiopulmonary response to inhaled toxicants.

The classic mouse genetic model is based upon the development and availability of numerous inbred mouse strains for research. For research purposes, these inbred strains are genetically homogeneous (99.9%) within a strain due to repeated brother-sister mating over many generations of breeding. Observation of different responses among inbred strains of mice implies that genetic factors control these inter-strain differences. These quantifiable inter-strain phenotypes are key to the utility of classic genetic studies and apply to inbred rat strains as well as mouse strains. Mouse models have significant advantages over rat models and have led to a far greater use of mice in the classic genetic approach and in genetically modified rodent models. These advantages include cost as well as the greater availability of molecular tools and sequence information.

The classic mouse genetic model utilizes a linkage analysis to identify quantitative trait loci (QTL, i.e., regions on chromosomes) that contain gene(s) which contribute to the response. Conducting a QTL analysis can be time and labor intensive, but the advent of powerful statistical packages has made the procedure fairly routine. Excellent reviews on this topic can be referenced elsewhere (3,5,6). This method depends upon clear, statistically significant phenotypic differences among strains and these inter-strain differences are heritable. Briefly, after identification of inbred strains which are sensitive and resistant to the cardiopulmonary effect of an inhaled article or gas, the heritability of the trait is first tested in an F1 generation of mice bred from the sensitive and resistant strains and the QTL analysis is typically performed in a segregation study in which F2 mice (bred from F1 mice) or backcross mice (bred from F1 mice and one of the parental strains) are phenotyped and genotyped after exposure to the air pollutant under study (3). The genotype and phenotype information is then entered into any one of a number of freely available statistical packages (http://www.biostat.jhsph.edu/~kbroman/qtl/) that identify chromosomal regions of the mouse genome that are significantly linked to the phenotype. The use of recombinant inbred (RI) mice is another approach to performing genetic linkage studies in air pollution studies. Recombinant inbred mice are produced by the selective breeding of two progenitor strains (e.g., A/J and C57BL/6 mice) to produce F1 mice which are randomly bred to produce inbred substrains of the F2 mice. Because RI mice are commercially available (The Jackson Laboratory, Bar Harbor, ME) and already genotyped, considerable time and money is saved when they can be used. After identification of QTLs (i.e., chromosomal regions statistically linked to the phenotype), additional experiments are then necessary to identify the gene(s) within that chromosome which contribute to the observed phenotype. This genome-wide approach has been used successfully in recent years by a limited number of laboratories to identify candidate genes involved in the pulmonary response of mice to inhaled particles and gases. This approach can also be used in other rodent species, such as the rat, as sufficient genotyping tools and genetic and phenotypic diversity become available.

A number of clinical studies have demonstrated that the inflammatory and physiologic responses to ozone, sulfur dioxide, and nitrogen dioxide are quite diverse in human subjects. Because both genetic and environmental factors can contribute to this heterogeneity, it is important to study these factors in studies which control as many variables as possible. Researchers have begun to examine the role of the genetic response to inhaled ozone in human subjects (7–9), but the majority of research examining the genetic susceptibility in the response to inhaled pollutants has been conducted in animal studies in which the genetic heterogeneity and uncontrolled environment of the human population can be avoided. These animal studies have verified the diversity in response of the mammalian cardiopulmonary system to inhaled pollutants.

A. Pulmonary Studies

Goldstein et al. (10) reported the first study which fully examined the inter-strain difference in response to an air pollutant. They exposed 19 inbred strains to lethal concentrations of ozone and observed significant inter-strain differences in survival time. In particular, the F1 mice bred from the resistant C57BL/6 and sensitive A strains had a response similar to the C57BL/6 mice indicating a heritable genetic response in which the resistant trait was dominant. A similar inter-strain response was seen in inbred mice exposed to lethal concentrations of nitrogen dioxide and the authors concluded that the two oxidant air pollutants could be working via similar mechanisms. Importantly, this genetic susceptibility study demonstrated the utility of inbred mice in air pollution studies and emphasized caution in the strain choice of rodents and the interpretation of study results obtained in limited inbred strains. Drew et al. (11) later determined that inbred strains of rats also demonstrate differences in response to ozone, thus confirming that genetic factors appear to contribute to the pulmonary response of rodents to ozone. Similarly, Ichinose et al. (12) demonstrated in 4 strains of mice that the pulmonary response to nitrogen dioxide was strain dependent and the effect on oxidative stress protective enzymes was generally greater in the pigmented (skin) strains.

The Goldstein ozone study was far ahead of its time and it was more than two decades before Leikauf, (2,13) and colleagues could utilize modern statistical analysis software and efficient genotyping methodologies to followup this ozone survival study. They demonstrated inter-strain differences in the survival response to ozone that were similar but not identical to the results of the Goldstein study. The inter-laboratory differences could have been due to methodological differences, but the differences also point toward the importance of controlling for the source of the inbred rodent strains (14) in such experiments. The first acute lung injury study from the Leikauf laboratory (2) demonstrated significant inter-strain differences in the survival time during continuous exposure to 10 ppm ozone, thus suggesting that susceptibility to ozone is genetically determined. A/J and C57BL/6 mice demonstrated sensitive and resistant survival phenotypes, respectively, and, therefore, RI mice were used to perform a segregation analysis for this phenotype. The investigators observed three QTLs (Ali 1, 2, and 3 - a̲cute l̲ung i̲njury) which harbored genes involved in the acute lung injury response to ozone. The investigators' second study used F2 mice as the segregant study population to validate the QTLs observed in the RI mouse study (13). They observed that Ali1 and Ali3 showed significant and suggestive linkage, respectively, to the survival phenotype whereas the observation of a QTL at Ali2 was not supported. Thus, the investigators were able to confirm the importance of two QTLs and to narrow their search for candidate genes which act as genetic determinants of the acute lung injury (survival) phenotype.

Kleeberger et al. (15) have also conducted a number of pioneering linkage studies examining the inflammatory and physiologic response to ozone. In their first ozone study, they demonstrated significant inter-strain differences in response to an acute exposure to 2 ppm ozone. Unlike the acute lung injury model of Leikauf and colleagues, C57BL/6 mice were sensitive to the inflammatory effects of ozone. Experiments with F1 and F2 mice (C57BL/6 and C3H/HeJ were the sensitive and resistant progenitor strains, respectively) suggested that a single gene inheritance pattern was responsible for the observed increase in PMNs in the lavage fluid of ozone-exposed mice. The linkage of a single chromosomal locus (Inf) to PMNs in lavage fluid was also observed in mice after subacute exposure to 0.3 ppm ozone (16). Experimental exposure of RI strains derived from C57BL/6 and C3H/HeJ mice, however, demonstrated that different loci regulated the response to the high dose and low dose exposures. The RI experiment also indicated that a modifying gene (Inf-2) contributed to the PMN phenotype. Thus, the use of relevant exposure concentrations of air pollutants is of paramount importance for utilizing genetic susceptibility studies to understand the mechanisms of response to inhaled toxicants. In an F2 linkage study, it was demonstrated that QTLs on chromosome 17 and 11 had significant contributions to the inflammatory response (1). These two loci contained many candidate genes including TNF-alpha and small inducible cytokines, respectively. The success of this classic genetics approach was made evident in subsequent experiments in which the candidate gene TNF-alpha was examined (17). It was observed that TNF receptor knockout mice had a significantly less inflammatory response than wild type mice exposed to 0.3 ppm ozone, thus strongly suggesting a role for TNF-alpha/TNF receptors in the inflammatory response to ozone.

Exposure to ozone is associated with many adverse endpoints and, therefore, a critical question to be asked in these linkage studies is whether other phenotypes (e.g., protein leakage or pulmonary function) are linked to the same QTLs identified for ozone-induced inflammation (i.e., PMNs in lavage fluid). In experiments from Kleeberger's lab, a number of additional phenotypes have been studied in mice exposed to ozone and include hyperpermeability (i.e., protein leakage into the alveolar spaces), airway responsiveness to methacholine (18), and tracheal electrophysiology (19). In determining the strain differences in the development of ozone-induced airway hyperresponsiveness, they observed that the murine strains which were susceptible and resistant to the inflammatory effects of ozone were the same strains that were resistant and sensitive to the induction of airway hyperresponsiveness. Such an observation suggests that similar events or pathways are involved in the pathogenesis of ozone-induced pulmonary inflammation and airway hyperresponsiveness.

Decrements in tracheal transepithelial potential were also strain dependent in mice acutely exposed to 2 ppm ozone (19). Unlike the similarity observed between inflammation and airway hyperresponsiveness, the susceptibility and resistance of the inbred strains in terms of an electrophysiologic response was discordant with the inflammatory response to ozone suggesting that different genetic control factors contributed to these endpoints. Protein leakage (a.k.a. hyperpermeability) was also determined along with inflammation in these genetic susceptibility studies. As with tracheal electrophysiology, susceptibility to ozone-induced hyperpermeability was discordant with the strain response pattern for the inflammation phenotype (15,20). A genome-wide screen with RI strains of mice (progenitor strains were the susceptible C57BL/6 and resistant C3H/HeJ mice) identified a single locus on mouse chromosome 4 which explained 70% of the total trait variance, while minor suggestive QTLs were observed on chromosome 11 and 3. Toll-like receptor 4 (Tlr4) was tested as a candidate gene within the chromosome 4 locus by exposing inbred strains, which are polymorphic for Tlr4, to ozone. Because a significantly greater protein response and different mRNA expression patterns were observed in

C3H/OuJ mice compared to the closely related C3H/HeJ mice (which have a polymorphism in Tlr4 which makes them resistant to endotoxin), Tlr4 appeared to be a strong candidate gene for controlling the hyperpermeability response to ozone. Recent work by Hollingsworth et al. (21), however, has demonstrated that Tlr4-deficient C57BL/6 mice are still susceptible to the adverse pulmonary effects of ozone. Because these mice are also sensitive to inhaled endotoxin, these results suggest that strain background can influence the role of Tlr4 in ozone-induced pulmonary effects.

Savov et al. (22) have also examined the strain-dependent response of mice to ozone using the 2 ppm × 3 hr protocol of Kleeberger et al. (15). Although some phenotype results were similar to the findings of Kleeberger et al. (e.g., C57BL/6J and C3H/HeJ mice were sensitive and resistant, respectively, to the ozone-induced influx of neutrophils), other strain-dependent responses differed. Interestingly, the strain-dependent data were analyzed using the *in silico* method of Peltz and colleagues (23). Unlike the classical QTL approach which determined important loci on chromosomes 4, 11, and 17 (16), the *in silico* approach utilized the genetic diversity of several inbred strains of mice and identified several new chromosomal loci which may contribute to the neutrophil and hyperpermeability response to ozone. In addition, the *in silico* approach did not always identify the same loci on chromosomes 4, 11, and 17 as did Kleeberger's QTL studies. It must be noted that inter-laboratory differences in animal handling and exposure, post-exposure observation time points, and strain differences may have contributed to these diverse findings. For example, the 129 murine strain has developed spontaneous mutations which can severely affect the phenotype (24) and different sublines were apparently used in the Savov and Kleeberger experiments. Indeed, in the author's laboratory, 129X1/SvJ mice were found to be the most resistant of eight strains, in terms of the neutrophil and protein response, at 24 hr after a 5 hr exposure to 0.8 ppm ozone. The phenotype produced by exposure to inhaled particles and gases is crucial in determining QTLs and, thus, it is critically important to consider all experimental variables when comparing QTLs from different studies.

Another important question to address in genetic susceptibility studies is whether the same genetic factors play a role in the response to different particulate or gaseous pollutants. Only one mouse study has examined the inter-strain susceptibility to ambient particles (25). No indices of pulmonary inflammation or injury were increased over control values in the lavage fluid of C57BL/6J and C3H/HeJ mice, although increases in cytokine mRNA expression were observed in both murine strains exposed to concentrated ambient particulate matter. The increases in lung tissue cytokine mRNA expression, however, were generally small (approximately twofold), but the effects on IL-6, TNF-alpha, TGF-beta2, and gamma-interferon were consistent.

In another comparative study, Wesselkamper et al.(26) exposed inbred strains of mice continuously to nickel sulfate, polytetrafluoroethylene fumes, or ozone. They observed nearly identical strain sensitivity patterns with the three inhaled toxicants, thus suggesting that a common genetic factor controlled the survival response to continuous exposure to these agents. As in the work from Kleeberger's lab (15,20), the survival phenotype was discordant with lavage protein and PMN phenotypes observed after exposure to lower concentrations of nickel sulfate.

In addition to ozone, Kleeberger and colleagues (27) have also studied the inflammation and hyperpermeability phenotypes in inbred strains of mice exposed to particles such as residual oil fly ash (ROFA), sulfate-coated carbon particles, and, although not pertinent to air pollution per se, common airborne allergens. In particular, the studies with the coated carbon particles have demonstrated that genetic factors contribute to the pulmonary response to surrogate particles (28). In the coated carbon study, macrophage function was altered in a strain-dependent manner by exposure to sulfate-coated carbon particles at concentrations which produced minimal (two of nine strains had very small but statistically significant increases in PMNs) to no (protein, total cells, lymphocytes, or epithelial cells) changes in lavage cellular and biochemical indices of inflammation and injury. Exposure of F1 mice bred from sensitive C57BL/6 and resistant C3H/HeJ mice demonstrated that sensitivity to the adverse effect of coated particles on macrophage Fc receptor-mediated phagocytosis was inherited in a recessive manner (alternatively, of course, it could be said that resistance to the adverse effect on phagocytosis was inherited in a dominant fashion). This manner of inheritance was observed to be similar to that observed for the effects of ozone and nitrogen dioxide on lavage indices of lung inflammation and injury. When the differential strain responses to ozone, nitrogen dioxide, and coated particles were compared in a rank order, it was determined that the rank pattern for coated particles was correlated with that for ozone but not for nitrogen dioxide. This finding suggested the potential for similar mechanisms of action for carbon coated particles and ozone (28) and this similarity was confirmed in a linkage analysis study in F2 mice, which demonstrated significant and suggestive QTLs on chromosomes 17 and 11, respectively (29). These QTLs overlap with those described for ozone lung inflammation (1) and acute lung injury (2). Thus, the genetic animal models from the Leikauf and Kleeberger laboratories provide solid, but preliminary, evidence that certain air pollutants may produce lung injury and inflammation via similar mechanisms.

Genetic susceptibility studies by Kleeberger have determined that Tlr4 appears to also play a role in the lung injury produced by ROFA particles (30). Significant inter-strain differences in PMNs and protein in lavage fluid strains were observed in mice instilled with ROFA. C3H/HeJ and C3H/HeOuJ have a functional polymorphism in the coding region of the Tlr4 gene and were found to have polar responses (resistant and sensitive, respectively). Based upon the significant role of Tlr4 in the murine response to ozone and lipopolysaccharide (21,31), Kleeberger and colleagues (30) were able to rapidly examine the contribution of Tlr4 and associated signaling genes to the innate immune response to ROFA. Tlr4 mRNA expression was higher in the lungs of C3H/HeOuJ mice and greater activation of downstream signaling molecules in the Tlr4 pathway, including MyD88, TRAF6, IRAK-1, and NFkB, were observed. One potential problem in drawing mechanistic conclusions from such studies, however, is that they are based upon the observation of strain differences between only two murine strains. Because a linkage study using two inbred strains of mice can only investigate mechanistic differences based upon the limited genetic differences between those two strains, there may be other unidentified genetic factors involved and it can be difficult to make the broader extrapolation of the murine response to the outbred human. In the case of the Tlr4 signaling pathway, however, its role in ROFA-induced pulmonary inflammation has also been observed in another species. Spontaneously hypertensive rats (SHR) have demonstrated greater pulmonary inflammation than Wistar–Kyoto control rats instilled with ROFA (32). The observed increase in PMNs was accompanied by increased expression of Tlr4 protein in pulmonary cells as well as a greater activation of NFkB in SHR rats. Thus, both ozone and particle studies (the latter in two species) suggest that innate immunity plays a role in the adverse effects of inhaled pollutants, although the mechanism(s) by which Tlr4, a highly conserved receptor for lipopolysaccharides, interacts with either particles or gases in the lung is unknown. Based upon this evidence in rodent species, understanding the role of innate immunity in the response to air pollutants could be studied in controlled clinical human studies which examine the association between gene polymorphisms and the response to inhaled pollutants (Dr. W. Michael Foster, personal communication).

Genetic host factors also appear to contribute to the development of tolerance to lung injury and inflammation after repeated exposure to inhaled particles. Zinc is present in ambient urban particulate matter and in occupational settings. The development of tolerance to the symptoms of metal fume fever to zinc oxide has been observed for more than a century and confirmed in a controlled clinical study (33). Gordon and colleagues (34) examined the role of host genetic factors in zinc oxide-induced tolerance using the classic genetic mouse model approach. As with other pollutants, significant inter-strain differences in the response to a single exposure to ultrafine zinc oxide particles were observed. Moreover, in the inbred strains of mice that responded to a single exposure to zinc oxide, all but one strain developed tolerance after five daily exposures to zinc oxide particles. A linkage study using an F2 intercross of BALB/CBy (tolerant) and DBA/2 (non-tolerant) mice identified a significant tolerance QTL on the distal portion of chromosome 1. Importantly, this loci has not been reported in any of the linkage studies examining the genetic susceptibility to single or continuous exposure to other air pollutants, thus suggesting a unique candidate gene which may control the development of tolerance to repeated exposure to zinc oxide. This QTL for tolerance to zinc oxide may not be applicable to all particles and gases, as repeated exposure to ozone produced tolerance in BALB/CBy but not in DBA/2 mice (similar to zinc oxide), whereas endotoxin produced tolerance in both inbred strains of mice.

The examination of genetic susceptibility to air pollutants in inbred mouse strains has been done almost exclusively in one gender of young adult mice in the range of 2–3 months old. Thus, little is known regarding the role of genetic host factors in the response to air pollutants at other, perhaps more sensitive, stations of life such as in children or the elderly or in one gender vs. the other. Work in the author's laboratory has begun to examine the potential for the interaction of age and gender with the genetic factors which control the response to ozone. The pulmonary response of neonatal (15 and 16 days old) mice to ozone was strain dependent and, as in other studies, the continuous nature in the magnitude of response among the inbred strains suggests that multiple genetic factors control the response (i.e., a complex trait). Interestingly, the strain-dependent response of neonatal mice exposed to ozone did not match that of adult (15 weeks old) male or female mice. In terms of the influx of PMNs, SJL, C3H/HeJ, and BALB/C neonatal mice were the most sensitive and AKR and 129 neonatal mice were the most resistant strains exposed to ozone. Yet, adult SJL mice had no increase in PMNs or total protein in lavage fluid suggesting that different mechanisms may underlie the pulmonary response to ozone in neonatal vs. adult mice. Interestingly, two of the eight inbred strains of mice showed gender specific responses, with female mice demonstrating greater inflammation than male mice. Although these findings have not been tested for other gases or particles, they have important implications for understanding the adverse health effects in children and adults exposed to air pollution.

B. Cardiovascular Studies

The use of genetic linkage studies in examining the adverse cardiovascular effects of air pollutants has been extremely limited. Research in the author's laboratory has examined the cardiopulmonary effect of the complex mixture of mainstream cigarette smoke in nine strains of inbred mice (Gordon and Nadziejko, unpublished results). The potential for classic genetic mouse studies to evaluate the cardiovascular effects of inhaled particles and gases was clearly demonstrated in our study by the observation of a strain-dependent differences in the pulmonary hypertension response to chronic cigarette smoke exposure, as quantified by the ratio of the weights of the right and left ventricles.

Although QTL studies in mice have not been conducted to study the cardiovascular effects of ambient air pollutants, investigators have utilized strain differences in rats and genetically modified mice to examine the cardiovascular effects of ambient particulate matter. Drew et al.(11) were the first to study the effect of gaseous pollutants in rodents with different cardiovascular backgrounds. In Dahl rats that were sensitive or resistant to salt-induced hypertension, chronic exposure to sulfur dioxide induced greater increases in systemic blood pressure in salt-sensitive compared to salt-resistant rats fed a high salt diet. Salt-sensitive Dahl rats also experienced mortality during a chronic exposure to ozone regardless of their salt intake. Thus, the genetic background of the Dahl rats contributed significantly to the cardiovascular and mortality effects of two gaseous air pollutants.

Spontaneous hypertension (SH) has been observed in a line of Wistar–Kyoto rats and these rats have been exposed to a variety of air pollutants and shown to have a greater cardiopulmonary response than a normotensive strain of Wistar–Kyoto rats. For example, daily inhalation exposure to ROFA for 3 days produced greater pulmonary injury and inflammation in SH rats compared to normotensive Wistar–Kyoto rats (35). These pulmonary changes were accompanied by exacerbated cardiac effects in the SH rats. An ST-segment area depression of the ECG waveform, monitored by radiotelemetry, was observed in ROFA-exposed SH but not normotensive Wistar–Kyoto rats. A thrombogenic response to instilled ROFA, as seen by increases in plasma fibrinogen, was also observed to be greater in SH rats compared to normotensive Wistar–Kyoto rats (36). Decreases in circulating lymphocytes and increases in circulating PMNs were also greater in SH rats. To begin to dissect out the role of particle components in cardiac toxicity, the increased sensitivity of the SH rat was used as a model to examine the cardiac effects of ROFA combustion particles with a low metal content (37). As previously observed with high metal content ROFA, instilled low-metal content ROFA induced dose-dependent decreases in heart rate and blood pressure. While these studies suggest that the SH rat is more susceptible to the cardiopulmonary effects of inhaled particles, a follow-up study examining the cardiac response to repeated inhalation exposure to ROFA particles surprisingly demonstrated that the normotensive Wistar–Kyoto rat, but not the SH or Sprague–Dawley strains of rat, showed cardiac lesions related to the ROFA particle exposure (38). Multi-focal myocardial degeneration, chronic inflammation, and fibrosis were present in Wistar–Kyoto rats exposed to ROFA but not filtered air. Thus, caution must be used in interpreting the role of genetic host factors and gene–environment interactions in the cardiopulmonary response to particulate matter and therefore, the dose, phenotype being studied, and pollutant must be carefully considered. In addition, most laboratory rat strains are derived from Wistar-related or Sprague–Dawley-related stocks and because these strains share a common origin, there is relatively little genetic diversity in common inbred rat strains (39). Thus, because genetic diversity is critical to the success of genetic susceptibility studies, the mouse may be more appropriate to such studies because of the greater resources.

III. Genetically Modified Mice

The term "genetically modified mouse" refers to a range of artificial, yet permanent, alterations in the genetic code of a mouse and covers transgenic, knock-out, knock-in, and mutagenized mice. The ever-growing availability of genetically modified mice (GMM) enables researchers to investigate the role of a single gene in a complex disease. Table 1 lists GMM which have been used in cardiopulmonary and air pollution studies. The addition or subtraction of a single gene, however, rarely produces a simple change in the genetic makeup of a mouse (or rat). Other genes may compensate for the removal of a single gene, for example, in the multiple pathways involved in inflammation. This problem, as well as lethal developmental issues related to the insertion or deletion of a gene, can be bypassed by the use of conditional activation of the targeted gene (40) later in life. Many other issues of concern must be addressed in the experimental use of GMM in air pollution research. The most critical problem for using GMM in air pollution studies is the choice of the correct control strain(s) to be used for comparison. In particular, FVB/N and 129 inbred strains are currently the most commonly used strains in the production of GMM. This is due to production efficiency: FVB/N females produce more mice per litter than other inbred strains (3) and several lines of 129-derived embryonic stem cells are available for targeted mutation (The Jackson Laboratory, http://jaxmice.jax.org). Unfortunately, FVB/N and 129 mice have been rarely used in inhalation studies. More importantly, there is the uncertainty of the genetic background of the host mouse on the penetrance (i.e., the phenotypic expression) of the transgene or knockout gene (41,42). Therefore, investigators typically backcross the GMM from the FVB/N or 129 founder stock onto one or more inbred strains such as C57BL/6. This additional effort, although shortened by speed congenic techniques (43), significantly increases the cost of production of GMM and makes the choice of control mice somewhat more difficult.

Regardless of the difficulties encountered in the generation and use of GMM, they can be critically important in examining the contribution of specific genes or pathways to the cardiopulmonary effects of inhaled particles and gases. Many investigators choose to maintain their GMM in a homozygous line of breeding stock, while others utilize mice bred from stock that is heterozygous for the transgene or knockout gene. This latter technique is

Table 1 Genetically Modified Mice Used in Inhalation Toxicology Studies

GMM strain	Use	Reference
Alpha-1-antitrypsin knockout	Cigarette smoke-induced emphysema	54
Neutrophil elastase	Cigarette smoke-induced emphysema	55
Macrophage metalloelastase knockout	Cigarette smoke-induced emphysema	56
Hras2 transgenic CB6F1	Diesel exhaust-induced airway hyperresponsiveness	57
Dominant-negative p53	Asbestos-induced fibrosis	58
Dominant-negative p53	Cigarette smoke and lung cancer	59
Big Blue	Peroxyacetyl nitrate-induced mutations	60
NF-kappaB luciferase reporter	Particle-induced inflammation	61
NF-kappaB p50 knockout	Ozone-induced inflammation and injury	62
iNOS knockout	Asbestos-induced lung injury	63
iNOS knockout	Macrophage function	64
iNOS knockout	Silica-induced fibrosis	65
iNOSII knockout	Ozone-induced inflammation	66
iNOS knockout	Ozone-induced inflammation and injury	62,67
iNOS knockout	Ozone-induced injury and inflammation	68
Apolipoprotein E knockout	Hypercholesterolemia	69
Apolipoprotein E knockout	Cigarette smoke-induced atherosclerosis	44
Superoxide dismutase transgenic	Ozone-induced inflammation and injury	62,70
Extracellular superoxide dismutase transgenic	ROFA-induced inflammation and injury	71
Extracellular-SOD null	Inflammation and injury	72
Manganese superoxide dismutase transgenic; copper–zinc superoxide dismutase knockout; cellular glutathione peroxidase knockout	Hyperoxia	73
TNF receptor knockout	Silica, asbestos, and bleomycin-induced fibrosis	74

(Continued)

Table 1 Genetically Modified Mice Used in Inhalation Toxicology Studies *(Continued)*

GMM strain	Use	Reference
TNF receptor knockout	Silica-induced inflammation	75
TNF receptor knockout	Ozone-induced airway hyperresponsiveness and inflammation	76
TNFR1/2 knockout	Ozone-induced inflammation, injury, and airway hyperresponsiveness; cigarette smoke-induced inflammation	17,77
IFN-gamma knockout	Silica-induced fibrosis	78
IL-1-beta knockout	Silica-induced inflammation and apoptosis	65
IL-5 transgenic	Diesel exhaust particles and allergic asthma	79
IL-6 knockout	Cigarette smoke and ozone-induced injury and inflammation	80
IL-9 transgenic	Silica-induced fibrosis	81
IL-10 knockout	Silica-induced fibrosis	82
IL-12 knockout	Silica-induced fibrosis	83
IL-13 transgenic	Asthma	84
Human platelet-derived growth factor B chain	Silica and bleomycin-induced fibrosis	41
TGF-alpha transgenic	Nickel sulfate lung injury	85
CCSP-beta transgenic	Ozone-induced airway hyperresponsiveness	86
Clara cell secretory protein (CCSP) knockout	Inflammation and chemokine response	87,88
Gamma delta-deficient	Ozone-induced inflammation	89
hsp70–1 promoter	Oxidative stress	90

more costly because each mouse has to be genotyped, but may be more favorable because littermate wildtype/wildtype and wildtype/variant mice can be used as controls and to investigate gene dosage, respectively.

Genetically modified mice have rarely been used in examining the cardiovascular effects of inhaled pollutants. Studies have used apoE knockout mice, however, to examine the cardiovascular effects of non-ambient air pollutants. For example, cigarette smoke was found to exacerbate the atherogenesis produced in apoE knockout mice (44). Chen and colleagues (45) have used an apoE knockout mouse model of cardiovascular disease to examine the cardiovascular response of mice repeatedly exposed to concentrated ambient particulate matter. They observed changes in heart rate and heart rate variance in apoE knockout mice but not identically-exposed C57BL/6 control mice. Thus, there is a great, largely untapped resource of GMM to study the adverse effects of inhaled pollutants. Table 1 lists a number of GMM models which have been used to study the adverse pulmonary effects of inhaled pollutant gases and particles. Generally, investigators have used these GMM models to answer specific mechanistic questions and not to address genetic susceptibility per se, but they have great utility in investigating the role of candidate genes identified by classic mouse genetic studies to play a role in the susceptibility to inhaled pollutants.

IV. Conclusion

The molecular tools that have become available over the last decade provide many opportunities to study genetic susceptibility. It is still difficult to extend the results of QTL studies directly into investigations of promising candidate genes, but molecular and statistical resources for rodent research are growing rapidly. Better statistical methods for identifying multiple QTLs are continually being updated (46) and will permit the discovery of multiple QTLs in complex traits as well as the examination of interaction between significant loci on the same or different chromosomes. In addition, methodologies are being developed to link the results of different methods, such as QTL studies and microarray expression assays, to more quickly focus on promising candidate genes (47–49).

Moreover, there are no hard and fast rules regarding the use of the QTL approach in examining genetic susceptibility and gene discovery. Although the classic genetic approach in mice is the predominant procedure used in air pollution studies, exciting new approaches have been developed to identify QTLs using expression data only (50). This method treats mRNA expression data as the phenotype and, thus, QTLs are examined for each gene in a backcross or intercross. Because of the large number of mRNA expression levels queried on a microarray, this expression QTL approach can be computationally intensive but doable (50). Two other new approaches focus on the issue of genetic diversity in mice. As mentioned previously, the *in silico* approach of Peltz and colleagues (23) utilizes the genetic differences in multiple inbred strains of mice, instead of the usual two strains, to identify chromosomal loci containing genes responsible for the observed phenotype. Wiltshire et al. (51) have also developed an *in silico* approach to examine SNP differences and haplotypes in over 40 inbred strains of mice. Strain comparison databases are available from both groups of investigators (http://mousesnp.roche.com and http://snp.gnf.org/). The second approach to increasing the genetic diversity of the mice used in genetic susceptibility studies is to utilize crosses of mice bred from more than two strains of mice. Heterogenous stocks of mice bred from as many as eight progenitor strains have been successfully used to identify QTLs in behavioral studies (52). An even more ambitious approach has recently been proposed and will use a heterogenous stock of progenitor mice to produce 1000 RI strains of mice (53, www.complextrait.org). A 1000 RI resource will have two major advantages: (1) as with other RI strains, once genotyping is done once, it will not need to be repeated; and (2) the resolution of phenotyping the 1000 RI strains will be approximately 0.1 centiMorgan which would contain from 1 to 5 candidate genes, which is a significant improvement on the resolution of a QTL determined by the classic mouse genetic approach.

In summary, the available animal models of genetic susceptibility, as presented in this review, offer exciting possibilities for identification of host factors that contribute to the adverse effects of air pollutants. Optimal experimental designs will permit the determination of the relative contribution of genetic and environmental factors to these adverse cardiopulmonary changes. Understanding the relative contributions of genes and environment is critical because the diseases associated with exposure to ambient pollutants appear to be as complex as the mixtures of particles and gases to which the mammalian cardiopulmonary system is exposed. Despite attempts to reduce environmental levels of particulate and gaseous air pollutants in developed countries, there continues to be concern over present and future ambient concentrations of these pollutants throughout the world.

References

1. Kleeberger SR, Levitt RC, Zhang LY, Longphre M, Harkema J, Jedlicka A, Eleff SM, DiSilvestre D, Holroyd KJ. Linkage analysis of susceptibility to ozone-induced lung inflammation in inbred mice. Nat Genet 1997; 17:475–478.
2. Prows DR, Shertzer HG, Daly MJ, Sidman CL, Leikauf GD. Genetic analysis of ozone-induced acute lung injury in sensitive and resistant strains of mice. Nat Genet 1997; 17:471–474.
3. Silver LM. . Mouse Genetics. Concepts and Applications. Oxford University Press, 1995.
4. Williams RW, Flaherty L, Threadgill DW. The math of making mutant mice. Genes Brain Behav 2003; 2:191–200.

5. Manly KF, Olson JM. Overview of QTL mapping software and introduction to map manager QT. Mamm Genome 1999; 10:327–334.

6. Doerge RW. Multifactorial genetics. Mapping and analysis of quantitative trait loci in experimental populations. Nature Rev Genet 2002; 3:43–52.

7. Romieu I, Sienra-Monge JJ, Ramirez-Aguilar M, Moreno-Macias H, Reyes-Ruiz NI, Estela del Rio-Navarro B, Hernandez-Avila M, London SJ. Genetic polymorphism of GSTM1 and antioxidant supplementation influence lung function in relation to ozone exposure in asthmatic children in Mexico City. Thorax 2004; 59:8–10.

8. Huang W, Wang G, Phelps DS, Al-Mondhiry H, Floros J. Human SP-A genetic variants and bleomycin-induced cytokine production by THP-1 cells: effect of ozone-induced SP-A oxidation. Am J Physiol Lung Cell Mol Physiol 2004; 286:L546–L553.

9. Otto-Knapp R, Jurgovsky K, Schierhorn K, Kunkel G. Antioxidative enzymes in human nasal mucosa after exposure to ozone. Possible role of GSTM1 deficiency. Inflamm Res 2003; 52:51–55.

10. Goldstein BD, Lai LY, Ross SR, Cuzzi-Spada R. Susceptibility of inbred mouse strains to ozone. Arch Environ Health 1973; 27:412–413.

11. Drew RT, Kutzman RS, Costa DL, Iwai J. Effects of sulfur dioxide and ozone on hypertension sensitive and resistant rats. Fundam Appl Toxicol 1983; 3:298–302.

12. Ichinose T, Suzuki AK, Tsubone H, Sagai M. Biochemical studies on strain differences of mice in the susceptibility to nitrogen dioxide. Life Sci 1982; 31:1963–1972.

13. Prows DR, Daly MJ, Shertzer HG, Leikauf GD. Ozone-induced acute lung injury: genetic analysis of F(2) mice generated from A/J and C57BL/6J strains. Am J Physiol 1999; 277:L372–L380.

14. Harkema JR, Weirenga CM, Herrera LK, Hotchkiss JA, Evans WA, Burt DG, Hobbs CH. Strain-related differences in ozone-induced secretory metaplasia in the nasal epithelium of rats. In: Miller FJ, ed. Nasal Toxicity and Dosimetry of Inhaled Xenobiotics: Implications for Human Health. Washington, DC: Taylor & Francis, 1995:220–222.

15. Kleeberger SR, Bassett DJ, Jakab GJ, Levitt RC. A genetic model for evaluation of susceptibility to ozone-induced inflammation. Am J Physiol 1990; 258:L313–L320.

16. Kleeberger SR, Levitt RC, Zhang LY. Susceptibility to ozone-induced inflammation. I. Genetic control of the response to subacute exposure. Am J Physiol 1993; 264:L15–L20.

17. Cho HY, Zhang LY, Kleeberger SR. Ozone-induced lung inflammation and hyperreactivity are mediated via tumor necrosis factor-alpha receptors. Am J Physiol Lung Cell Mol Physiol 2001; 280:L537–L546.

18. Zhang LY, Levitt RC, Kleeberger SR. Differential susceptibility to ozone-induced airways hyperreactivity in inbred strains of mice. Exp Lung Res 1995; 21:503–518.

19. Takahashi M, Kleeberger SR, Croxton TL. Genetic control of susceptibility to ozone-induced changes in mouse tracheal electrophysiology. Am J Physiol 1995; 269:L6–L10.

20. Kleeberger SR. Genetic aspects of susceptibility to air pollution. Eur Respir J Suppl 2003; 40:52s–56s.

21. Hollingsworth JW II, Cook DN, Brass DM, Walker JK, Morgan DL, Foster WM, Schwartz DA. The role of Toll-like receptor 4 in environmental airway injury in mice. Am J Respir Crit Care Med 2004; 170:126–132.

22. Savov JD, Whitehead GS, Wang J, Liao G, Usuka J, Peltz G, Foster WM, Schwartz DA. Ozone-induced acute pulmonary injury in inbred mouse strains. Am J Respir Cell Mol Biol 2004; 31:69–77.

23. Grupe A, Germer S, Usuka J, Aud D, Belknap JK, Klein RF, Ahluwalia MK, Higuchi R, Peltz G. In silico mapping of complex disease-related traits in mice. Science 2001; 292:1915–1918.

24. Threadgill DW, Yee D, Matin A, Nadeau JH, Magnuson T. Genealogy of the 129 inbred strains: 129/SvJ is a contaminated inbred strain. Mamm Genome 1997; 8:390–393.

25. Shukla A, Timblin C, BeruBe K, Gordon T, McKinney W, Driscoll K, Vacek P, Mossman B. Inhaled particulate matter causes expression of NF-kappaB-related genes and oxidant-dependent NF-kappaB activation in vitro. Am J Respir Cell Mol Biol 2000; 23:182–187.

26. Wesselkamper SC, Prows DR, Biswas P, Willeke K, Bingham E, Leikauf GD. Genetic susceptibility to irritant-induced acute lung injury in mice. Am J Physiol Lung Cell Mol Physiol 2000; 279:L575–L582.

27. Sarpong SB, Zhang LY, Kleeberger SR. A novel mouse model of experimental asthma. Int Arch Allergy Immunol 2003; 132:346–354.

28. Ohtsuka Y, Clarke RW, Mitzner W, Brunson K, Jakab GJ, Kleeberger SR. Interstrain variation in murine susceptibility to inhaled acid-coated particles. Am J Physiol Lung Cell Mol Physiol 2000; 278:L469–L476.

29. Ohtsuka Y, Brunson KJ, Jedlicka AE, Mitzner W, Clarke RW, Zhang LY, Eleff SM, Kleeberger SR. Genetic linkage analysis of susceptibility to particle exposure in mice. Am J Respir Cell Mol Biol 2000; 22:574–581.

30. Cho HY, Jedlicka AE, Zhang L-Y, Clarke R, Kleeberger SR. Residual oil fly ash (ROFA)-induced lung injury in mice: role of toll-like receptor 4 (TLR4) signaling. Am J Respir Crit Care Med 2002; 165:A46.

31. Kleeberger SR, Reddy S, Zhang LY, Jedlicka AE. Genetic susceptibility to ozone-induced lung hyperpermeability: role of toll-like receptor 4. Am J Respir Cell Mol Biol 2000; 22:620–627.

32. Gilmour PS, Schladweiler MC, Richards JH, Ledbetter AD, Kodavanti UP. Hypertensive rats are susceptible to TLR4-mediated signaling following exposure to combustion source particulate matter. Inhal Toxicol 2004; 16(suppl 1):5–18.

33. Fine JM, Gordon T, Chen LC, Kinney P, Falcone G, Sparer J, Beckett WS. Characterization of clinical tolerance to inhaled zinc oxide in naive subjects and sheet metal workers. J Occup Environ Med 2000; 42:1085–1091.

34. Wesselkamper SC, Chen LC, Kleeberger SR, Gordon T. Genetic variability in the development of pulmonary tolerance to inhaled pollutants in inbred mice. Am J Physiol Lung Cell Mol Physiol 2001; 281:L1200–L1209.

35. Kodavanti UP, Schladweiler MC, Ledbetter AD, Watkinson WP, Campen MJ, Winsett DW, Richards JR, Crissman KM, Hatch GE, Costa DL. The spontaneously hypertensive rat as a model of human cardiovascular disease: evidence

of exacerbated cardiopulmonary injury and oxidative stress from inhaled emission particulate matter. Toxicol Appl Pharmacol 2000; 164:250–263.

36. Kodavanti UP, Schladweiler MC, Ledbetter AD, Hauser R, Christiani DC, McGee J, Richards JR, Costa DL. Temporal association between pulmonary and systemic effects of particulate matter in healthy and cardiovascular compromised rats. J Toxicol Environ Health A 2002; 65:1545–1569.

37. Wichers LB, Nolan JP, Winsett DW, Ledbetter AD, Kodavanti UP, Schladweiler MC, Costa DL, Watkinson WP. Effects of instilled combustion-derived particles in spontaneously hypertensive rats. Part I: Cardiovascular responses. Inhal Toxicol 2004; 16:391–405.

38. Kodavanti UP, Moyer CF, Ledbetter AD, Schladweiler MC, Costa DL, Hauser R, Christiani DC, Nyska A. Inhaled environmental combustion particles cause myocardial injury in the Wistar Kyoto rat. Toxicol Sci 2003; 71:237–245.

39. McBride MW, Charchar FJ, Graham D, Miller WH, Strahorn P, Carr FJ, Dominiczak AF. Functional genomics in rodent models of hypertension. J Physiol 2004; 554:56–63.

40. Matsuda I, Aiba A. Receptor knock-out and knock-in strategies. Methods Mol Biol 2004; 259:379–390.

41. Li J, Ortiz LA, Hoyle GW. Lung pathology in platelet-derived growth factor transgenic mice: effects of genetic background and fibrogenic agents. Exp Lung Res 2002; 28:507–522.

42. Wolfer DP, Crusio WE, Lipp HP. Knockout mice: simple solutions to the problems of genetic background and flanking genes. Trends Neurosci 2002; 25:336–340.

43. Wakeland E, Morel L, Achey K, Yui M, Longmate J. Speed congenics: a classic technique in the fast lane (relatively speaking). Immunol Today 1997; 18:472–477.

44. Gairola CG, Drawdy ML, Block AE, Daugherty A. Sidestream cigarette smoke accelerates atherogenesis in apolipoprotein E-/- mice. Atherosclerosis 2001; 156:49–55.

45. Hwang J-S, Nadziejko C, Chen LC. Effects of subchronic exposure to concentrated ambient particles in mice: III. Acute and chronic effects of CAPs on heart rate, heart rate variance, and body temperature. Inhal Toxicol. In press.

46. Broman KW, Wu H, Sen S, Churchill GA. R/qtl: QTL mapping in experimental crosses. Bioinformatics 2003; 19:889–890.

47. Leikauf GD, McDowell SA, Wesselkamper SC, Hardie WD, Leikauf JE, Korfhagen TR, Prows DR. Acute lung injury: functional genomics and genetic susceptibility. Chest 2002; 121(suppl 3):70S–75S.

48. Gohil K, Cross CE, Last JA. Ozone-induced disruptions of lung transcriptomes. Biochem Biophys Res Commun 2003; 305:719–728.

49. Cook DN, Wang S, Wang Y, Howles GP, Whitehead GS, Berman KG, Church TD, Frank BC, Gaspard RM, Yu Y, Quackenbush J, Schwartz DA. Genetic regulation of endotoxin-induced airway disease. Genomics 2004; 83:961–969.

50. Schadt EE, Monks SA, Drake TA, Lusis AJ, Che N, Colinayo V, Ruff TG, Milligan SB, Lamb JR, Cavet G, Linsley PS, Mao M, Soughton RB, Friend SH. Genetics of gene expression surveyed in maize, mouse and ma. Nature 2003; 422:297–302.

51. Wiltshire T, Pletcher MT, Batalov S, Barnes W, Tarantino LM, Cooke MP, Wu H, Smylie K, Santrosyan A, Copeland NG, Jenkins NA, Kalush F, Mural RJ, Glynne RJ, Kay SA, Adams MD, Fletcher CF. Genome-wide single-nucleotide polymorphism analysis defines haplotype patterns in mouse. Proc Natl Acad Sci USA 2003; 100:3380–3385.

52. Mott R, Flint J. Simultaneous detection and fine mapping of quantitative trait loci in mice using heterogeneous stocks. Genetics 2002; 160:1609–1618.

53. Vogel G. Scientists dream of 1001 complex mice. Science 2003; 301:456–457.

54. Churg A, Wang RD, Xie C, Wright JL. Alpha-1-Antitrypsin ameliorates cigarette smoke-induced emphysema in the mouse. Am J Respir Crit Care Med 2003; 168:199–207.

55. Shapiro SD, Goldstein NM, Houghton AM, Kobayashi DK, Kelley D, Belaaouaj A. Neutrophil elastase contributes to cigarette smoke-induced emphysema in mice. Am J Pathol 2003; 163:2329–2335.

56. Churg A, Zay K, Shay S, Xie C, Shapiro SD, Hendricks R, Wright JL. Acute cigarette smoke-induced connective tissue breakdown requires both neutrophils and macrophage metalloelastase in mice. Am J Respir Cell Mol Biol 2002; 27:368–374.

57. Birumachi J, Suzuki AK, Itoh K, Hioki K, Maruyama C, Ohnishi Y. Diesel exhaust-induced airway hyperresponsiveness in c-Ha-ras transgenic mice. Toxicology 2001; 163:145–152.

58. Nelson A, Mendoza T, Hoyle GW, Brody AR, Fermin C, Morris GF. Enhancement of fibrogenesis by the p53 tumor suppressor protein in asbestos-exposed rodents. Chest 2001; 120(suppl 1):33S–34S.

59. De Flora S, Balansky RM, D'Agostini F, Izzotti A, Camoirano A, Bennicelli C, Zhang Z, Wang Y, Lubet RA, You M. Molecular alterations and lung tumors in p53 mutant mice exposed to cigarette smoke. Cancer Res 2003; 63: 793–800.

60. DeMarini DM, Shelton ML, Kohan MJ, Hudgens EE, Kleindienst TE, Ball LM, Walsh D, de Boer JG, Lewis-Bevan L, Rabinowitz JR, Claxton LD, Lewtas J. Mutagenicity in lung of big Blue((R)) mice and induction of tandem-base substitutions in Salmonella by the air pollutant peroxyacetyl nitrate (PAN): predicted formation of intrastrand cross-links. Mutat Res 2000; 457:41–55.

61. Hubbard AK, Timblin CR, Shukla A, Rincon M, Mossman BT. Activation of NF-kappaB-dependent gene expression by silica in lungs of luciferase reporter mice. Am J Physiol Lung Cell Mol Physiol 2002; 282:L968–L975.

62. Laskin DL, Fakhrzadeh L, Heck DE, Gerecke D, Laskin JD. Upregulation of phosphoinositide 3-kinase and protein kinase B in alveolar macrophages following ozone inhalation. Role of NF-kappaB and STAT-1 in ozone-induced nitric oxide production and toxicity. Mol Cell Biochem 2002; 234–235: 91–98.

63. Dorger M, Allmeling AM, Kiefmann R, Schropp A, Krombach F. Dual role of inducible nitric oxide synthase in acute asbestos-induced lung injury. Free Radic Biol Med 2002; 33:491–501.

64. Zeidler PC, Roberts JR, Castranova V, Chen F, Butterworth L, Andrew ME, Robinson VA, Porter DW. Response of alveolar macrophages from indu-cible

nitric oxide synthase knockout or wild-type mice to an in vitro lipopolysaccharide or silica exposure. J Toxicol Environ Health A 2003; 66:995–1013.

65. Srivastava KD, Rom WN, Jagirdar J, Yie TA, Gordon T, Tchou-Wong KM. Crucial role of interleukin-1beta and nitric oxide synthase in silica-induced inflammation and apoptosis in mice. Am J Respir Crit Care Med 2002; 165:527–533.

66. Laskin DL, Fakhrzadeh L, Laskin JD. Nitric oxide and peroxynitrite in ozone-induced lung injury. Adv Exp Med Biol 2001; 500:183–190.

67. Fakhrzadeh L, Laskin JD, Laskin DL. Deficiency in inducible nitric oxide synthase protects mice from ozone-induced lung inflammation and tissue injury. Am J Respir Cell Mol Biol 2002; 26:413–419.

68. Kenyon NJ, van der Vliet A, Schock BC, Okamoto T, McGrew GM, Last JA. Susceptibility to ozone-induced acute lung injury in iNOS-deficient mice. Am J Physiol Lung Cell Mol Physiol 2002; 282:L540–L545.

69. Knight-Lozano CA, Young CG, Burow DL, Hu ZY, Uyeminami D, Pinkerton KE, Ischiropoulos H, Ballinger SW. Cigarette smoke exposure and hypercholesterolemia increase mitochondrial damage in cardiovascular tissues. Circulation 2002; 105:849–854.

70. Fakhrzadeh L, Laskin JD, Gardner CR, Laskin DL. Superoxide dismutase-overexpressing mice are resistant to ozone-induced tissue injury and increases in nitric oxide and tumor necrosis factor-alpha. Am J Respir Cell Mol Biol 2004; 30:280–287.

71. Ghio AJ, Suliman HB, Carter JD, Abushamaa AM, Folz RJ. Overexpression of extracellular superoxide dismutase decreases lung injury after exposure to oil fly ash. Am J Physiol Lung Cell Mol Physiol 2002; 283:L211–L218.

72. Jonsson LM, Edlund T, Marklund SL, Sandstrom T. Increased ozone-induced airway neutrophilic inflammation in extracellular-superoxide dismutase null mice. Respir Med 2002; 96:209–214.

73. Ho YS. Transgenic and knockout models for studying the role of lung antioxidant enzymes in defense against hyperoxia. Am J Respir Crit Care Med 2002; 166:S51–S56.

74. Liu JY, Sime PJ, Wu T, Warshamana GS, Pociask D, Tsai SY, Brody AR. Transforming growth factor-beta(1) overexpression in tumor necrosis factor-alpha receptor knockout mice induces fibroproliferative lung disease. Am J Respir Cell Mol Biol 2001; 25:3–7.

75. Pryhuber GS, Huyck HL, Baggs R, Oberdorster G, Finkelstein JN. Induction of chemokines by low-dose intratracheal silica is reduced in TNFR I (p55) null mice. Toxicol Sci 2003; 72:150–157.

76. Shore SA, Schwartzman IN, Le Blanc B, Murthy GG, Doerschuk CM. Tumor necrosis factor receptor 2 contributes to ozone-induced airway hyperresponsiveness in mice. Am J Respir Crit Care Med 2001; 164:602–607.

77. Churg A, Dai J, Tai H, Xie C, Wright JL. Tumor necrosis factor-alpha is central to acute cigarette smoke-induced inflammation and connective tissue breakdown. Am J Respir Crit Care Med 2002; 166:849–854.

78. Desaki M, Sugawara I, Iwakura Y, Yamamoto K, Takizawa H. Role of interferon-gamma in the development of murine bronchus-associated lymphoid tissues induced by silica in vivo. Toxicol Appl Pharmacol 2002; 185:1–7.

79. Hao M, Comier S, Wang M, Lee JJ, Nel A. Diesel exhaust particles exert acute effects on airway inflammation and function in murine allergen provocation models. J Allergy Clin Immunol 2003; 112:905–914.

80. Yu M, Zheng X, Witschi H, Pinkerton KE. The role of interleukin-6 in pulmonary inflammation and injury induced by exposure to environmental air pollutants. Toxicol Sci 2002; 68:488–497.

81. Arras M, Huaux F, Vink A, Delos M, Coutelier JP, Many MC, Barbarin V, Renauld JC, Lison D. Interleukin-9 reduces lung fibrosis and type 2 immune polarization induced by silica particles in a murine model. Am J Respir Cell Mol Biol 2001; 24:368–375.

82. Huaux F, Louahed J, Hudspith B, Meredith C, Delos M, Renauld JC, Lison D. Role of interleukin-10 in the lung response to silica in mice. Am J Respir Cell Mol Biol 1998; 18:51–59.

83. Huaux F, Arras M, Tomasi D, Barbarin V, Delos M, Coutelier JP, Vink A, Phan SH, Renauld JC, Lison D. A profibrotic function of IL-12p40 in experimental pulmonary fibrosis. J Immunol 2002; 169:2653–2661.

84. Elias JA, Zheng T, Lee CG, Homer RJ, Chen Q, Ma B, Blackburn M, Zhu Z. Transgenic modeling of interleukin-13 in the lung. Chest 2003; 123(suppl 3): 339S–345S.

85. Leikauf GD, McDowell SA, Wesselkamper SC, Miller CR, Hardie WD, Gammon K, Biswas PP, Korfhagen TR, Bachurski CJ, Wiest JS, Willeke K, Bingham E, Leikauf JE, Aronow BJ, Prows DR. Pathogenomic mechanisms for particulate matter induction of acute lung injury and inflammation in mice. Res Rep Health Eff Inst 2001; 105:5–58.

86. McGraw DW, Forbes SL, Mak JC, Witte DP, Carrigan PE, Leikauf GD, Liggett SB. Transgenic overexpression of beta(2)-adrenergic receptors in airway epithelial cells decreases bronchoconstriction. Am J Physiol Lung Cell Mol Physiol 2000; 279:L379–L389.

87. Mango GW, Johnston CJ, Reynolds SD, Finkelstein JN, Plopper CG, Stripp BR. Clara cell secretory protein deficiency increases oxidant stress response in conducting airways. Am J Physiol 1998; 275:L348–L356.

88. Johnston CJ, Finkelstein JN, Oberdorster G, Reynolds SD, Stripp BR. Clara cell secretory protein-deficient mice differ from wild-type mice in inflammatory chemokine expression to oxygen and ozone, but not to endotoxin. Exp Lung Res 1999; 25:7–21.

89. King DP, Hyde DM, Jackson KA, Novosad DM, Ellis TN, Putney L, Stovall MY, Van Winkle LS, Beaman BL, Ferrick DA. Cutting edge: protective response to pulmonary injury requires gamma delta T lymphocytes. J Immunol 1999; 162:5033–5036.

90. Wirth D, Christians E, Munaut C, Dessy C, Foidart JM, Gustin P. Differential heat shock gene hsp70-1 response to toxicants revealed by in vivo study of lungs in transgenic mice. Cell Stress Chaperones 2002; 7:387–395.

5

Air Pollutants, Epithelial Surfaces, and Lung Disease

JEFFREY G. SHERMAN, JANICE L. PEAKE, VIVIANA J. WONG, and
KENT E. PINKERTON

Center for Health and the Environment, University of California,
Davis, California, U.S.A.

I. Introduction

The epithelial cells of the respiratory system are composed of numerous types, which vary as a function of location. Each cell type provides for specific needs required at each site along the upper and lower airways and alveoli. The primary function of epithelial cells is to provide an appropriate interface with the environment, which will allow a number of processes to be completed. One of these is to condition the air through warming and humidification during transport through the nasal cavity and tracheobronchial tree. In these same regions, a combination of epithelial cells work in concert to provide a protective lining layer (mucous) and movement of this layer along the airways (ciliary beating). The epithelium beyond the conducting airways serves to facilitate the rapid passage and exchange of gases from alveolar air spaces to the blood by forming a portion of the air-to-blood tissue barrier. Specific epithelial cells of the distal lung also secrete a complex of phospholipids, proteins, and carbohydrates (known as surfactant) to form a liquid lining layer over the alveolar surfaces to create a low surface tension at the air–tissue interface. Surfactant maintains open alveolar air spaces during ventilation and the appropriate conditions to prevent desiccation of delicate epithelial cells. Both surfactant functions derived from the epithelium are critical in facilitating gas exchange. In essence, the role of the epithelium is to provide a highly effective barrier while also maintaining conditions that will not subject the respiratory tract to damage due to its interaction with the external environment.

Although epithelial cells are designed to create the most optimal interface for the respiratory system as the portal of air delivery to the body, these cells must also serve to protect against the invasion of airborne substances that could potentially damage or alter the respiratory tract. This protection is provided by immune, neural, and endocrine systems that are intimately associated with epithelial cells. As a consequence, cells of the immune, neural, and endocrine systems are also present in the epithelial lining. Only vascular tissues do not penetrate the epithelium but are in close apposition.

The purpose of this chapter is to describe the respiratory epithelium of humans and the effects of air pollutants on epithelial surfaces in normal and diseased states. Much of our current knowledge of air pollutants and the epithelium are derived from animals which may not always extrapolate to the human epithelium. However, many of the similarities across species can provide critical information to better understand the impact of air pollutants on epithelial surfaces in the respiratory tract. Table 1 provides a simple comparison of epithelial cell types across a number of species with further details given throughout the chapter.

II. Nasal Passages

The nasal vestibule is lined with a keratinizing stratified squamous epithelium and, in most species, contains hair from follicles in the underlying dermis to enhance the deposition of large particles. Langerhans or dendritic cells have been reported in the squamous epithelium of the nasal cavity (1,2). The anterior nasal cavity contains regions with squamous epithelium near the nares, whereas cuboidal to columnar respiratory epithelium is found more distally in the nasal cavity. Olfactory epithelium is found within the more posterior and superior regions of the nasal cavity. The respiratory epithelium of the nasal cavity lines the walls and extends into the choanae that connects with the pharyngeal region of the oral cavity. Cell types within the nasal respiratory epithelium include ciliated cells, mucous goblet cells, basal cells, and brush cells (3). Metaplastic squamous epithelium can also be present. Paranasal sinuses are covered with a respiratory epithelium similar to that found in the nasal sinus. The olfactory epithelium is composed of sustentacular cells (columnar supporting cells), bipolar olfactory cells, basal cells, and occasional brush cells. Nasal-associated lymphoid tissue (NALT) is located in the nasopharyngeal mucosa of humans and

Table 1   Epithelial Cells of the Respiratory System

Anatomic location	Human	Rodent	Dog
Nasal cavity			
Squamous	+	+	+
Respiratory	+	+	+
Ciliated	+	+	+
Mucus	+	+	+
Olfactory			
Supporting	+	+	+
Olfactory	+	+	+
Basal	+	+	+
Nasopharynx			
Squamous	+	+	+
Trachea and bronchi			
Ciliated	+	+	+
Mucus	+	+	+
Basal	+	+	+
Secretory	+	+	+
Neuroendocrine	+	+	+
Kulchitsky	+	+	+
Small granule	+	+	+
Brush	+	+	+
Clara	−	+[a]	−
Bronchioles			
Ciliated	+	+	+
Clara	+	+	+
Respiratory bronchioles			
Ciliated	+	NA	+
Clara	+	NA	+
Type I	+	NA	+
Type II	+	NA	+
Alveolar ducts and alveoli			
Type I	+	+	+
Type II	+	+	+
Type III	?	+	?

[a]In mice and hamsters, Clara cells are found in the trachea and bronchi (15–60% of the total epithelial cell population). In rats, Clara cells are occasionally found in bronchi but not in the trachea.

Note: "+" denotes cell type is present at this level of the respiratory system. "−" denotes cell type is absent at this level of the respiratory system. NA: not applicable, as rodents do not have respiratory bronchioles.

animals (4). A lymphoepithelium covers those surfaces where NALT is found in the underlying interstitium.

III. Nasopharynx and Larynx

The nasopharynx serves a dual respiratory and gastrointestinal function with most surfaces covered by stratified squamous epithelium. This type of epithelium is found in areas with a significant degree of friction due to the passage of liquids and solids (i.e., food). The epiglottis, vocal folds, and proximal surfaces entering the larynx are also covered by stratified squamous epithelium, whereas ciliated pseudostratified columnar epithelium is found in more distal portions of the larynx. Small numbers of mast cells and lymphocytes can also be found in the epithelium of the larynx (5).

IV. Tracheobronchial Tree

The conducting airway extending from the proximal trachea to the terminal bronchioles contains up to eight differentiated epithelial cell types. Epithelial thickness becomes progressively thinner from proximal to distal generations, changing from a ciliated pseudostratified columnar epithelium in the proximal airways to a low cuboidal epithelium in the distal airways (Fig. 1). In general, the proportion of ciliated cells decreases in distal and respiratory bronchioles while nonciliated cells increase (Fig. 2).

The cell types of the epithelium found in the tracheobronchial tree are ciliated cells, mucous or goblet cells, serous cells, small granule or Kulchitsky cells, basal cells, brush cells, neuroendocrine cells, and Clara cells. Intermediate or undifferentiated cells are also present (6). Epithelial invaginations of the larger airways form submucosal glands containing mucous and serous cells. In terminal bronchioles, the epithelium is composed of ciliated cells, Clara cells, and occasional granule and brush cells. In those locations along the tracheobronchial tree where bronchus-associated lymphoid tissue is present in the airway wall, the epithelium overlying these regions is typically covered with a low-to-cuboidal, nonciliated lymphoepithelium (7). This type of epithelium is thought to facilitate the presentation of inhaled antigens to the underlying lymphoid tissues.

V. Respiratory Bronchioles

In respiratory bronchioles, the epithelium transitions to a simple cuboidal epithelium composed of a mixture of ciliated and numerous nonciliated bronchiolar (Clara) cells. Occasional brush cells and small granule cells may be present but are rare in occurrence. Alveolar out pockets within the walls are lined by squamous epithelial type I and cuboidal epithelial

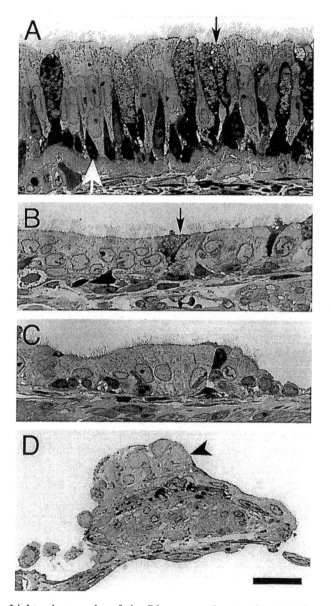

Figure 1 Light micrographs of the Rhesus monkey trachea (A), bronchus (B), bronchiole (C), and respiratory bronchiole (D). Ciliated cells are present in the trachea, bronchus, and bronchiole, whereas cuboidal cells line the nonalveolated portions of the respiratory bronchioles. Mucous goblet cells (black arrows) are present in the trachea and bronchus, whereas Clara cells (arrowhead) are found in the bronchiole and respiratory bronchiole. Basal cells (white arrow) are prevalent in the trachea and bronchus while less frequent in the bronchiole and respiratory bronchiole. Scale bar is 20 μm.

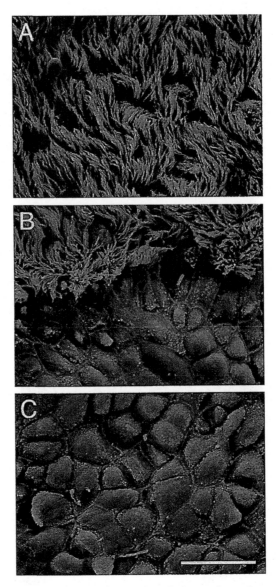

Figure 2 Scanning electron micrographs of the surface characteristics of the bronchus (primarily ciliated cells) (A), bronchiole junction with the respiratory bronchiole (showing the transition from ciliated to nonciliated cells) (B), and the respiratory bronchiole (primarily Clara cells) (C) of Rhesus monkey airways. Scale bar is 20 μm.

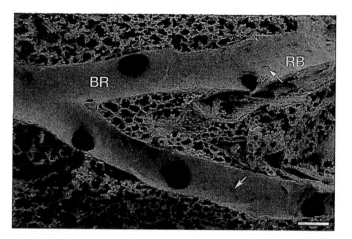

Figure 3 Scanning electron micrograph of bronchioles (BR) transitioning into respiratory bronchioles (RB) in the lung of a Rhesus monkey. The branching geometry of the lower airways gives rise to the more peripheral RB with alveolar outpocketings (arrows) along the walls. Scale bar is 500 μm.

type II cells. Owing to the interdigitation of these anatomical structures, respiratory bronchioles are involved in both air conduction and gas exchange. Respiratory bronchioles are found in humans, monkeys, dogs, cats, and ferrets (Fig. 3) but are absent in mice, rats, hamsters, guinea pigs, cows, and horses (Fig. 4).

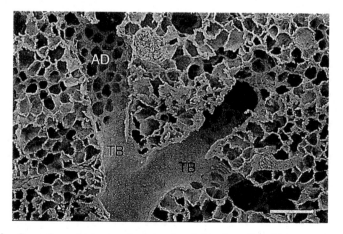

Figure 4 Scanning electron micrograph of the junction between the terminal bronchiole and alveolar duct in the lung of a rat. In contrast to the monkey, the transition from conducting airways to gas exchange regions is abrupt without an intervening respiratory bronchiole. Scale bar is 200 μm.

VI. Lung Parenchyma

The epithelium of alveolar ducts, sacs, and alveoli consists of epithelial type I cells (also known as pneumocytes), covering 95% of the total surface area, and epithelial type II cells, covering the remaining 2–5% of alveolar surfaces (Fig. 5). Epithelial type III cells have also been described but are not well characterized. These cells, also known as brush cells, are present in low numbers in the alveoli near terminal bronchioles (8).

VII. Functions of the Epithelium

Stratified squamous epithelium is found in areas subject to trauma and serves primarily as a protective barrier. Sustentacular cells are the supporting cells of the olfactory epithelium. Bipolar olfactory cells are sensory epithelium with nonmotile cilia in the rostral portion of the nasal cavity to facilitate the sense of smell via neural connections to the olfactory bulb of the brain.

Ciliated cells possess motile apical cilia important for the function of the mucociliary escalator. Goblet cells are the mucous secreting cells that produce the protective viscous layer of the airway lining. Serous cells are less numerous but phenotypically similar to mucous cells. Serous cells provide the liquid lining found beneath the mucous lining of the airways to facilitate free movement of the cilia. This periciliary fluid is frequently referred to as the sol layer, whereas the overlying mucous is the gel layer. Nonciliated bronchiolar epithelial cells (Clara cells) are found in place of goblet cells in the distal airways. Clara cells serve both as a secretory function and as a stem cell function in the bronchioles of most species. Clara cells are also important in xenobiotic metabolism.

Brush cells phenotypically have relatively thick, short microvilli. These cells are thought to have a sensory function. Brush cells of the nasal olfactory epithelium have synaptic contact with sensory fibers of trigeminal nerve origin in contact with their basal surface (9). In the rat, brush cells are most numerous in the trachea and the bifurcations of alveolar ducts (8). Neuroepithelial cells form neuroepithelial bodies (Fig. 6) and appear to be more numerous in the fetus than in the adult. Neuroepithelial bodies are believed to have a sensory function through the release of substance P and other neurokinins. These cells are found to the level of respiratory bronchioles in adults but only in the tracheal epithelium in the fetus at gestational week 20 (10).

Basal cells may serve as progenitor cells, although some findings dispute this theory. Basal cells have an important function in anchoring the epithelium to the basal lamina. Hemidesmosomes and anchoring fibrils are found on their basal surfaces in large airways (11,12). Small granule

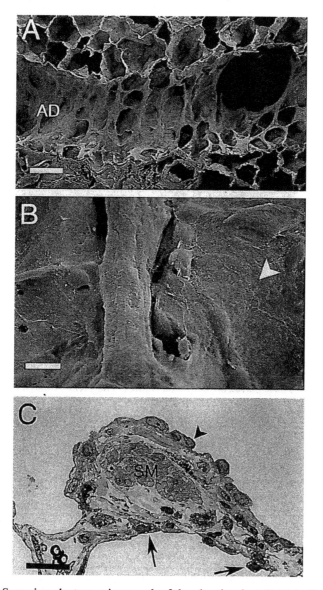

Figure 5   Scanning electron micrograph of the alveolar duct (AD) in the lung of a Rhesus monkey (A). A higher scanning magnification of two alveoli with an intervening alveolar septal ridge is shown in panel B. The majority of alveolar surfaces shown in panels A and B are covered by epithelial type I cells (arrowhead). Panel C is a light micrograph of an alveolar septal tip (ridge) located between two adjacent alveoli in the Rhesus lung. The epithelial lining is formed by alveolar type I (arrowhead) and type II (arrows) cells. Within the alveolar septal tip is a prominent smooth muscle (SM) bundle. Scale bar is 50 μm (A), 5 μm (B), and 20 μm (C).

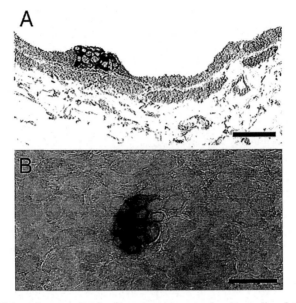

Figure 6   Light micrograph of pulmonary neuroendocrine cells of the airways in the mouse lung. Panel A is a paraffin section. Panel B is a whole mount airway preparation showing the epithelium from an en face (airway lumen) view. In both panels, neuroendocrine cells have been stained with an antibody specific for calcitonin gene-related protein (CGRP). Neuroendocrine cells forming clusters in the airways are known as neuroepithelial bodies. The proportion of airway epithelium composed of this cell type is 0.4%. Scale bar is 20 μm.

or Kulchitsky cells possess small apical granules and may be neuroendocrine cells. Intermediate cells are thought to represent developing ciliated cells or goblet cells that have discharged their mucous.

Type I cells are simple squamous epithelia that facilitate in gas exchange. Type II cells have a dual function as progenitor cells and important sources of pulmonary surfactant found within intracellular lamellar bodies. Type II cells are the major cells involved in epithelial repair of the alveoli and transdifferentiation into epithelial type I cells (13). The differentiation of type II cells into type I cells has been demonstrated to be influenced by lung expansion in fetal sheep (14).

VIII.   Epithelial Cell Metabolism

The respiratory system is the primary site for the entrance of airborne toxicants. It receives 100% of the cardiac output and is therefore also exposed to toxicants entering the circulation by alternate routes (15).

Numerous endogenous and inducible cytochrome P450 families of enzymes have been reported in human bronchial epithelium and in alveolar macrophages (16). The lung can contribute significantly to first-pass metabolism of inhaled xenobiotics (17). Xenobiotic metabolizing enzymes are expressed throughout the respiratory epithelium. Clara cells, epithelial type II cells, and alveolar macrophages are principal targets for xenobiotic toxicants activated by cytochrome P450 isozymes (15,18). Xenobiotic toxicity has been shown to be specific to respiratory microenvironments. Responses to xenobiotics are influenced by the metabolic potential of the cell, local inflammatory responses, age, gender, species, and prior exposure (19). For example, Clara cells located in the bronchiolar airways have been shown to be highly susceptible to toxicants due to the presence of cytochrome P450 xenobiotic metabolizing isozymes in these cells that bioactivate the toxins (20,21).

The nasal mucosa is the first tissue to contact xenobiotics entering the respiratory tract and possesses extensive xenobiotic-metabolizing capacity. In hamster and rat nasal mucosa, cytochrome P450 isoforms are found in nonciliated cells of the nonolfactory epithelium and the sustentacular cells of the olfactory epithelium (22,23). In the rabbit, nasal cytochrome P450 2A, responsible for the activation of some xenobiotic carcinogens, is present in ciliated cells of the nasal respiratory epithelium and olfactory sustentacular cells but is absent in squamous epithelial cells (17).

Xenobiotics further induce P450 metabolizing capability in respiratory epithelial cells, which may alter the susceptibility of these cells to toxicity. In rats, intratracheal instillation of diesel-exhaust particles induces cytochrome P450 1A1 (24). In humans, cigarette smoke induces numerous P450 isoforms in epithelial cells.

Phase II enzymes are also present in the respiratory epithelium and serve as an important function in the detoxification of xenobiotics. These enzymes are expressed heterogeneously throughout the respiratory system. In the rat, some UDP-glucuronosyl transferases are predominantly expressed in the nasal epithelium (25). Xenobiotic toxicity can be dependent on a balance between activation and detoxification enzymes and varies by cell type and location. Glutathione (GSH) and other antioxidants are important components of both the mucous/sol lining layer and the respiratory epithelial cells. GSH can function in the detoxification of xenobiotics and depletion of GSH increases oxidative injury to the epithelium (26). In mouse, glutathione-*S*-transferase activity increases with age. Neonates are more susceptible to injury from bioactivated pulmonary toxicants despite lower P450 activity. Lower glutathione-*S*-transferase activity may hinder the detoxification of electrophilic intermediates in neonates (27). Significant variation in the expression of phase I and phase II metabolizing enzymes exists in different regions of the respiratory system. Significant species variation has also been reported (28).

Multiple drug resistance transporter genes have been demonstrated in epithelial type I cells and may serve as an important barrier to xenobiotic transfer across the alveolar epithelium (29). The primary stem cells available for repair following xenobiotic-induced toxicity are thought to be the basal and goblet cell of the trachea and bronchi, the Clara cell in the bronchioles, and epithelial type II cells in the alveoli. Some Clara cells appear to be spared toxic insult by lacking P450 enzymes (30). In neonatal calves, differentiation of Clara cells into ciliated cells involves a transitional stage during which glycogen is lost and polyribosomes are synthesized. This is followed by the synthesis of basal bodies and cilia (31).

The site and level of deposition of inhaled particulate matter (PM) are highly dependent on particle size, shape, density, chemical reactivity, and air flow rates (32) (see Chapter 2, which covers in-depth mechanisms and factors influential to particle deposition in the lung). In the rat, chronic exposure to high concentrations of particles has been shown to cause inflammation, proliferation, and impaired clearance. Alveolar macrophage function was also decreased (33). Clearance of insoluble and slightly soluble particles have been shown to have both a rapid and a slow phase and is affected by disease processes, as well as the original site of deposition (34,35). Clearance velocity is dependent on airway diameter, length and mucous volume, and ciliary beat frequency of epithelial lining cells. The slow phase represents clearance of particles from small distal airways and alveoli (36). Increasing particle solubility and/or bronchial blood flow increases retention of particles in the lung (37,38). In the dog, long-term retention of particles was in airways at the level of the bronchioles (39).

Human ciliary beat frequency is similar in nasal and tracheal mucosa. In sheep, the mucociliary apparatus can clear particles deposited in central airways within 2–4 hr while most particles are cleared from the more peripheral bronchioles within 72 hr (40). Epithelial transport processes are important in the maintenance of airway surface liquid. Proper depth and osmolality are critical for normal function of the mucociliary apparatus. Alterations in the normal homeostasis of ion transport by epithelial cells can play a significant role in epithelial pathologic states caused by disease or toxicity (41,42).

Polarized epithelium is dependent on tight junctions to maintain the integrity of the epithelial wall (43). Alterations in tight junctions appear to be integral to many disease processes. Epithelial cell wall adhesion to the underlying basement membrane is essential for normal growth and development and preservation of the epithelium as a protective barrier. Hemidesmosomes through cell surface integrins attach the epithelium to the underlying extracellular matrix (44).

The pulmonary immune system is a specialized and compartmentalized system capable of both local and systemic responses (45). A functioning immune system is essential to host defenses and the maintenance of a functional respiratory epithelium. The respiratory epithelium, in acting as a barrier, is a part of the innate host resistance to disease. Respiratory epithelium is believed to directly influence immunological responses initiated in the airways through the release of cytokines that have both local and systemic effects. In man and animals, substantial numbers of mast cells are found in the epithelium (46).

The airways receive their principal innervations from the vagus nerve (47) (see Chapter 6, for in-depth review of neural innervation of the respiratory tract). The epithelium lining the airways contains sensory innervations composed of varicose unmyelinated C-fibers. Nerve endings in the epithelia respond to stimulation by releasing neuropeptides. Neuropeptides have been shown to increase vascular permeability and dilation, increase mucous secretion, and recruit inflammatory cells (48).

Neuroepithelial bodies in the respiratory epithelium serve as an additional source of neuropeptides (Fig. 6). In the rat, a second sensory unmyelinated nerve fiber population innervates neuroepithelial bodies. Neuroepithelial bodies may serve as sensory end organs in the lung and are dispersed throughout the epithelium at all levels of the airways with a preference for bifurcations. While C-fibers react to noxious chemical stimuli and are weakly mechanosensitive, neuroepithelial bodies may be directly activated by hypoxic stimuli (49,50).

IX. Epithelial Surfaces, Air Pollutants, and Lung Disease

Numerous respiratory diseases are characterized by alterations in the epithelial surface. Morphologic and physiologic changes to airway lining cells may result in alterations in lung function, airway sensitivity, immune response, and the airway lining fluid. Changes in antioxidant levels, mucous secretions, and levels of cytokines and other mediators or biochemical signals arising from the epithelium are common findings in respiratory disease. Changes in gene expression, as a consequence of exposure to genetic, toxic, infectious, and metabolic etiologies, also appear to play a central role for many of these diseases.

A variety of air pollutants can interact directly or indirectly with the epithelial surface. Some air pollutants can further exacerbate respiratory diseases such as chronic obstructive pulmonary disease (COPD), pneumoconiosis, and cancer. Air pollutants may exacerbate existing disease conditions through their impact on epithelial (as well as interstitial) events (Figs. 7 and 8). In fact, cross-talk between the epithelial and interstitial compartments may be a driving force in disease progression. In this section, a number of pollutants and their impact on the epithelium and the disease process will be discussed with the goal of better understanding of what happens in humans. Numerous studies using animals will be referenced. These

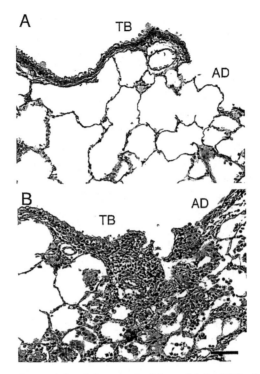

Figure 7   Light micrograph of the terminal bronchiole (TB)–alveolar duct (AD) junction in the lungs of a normal rat (A) and a rat with significant influx of inflammatory cells in the alveolar air spaces (B). Associated with this influx of inflammatory cells is a subtle, but significant alteration of the epithelium. Scale bar is 50 μm.

animal studies serve as models of a specific disease process and how a given pollutant may influence the disease. In a number of instances, the concentration of the pollutant studied will not reflect environmental conditions but can still provide important insights on epithelial–pollutant interactions and disease outcomes.

Chronic obstructive pulmonary disease, or emphysema, involves irreversible enlargement of airspaces distal to terminal bronchioles due to alveolar wall destruction. Change in antiprotease activity (αAT) is thought to be the predominant mechanism for increased alveolar wall destruction and occurs as a direct consequence of the inhalation of toxicants in tobacco smoke and other pollutants (51).

Exposure to ozone can exacerbate COPD in humans. In a recent study, Desqueyroux et al. (52) found that each 10 μg/m^3 increase in ozone concentration was significantly associated with a worsening of respiratory conditions for COPD. The COPD lesions are known to be caused by tobacco smoke and may also be caused by silica (53,54). In addition,

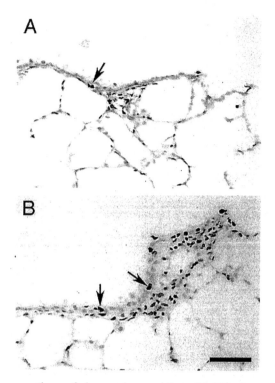

Figure 8 Incorporation of bromodeoxyuridine (BrdU) into epithelial cells (arrows) and underlying interstitial cells at the bronchiole–alveolar duct junction in the lungs of Brown-Norway (BN) rats sensitized and challenged with ovalbumin. Ovalbumin treatment leads to a pattern of airway sensitization and inflammation in this strain of rats. Panel A is taken from the lung of a BN rat exposed to filtered air only, whereas panel B is taken from the lung of a BN rat exposed to ammonium nitrate and carbon black particles. The BrdU uptake into cells is reflective of ongoing DNA synthesis. It is interesting to note the involvement of both epithelial and underlying interstitial cells, suggesting a process of cellular cross-talk during pulmonary inflammation. Scale bar is 50 μm.

tobacco smoke increases release of cytokines interleukin (IL)-8 and IL-1β by epithelial cells and, therefore, increases the influx of inflammatory cells (55). However, concurrent exposure to ozone (0.3 ppm for 8 hr/day for up to 13 months) did not significantly alter COPD pathology due to tobacco smoke exposure in mice (56).

Epidemiological studies have implicated some forms of PM to exacerbate COPD (57,58). Similar to ozone, PM can possess oxidant properties. Transition metals associated with PM are known to cause oxidative stress. Ultrafine carbon black can generate free radicals in the absence of metals. Particulate matter induced oxidative stress results in neutrophil influx, increased epithelial permeability, and increased transcription of proinflammatory genes, potentially exacerbating COPD (57,59). Concurrent adenoviral infection in individuals with COPD may amplify proinflammatory responses following exposure to PM (60). Changes in lung function and surface area, however, were found to have a sparing effect on a COPD model in rats exposed to diesel-exhaust particles (61) at a concentration of 3 mg/m³ for 7 hr/day, 5 days/week for up to 24 months.

Acute exposure to NO_2 or ozone at high concentrations (5–10 ppm NO_2 and 0.2–1.0 ppm ozone) causes epithelial necrosis and inflammation (Fig. 9) (62). Acute NO_2 exposure at 10 ppm in the rat recruits elastase-positive neutrophils causing mild centriacinar airspace enlargement with mild interstitial fibrosis. However, with continued exposure to NO_2, lesions did not progress (63,64). The NO_2 exposure in a protease-induced model of COPD failed to exacerbate protease destruction of alveolar walls (65).

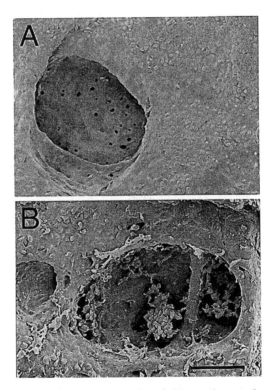

Figure 9   Scanning electron micrographs of the respiratory bronchiole with an alveolar outpocketing present in a Rhesus monkey lung exposed to filtered air (A) or to 1.0 ppm of ozone for 8 hr (B). Inflammatory cells and epithelial debris litter the surfaces of the respiratory bronchiole following acute exposure to high levels of ozone. Scale bar is 50 μm.

Chronic low-level NO_2 exposure (2 ppm) in elastase-induced COPD hamsters resulted in seemingly contradictory findings of increased alveolar mean linear intercept length and internal surface area (ISA) (66). Prolonged NO_2 exposure (9.5 ppm for 7 hr/day, 5 days/week for up to 24 months) is associated with epithelial hyperplasia and extension of cuboidal bronchiolar epithelium into proximal alveoli (67). Similar changes, should they occur in COPD lungs, would be expected to exacerbate symptoms due to interference with gas exchange, but supporting data are lacking. Mixed inflammatory cell infiltrates and enlargement of airspaces typical of COPD has been reported following combined NO_2 (0.2–2.96 ppm) and diesel particle exposure in Wistar rats (68). Nitrogen dioxide may cause COPD-like alveolar wall destruction by recruiting inflammatory cells producing proteases, as well as through free radical oxidant injury (69). Respiratory bronchioles appear to be particularly sensitive to the effects of NO_2 at high concentration. Narrowing of terminal bronchioles has been reported (69,70) following exposure to 15 ppm NO_2 for 17 months.

Sulfur dioxide (SO_2) has also been implicated in acute COPD exacerbations (58). A rat model of COPD has been developed using exposure to a high level of SO_2 of 250 ppm for 5 hr/day, 5 days/week for 7 weeks (71). Bronchiolar epithelial hyperplasia, with enlargement of airspaces and epithelial damage, goblet cell hyperplasia, and inflammatory cell infiltration of large airways, have been reported in rats following SO_2 exposure at 1 ppm for 4 months (72). Exposure to high levels of SO_2 (250 ppm) can produce pathologic changes that initially resemble chronic bronchitis which often progress to emphysematous and obstructive changes in the lungs (73).

Chronic bronchitis commonly results from long-term exposure to air pollutants including tobacco smoke and industrial air pollutants. Airway epithelial changes include mucous cell hyperplasia and hypertrophy in large and small airways with increased secretion of mucous into the airway lumen (74,75). This may progress to goblet cell metaplasia and mucous plugging of airways, in severe cases obliterating the airway lumen (bronchiolitis obliterans). Infiltration of epithelial and interstitial areas with inflammatory cells is common. Persistent small airway obstruction can lead to emphysematous changes. Bronchial epithelium may develop squamous metaplasia and dysplasia (76,77).

Epidemiology studies have demonstrated an association between the development of chronic bronchitis and ambient air pollution (75,78). Animal models of chronic bronchitis have been developed in rats, hamsters, and dogs using ozone, SO_2, tobacco smoke, and endotoxin lipopolysaccharide (LPS) from gram-negative bacteria (79). Mucous cell metaplasia in these models may be selectively localized in nasal (ozone) or bronchial (endotoxin) epithelium with some toxicants (74,80).

Particulate matter from a number of sources is known to induce airway inflammation. Wool dust can activate complement through generation of chemotaxins in mill workers (81). Coal dust infiltrates bronchial walls at all levels causing chronic bronchitis in many exposed workers and pneumoconiosis in some others (82). Cotton dust (5.3–14.5 mg/m³), diesel-exhaust particles (10 µg/mL), concentrated ambient particles (CAPs) (607 µg/m³), and SO_2 (200 ppm) have all been shown to cause bronchitis in the rat (83–85). Bronchitic rats exposed to CAPs demonstrated increased inflammation during selected periods while nothing in other periods, suggesting that CAPs can exacerbate chronic bronchitis depending on its constituents. Bronchitic rats retain more particles in their lungs following inhalation than normal rats (75).

A leading cause of chronic bronchitis is tobacco smoke. Mucous cell hyperplasia and inflammatory infiltration of airway epithelium are common (76). In rats, mucous cell hyperplasia appears to be more severe in females accompanied by a shift from periodic acid Schiff positive to Alcian blue positive goblet cells (86).

Chronic bronchitis develops in dogs exposed to 50 ppm of SO_2 for up to 18 months (87,88). Mucous hypersecretion and mucous gland hypertrophy, without increases in inflammatory cell infiltrates or increases in airway sensitivity, were noted in the lungs of these dogs (87,88). In rats exposed to SO_2, inflammation develops in hilar and peripheral regions of the bronchial tree characterized by loss of goblet cells and ciliated cells and by the development of epithelial metaplasia. Dysplasia of the epithelium has been noted in the central or proximal airways. Clara cells were preserved in the bronchiolar epithelium (89). Surfactant production by epithelial type II cells has also been noted to increase in rats exposed to SO_2 (90).

Asthma is an obstructive immune-mediated disease that appears to be exacerbated by air pollutants. The epithelium exhibits mucous cell hyperplasia including an increase in the size of the submucosal glands. Mucous plugs contain whorls of shed epithelium in severe cases (Curschmann spirals). A predominantly eosinophilic infiltration of the epithelium and basement membrane thickening is present. Hypertrophy of the smooth muscle in the airway wall, airway hypersensitivity, and reversible bronchoconstriction are the hallmarks of asthma (91,92).

Numerous epidemiological studies have demonstrated an association between increased morbidity in asthmatics and increased ambient levels of a variety of air pollutants. Asthma is common in children. An animal study utilizing a neonatal mouse suggested that pollutants disrupt resistance to allergens and promote airway hypersensitivity. The epithelium was found to contain increased numbers of dendritic cells following exposure to allergens and residual oil fly ash (ROFA). Whether changes in the epithelium are responsible for increased susceptibility in this study is not known (93). Numerous studies have demonstrated an adjuvant effect from exposure to air pollutants (94).

Epidemiological studies have shown that asthmatics may be at increased risk with exposure to ozone. Ozone is one of the most common oxidant pollutants and has been shown to have variable impacts on lung function in subjects with asthma (95,96). Ozone-induced inflammation has been shown to increase airway resistance in asthmatics (97,98). Responses to ozone differ between individuals and may not be dependent on asthma severity (99,100). Ozone has been shown to increase inflammation in the upper respiratory tract of asthmatics and is associated with increases in neutrophils, eosinophils, and epithelial cells in nasal lavage, signaling changes in nasal mucosa. These changes parallel the exacerbation of asthma symptoms (101).

Acute ozone exposure (0.1 ppm for 2 hr) causes an acute neutrophilic inflammation of airways and potentiates the late phase eosinophilic response following allergen exposure in atopic individuals (102). Some researchers have not found increased adhesion factors (P-selectin, ICAM-1) or neutrophil recruitment to be more severe in asthmatics following ozone exposure at 0.2 ppm for 2 hr (103). Cultured human epithelial cells (HBECs) from asthmatic and nonasthmatic subjects in the presence of 0.1 ppm ozone for 6 hr demonstrated in cells from asthmatics to have increased levels of IL-8, granulocyte/macrophage colony stimulating factor (GMCSF) and the adhesion factor ICAM-1 (104). HBECs from asthmatics also showed increased expression of the chemokine RANTES, not seen in HBECs from normal individuals (104). Increased expression of RANTES may increase eosinophilic inflammation and lead to an exacerbation of asthma symptoms and pathologic changes in the epithelium (104). Prolonged acute exposure to ozone at 0.16 ppm in human asthmatic subjects has been shown to increase eosinophilic inflammation in lower airways (105). Epithelial cytokine expression of IL-5, GMCSF, and IL-8 has also been found to be higher in asthmatics exposed for 2 hr to 0.2 ppm of ozone (106).

Bronchoconstriction following nonspecific stimulation of M3 receptors resulting in significant decreases in airway diameter has been shown following ozone exposure at 0.4 ppm for 2 hr in both asthmatic and nonasthmatic subjects (107). Ozone is believed to exhibit toxicity due to its potent oxidant properties by initially interacting with the lung lining fluid. Secondary oxidation products can transmit signals to underlining pulmonary epithelium resulting in changes in cytokines, adhesion molecule expression and tight junctions, resulting in edema and inflammatory influx. Bronchial C-fibers in the epithelium may be secondarily stimulated by ozone, resulting in changes in neuropeptide release (substance P). It is unclear whether any of these epithelial factors are responsible for increased bronchoconstriction and increased susceptibility to ozone (108). Substance P levels are increased in asthmatics. There is no evidence of increased M3 receptor function in asthma or from exposure to ozone. Hypersensitivity may be related to decreased M2 receptor function and subsequent decrease in M2 inhibition of β-adrenergic nerves (109). Calcitonin gene-related peptide and neuroepithelial bodies are also increased in the terminal bronchioles of rats following ozone exposure. Epithelial cells were also found to have increased granules presumably lipofusion (110).

Epidemiological studies have demonstrated a strong correlation between exposure to PM and increased asthma morbidity (111,112). The PM effects may be dependant on composition. The PM deposition on airway epithelium can cause inflammation, airway hypersensitivity, epithelial damage, and increases in epithelial permeability. Particle mass, metals, organic compounds, pollen, infectious organisms, and reactive oxygen species have all been shown to be responsible to varying degrees (113). Endotoxins carried by inhaled particles may also play a role in PM-generated inflammatory responses (114).

Exposure to ROFA by intratracheal instillation (1000 μg) in a Brown-Norway (BN) rat allergic model has shown an adjuvant effect to enhance sensitization (94). Particulate matter from combustion oils (100 μg/mL) inhibits cell proliferation and metabolism in cultured rat epithelial cells (113). Diesel-exhaust particulate increased release of TH2 cytokines through activation of p38 MAP kinase culminating with infiltration of inflammatory cells, increased mucous secretion, and serum leakage (115,116). Increased airway responses to CAPs in the presence or absence of ozone have also been noted in an allergic murine model (117). Chronic exposure to ambient PM in Mexico City results in small airway remodeling (118). Some believe PM may stimulate irritant C-fibers (119). These findings suggest that PM from various sources could further augment epithelial pathology present in asthmatics.

Epithelial tissue injury, following exposure to NO_2, is dependent on dose and anatomic site and is characterized by loss of epithelial cells. Compensatory cell proliferation is most persistent, following exposure in terminal bronchioles and, in severe cases, can resemble bronchiolitis obliterans. The mechanism of toxicity to epithelial cells probably involves free radical formation similar to that seen from ozone. Lung ISA is decreased, and lung phospholipids and protein synthesis appear to be depressed (69). High NO_2 concentrations ranging from 10 to 20 ppm cause epithelial necrosis, interstitial edema, and inflammatory influx. Repeated exposure at these concentrations can lead to centrilobular fibrosis and remodeling (62,120). Loss of cilia and replacement of squamous epithelial type I cells with cuboidal type II cells, along with the hypertrophy and hyperplasia of bronchial epithelium, have also been seen in rats following NO_2 exposure at a concentration of 20 mg/m^3 for 4 weeks (121).

The epithelium in the lungs of asthmatics may be more susceptible to NO_2, although no studies have confirmed this. In asthmatic subjects, experimental exposure to NO_2 at 500 μg/m^3 for 30 min did not affect respiratory symptoms but was associated with inflammation (122). The adjuvant effects seen with ozone and PM have been demonstrated in nonsensitized BN rats exposed to NO_2 in combination with ovalbumin. Antigen-specific IgE was 10-fold higher following combined exposure; however, it is not known if elevated IgE correlates with asthma exacerbation or epithelial changes (123).

Sulfur dioxide has also been shown to induce bronchoconstriction in asthmatics. The SO_2 inhalation at 0.05–0.15 ppm during exercise increases airway resistance and, therefore, may exacerbate asthma symptoms (124,125). Effects of SO_2 on the epithelium are likely to involve injury, repair, and eventual adaptive factors that may include extension of bronchiolar epithelium into the gas exchange portions of the lungs.

In idiopathic pulmonary fibrosis (IPF), hyaline membranes and mononuclear cell infiltration of the alveolar septa accompanied by hyperplasia of epithelial type II cells can progress to complete obliteration of alveoli with fibrous tissue. Idiopathic pulmonary fibrosis is one form of interstitial pneumonia with fibrosis as a central feature. Conditions with similar pathology include diseases such as desquamative interstitial pneumonia, respiratory bronchiolitis interstitial lung disease, and cryptogenic organizing pneumonia (126). Epidemiological studies suggest that inorganic dusts and tobacco smoke are risk factors for IPF and other interstitial disorders resulting in fibrosis (127–129).

In rats, ozone exposure causes hyperplasia of epithelial type II cells, along with interstitial changes in cells making collagen. Increased turnover of extracellular collagen in the presence of decreased degradation of intracellular collagen can lead to fibrosis within alveolar ducts (130,131). Epithelial and interstitial thickening can further lead to bronchiolar epithelial cell metaplasia in proximal alveolar regions, as well as further fibrotic change in the lungs of rats. These bronchiolar epithelial cells may exhibit swollen, abnormal cilia. The increase in the interstitial compartment is due to an increased volume of fibroblasts and noncellular components. Basement membrane volume is also increased with ozone exposure (132). Airway inflammation typically decreases following repeated exposure to ozone. For humans repeatedly exposed to laboratory-generated ozone, the data as to whether inflammation attenuates with re-exposure is somewhat controversial with the attenuation of BALF levels of PMNs in some studies (133), but not others (134), whereas airway biopsy of humans reflects no attenuation of inflammatory cell infiltration (135). For rodents, chronic ozone exposure (1.0 ppm) typically results in continued epithelial and fibrotic changes in airways and the proximal alveolar regions of the lungs (Fig. 10) (136).

Exposure to ozone and NO_2 leads to airway remodeling in rats and increased expression of type I and type III collagens. Increased inflammatory infiltration of macrophages and neutrophils in airway epithelium

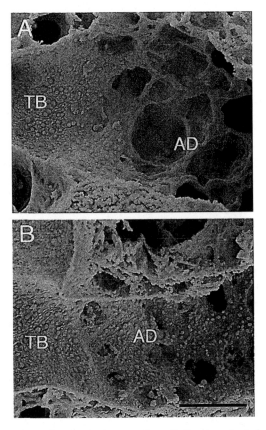

Figure 10 Scanning electron micrographs of the terminal bronchiole (TB)–alveolar duct (AD) junction from the lung of a filtered air control rat (A) and a rat exposed to ozone (1.0 ppm) for 6 hr/day, 5 days/week for 20 months (B). Bronchiolar epithelial cells have extended into the alveolar air spaces and now line alveolar surfaces. Scale bar is 100 μm.

may increase oxidative stress and increase levels of tumor necrosis factor alpha (TNFα) and transforming growth factor beta (TGFβ) known to activate fibroblasts (95,137). Interestingly, simultaneous exposure of mice to silica and NO_2 delayed fibrotic changes but did not alter chronic cellular inflammation (138).

Particulate matter, especially mineral dusts, is known to cause fibrotic changes in the walls of airways. Dusts that contain iron on their surfaces activate the transcription factor NF-κB via oxidant stimulation. Asbestos, silica, aluminum oxide, diesel-exhaust particles, and titanium oxide are the examples of PM that cause fibrotic changes (118,139–142). Asbestos fibers, iron particles, and many other fine and ultrafine particles penetrate the epithelium. Penetration may be required to initiate fibrosis (143). Mineral dusts directly induce epithelial and interstitial fibrogenic mediators, platelet-derived growth factor (PDGF), and TGFβ and matrix components, in the airway wall (144) (see Chapter 7, for in-depth review of airway remodeling, growth factors, and airway fibrosis).

In cats exposed to diesel-exhaust particles (6–11 mg/m^3 for 8 hr/day, 7 days/week for 27 months), peribronchial fibrosis has been associated with increases in lymphocytes, fibroblasts, and particle-laden macrophages. Bronchiolar metaplasia was reversible following termination of exposure, whereas fibrogenesis was found to be persistent (145).

Studies of epithelial changes in diseased lungs of individuals or animal models with IPF or other interstitial fibrotic disorders, or exacerbation of these diseases from additional exposure to airborne pollutants, are lacking. Despite this fact, it is presumed that exposure to airborne pollutants that stimulate epithelial and interstitial change in normal lungs would further exacerbate the fibrotic condition of diseased lungs.

Dust-related diseases, or pneumoconiosis, are clearly due to inhalation of air pollutants such as coal dust, silica, and silicates (146,147). Particulate air pollution has also been suggested to cause other deleterious effects to the pulmonary epithelium. Macrophage activation leads to epithelial type I cell damage lining alveoli followed by epithelial type II cell hypertrophy and hyperplasia. Lesions progress, as particle-laden macrophages form granulomas with fibrosis. Pneumoconiosis from welder's fumes was found to be reversible (148). Coal dust causes oxidative stress and upregulates PDGF, LTB4, TNFα, and other inflammatory cytokines and adhesion molecules. Activation of macrophages results in damaged epithelium, hyperplasia of mucous cells, and impaired mucociliary clearance. Loss of epithelial type I cells results in proliferation of epithelial type II cells. Epithelial cells produce matrix resulting in thickening of the basement membrane. Stimulated pulmonary fibroblasts cause interstitial fibrosis (147). Chronic exposure and subsequent ongoing inflammatory cell infiltration result in granuloma formation in the lungs.

Cystic fibrosis (CF) is an inherited disorder in epithelial cell chloride transport affecting the fluid lining layer in respiratory airways. Abnormally thick mucous secretions due to decreased water content lead to defective mucociliary clearance and secondary obstruction of airways with mucous. Distention of bronchioles and mucous cell hyperplasia and hypertrophy are seen. Secondary infections can cause additional pathology resembling chronic bronchitis and bronchiectasis (chronic necrotizing infection of large and small airways with abnormal airway dilation).

Adverse effects from environmental tobacco smoke (ETS) in children with CF have been reported. Growth rates and pulmonary function are decreased by ETS exposure despite lower urine cotinine levels in children with CF (149–151). Some epidemiological studies have failed to demonstrate a decrease in function in children with CF exposed to ETS (152). The specific effects of ETS and other air pollutants have not been adequately studied.

Infectious inflammation of the airways and lung parenchyma can, in some cases, be attributed to alterations in innate and adaptive immunity, the mucous lining layer of the airways, as well as to defective mucociliary clearance. Exposure to environmental air pollutants can further drive these changes in the respiratory system. Destruction of the respiratory epithelium by toxicants can further subject the upper and lower respiratory tract to infectious disease. Changes in the surface epithelium, which affect inflammatory cell infiltration and increase mucous secretion arising from immune mediated defenses, can occur. Epithelial injury and repair with transient or irreversible metastatic change and/or fibrosis can result from either the infectious agent or the immune response to the pathogen, thus representing a double-edged sword.

The mammalian respiratory epithelium defends itself from microbial invasion with both innate defenses and acquired immunity. Mucociliary clearance is an important first line of defense that may be significantly depressed by ozone, NO_2, SO_2, or tobacco smoke. Mucociliary clearance may also be depressed in diseases such as asthma, chronic bronchitis, and CF. Exposure to air pollutants in individuals compromised by these diseases could increase susceptibility to infection (153,154). In addition, continuous ozone exposure (0.5 ppm) has been shown to potentiate post-influenza inflammation (155).

Epidemiological studies suggest that environmental pollutants increase susceptibility to respiratory infections. Increases in acute respiratory infections following ozone and NO_2 exposure have been reported in children (156). Exposure to diesel-exhaust particles as low as 30 $\mu g/m^3$ for 6 hr/day for 7 days was found to increase respiratory syncytical virus-induced inflammation in C57B1/6 mice (157). Conversely, SO_2 exposure in hamsters with emphysematous-like changes decreased *Listeria* infection in the lungs 1 week postinfection (158). Individuals compromised with asthma or chronic bronchitis develop airflow obstruction at lower concentrations of inhaled LPS suggesting increased risk from gram-negative infection (159).

Neoplastic changes to the epithelium are varied and dependent on the neoplastic cell type and location. Tobacco smoke is believed to be the primary cause of lung cancer. Exposure to tobacco smoke is highly associated with pulmonary neoplasia in humans, although this has been difficult to demonstrate in animal models (160–162). Atmospheric toxicants are believed to be causative in some cases. Exposure to ozone and/or NO_2 may decrease tumor incidence in experimental animals possibly due to their cytotoxic effects (163,164). Human cancer cells may also have increased susceptibility to ozone (165).

Chronic ozone exposure (1.0 ppm) for up to 30 months induced lung neoplasia with a high percentage of K-ras mutations in B6C3F1 mice but not in F344 rats (166). Further studies in A/J mice exposed to ozone (0.8 ppm) for 32 weeks demonstrated no enhanced tumorigenic effects (167). Interestingly, ozone as low as 0.1 ppm in concentration increased the rate of pulmonary metastasis in mice infused with NR-FS fibrosarcoma cells (168). Exposure to NO_2, but not to ozone, demonstrated a similar effect in a B16 melanoma model (169). Exposure to ozone (0.1 ppm) was shown to increase tumorigenesis of *N-bis*-(2-hydroxypropyl nitrosamine) in Wistar rats (170). Combined exposure to ozone (0.1 ppm), sulfuric acid (H_2SO_4) (1 mg/m^3), and NO_2 (0.4 ppm) had an even greater effect (170). Because the tumors that formed were adenomas and adenocarcinomas, significant disruption of epithelial surfaces by tumor cells could be expected to further exacerbate epithelial changes due to other respiratory diseases (170). It has been shown that repeated 6-week exposure to low levels of cyclic ozone rising to a daily peak of 0.25 ppm can impair the clearance of asbestos fibers, a known carcinogen, from the lungs of Fisher 344 rats (171).

Exposure to high levels of diesel-exhaust particles has been associated with pulmonary tumors in the rat where epithelial type II cells may have increased susceptibility to change. As found with ozone, K-ras mutations have also been found in neoplasms associated with heavy diesel-exhaust particle exposure at 4 mg/m^3 or by intratracheal instillation of diesel particles (172,173). However, it has been suggested that particle-associated tumorigenesis following chronic epithelial hypertrophy, hyperplasia, and metaplasia may be specific to rats (174,175). In hamsters, diesel-exhaust particles, NO_2 (5 ppm), and SO_2 (10 ppm) were found to cause loss of cilia from epithelial cells and to induce focal metaplasia and dysplasia. However, none of these exposures increased tumor incidence following additional exposure to diethyl nitrosamine, a known carcinogen (176).

The cytotoxic effects of exposure to NO_2 (0.25 ppm for 7 hr/day, 5 days/week for up to 181 days) to the epithelium and other cells of the lungs may decrease tumor progression of spontaneous T-cell lymphoma in mice by adversely affecting the immune system (177). However, NO_2 exposure at 0.35 ppm for 6 weeks can induce endothelial injury, the formation of microthrombi, and tumor metastasis of murine B16 melanoma (178).

Cancer has also been induced in mice following inhalation of various organic compounds including carbon disulfide, 1,2-dibromomethane, ethylene oxide, and vinyl chloride. Disruption and alteration of epithelial surfaces have been found in these lungs associated with the tumors formed (179).

In adult respiratory distress syndrome (ARDS), alveolar walls become lined with fibrinous (hyaline) exudates and necrotic epithelial cells. Epithelial type II cells proliferate, and intra-alveolar fibrosis with thickening of alveolar walls due to the infiltration of inflammatory cells and deposition of collagen frequently leads to death in affected individuals. Air pollutants such as smoke and other irritant gases have been shown to cause ARDS, although numerous other etiologies have also been identified (77).

Other respiratory diseases such as hypersensitivity pneumonitis, eosinophilic pneumonitis, and Goodpasture syndrome are potential candidates for exacerbation by air pollutants, and in some cases, airborne toxicants are suspected to be the etiologic agents responsible for the development of the disease condition. In other cases the cause is unknown.

X. Conclusions

In the respiratory system, the epithelium is the first line of defense to the external environment. Epithelial cell types change as a function of location in the lung. Air pollutants can have different effects on epithelial cells depending on species, location within the lung, and pre-existing disease. Animal models can provide critical insights regarding the impact of air pollutants on epithelial cells, but all these effects do not necessarily extrapolate to humans. Epidemiological studies have demonstrated that in many situations, air pollutants can cause or exacerbate lung disease in humans. Although much is known, more is needed to fully understand the long-term impact of air pollutants on the epithelium and human lung disease.

References

1. Esrefoglu M, Selimoglu E, Esrefoglu M, Vuraler Ö. The influence of cigarette smoke on the epithelium of the vestibule: an electron microscopic study. Yonsei Med J 2002; 44.
2. Yoshimi R, Takamura H, Takasaki K, Kumagami H. Immunohistologic study of the nasal mucosa with reference to langerhans cells [in Japanese]. Nippon Jibiinkoka Gakkai Kaiho 1993; 96:1252–1257.
3. Poulsen J, Tos M. Goblet cells in the developing human nose. Acta Otolaryngol 1975; 6:442.
4. Harkema J, Plopper C, Hyde D, Wilson D, St George J, Wong V. Non-olfactory surface epithelium of the nasal cavity of the bonnet monkey: a morphologic and morphometric study of the transitional and respiratory epithelium. Am J Anat 1987; 180:266–279.
5. Maronian N, Haggitt R, Oelschlager BK, Bronner M, Yang J, Reyes V, Hillel A, Eubanks T, Pellegrini CA, Pope CE. Histologic features of reflux-attributed laryngeal lesions. Am J Med 2003; 115:105–108.
6. Reid L, Jones R. Bronchial mucosal cells. Fed Proc 1979; 38:191–196.
7. Harkema J, Plopper C, Pinkerton K. Comparative structure of the respiratory tract: airway architecture in humans and animals. In: Cohen M, Zelikoff J, Schlessinger RB, eds. Pulmonary Immunotoxicology. Boston: Kluwer Academic Publishers, 2000:1–59.

8. Chang LY, Mercer RR, Crapo JD. Differential distribution of brush cells in the rat lung. Anat Rec 1986.
9. Ross MH, Reith EJ, Romrell LJ. Histology: A Text and Atlas. 2d ed. Baltimore: Williams & Wilkins, 1989.
10. DiMaio MF, Kattan M, Ciurea D, Gil J, Dische R. Brush cells in the human fetal trachea. Pediatr Pulmonol 1990.
11. Evans MJ, Van Winkle LS, Fanucchi MV, Plopper CG. Cellular and molecular characteristics of basal cells in airway epithelium. Exp Lung Res 2001.
12. Nakajima M, Kawanami O, Jin E, Ghazizadeh M, Honda M, Asano G, Horiba K, Ferrans VJ. Immunohistochemical and ultrastructural studies of basal cells, Clara cells and bronchiolar cuboidal cells in normal human airways. Pathol Int 1998; 48:944–953.
13. Flecknoe SJ, Wallace MJ, Cock ML, Harding R, Hooper SB. Changes in alveolar epithelial cell proportions during fetal and postnatal development in sheep. Am J Physiol Lung Cell Mol Physiol 2003; 285:664–670.
14. Flecknoe SJ, Wallace MJ, Harding R, Hooper SB. Determination of alveolar epithelial cell phenotypes in fetal sheep: evidence for the involvement of basal lung expansion. J Physiol 2002.
15. Dimova S, Hoet PHM, Nemery B. Xenobiotic-metabolizing enzyme activities in primary cultures of rat type II pneumocytes and alveolar macrophages. Am Soc Pharmacol Exp Ther 2001; 29.
16. Willey JC, Coy E, Brolly C, Utell MJ, Frampton MW, Hammersley J, Thilly WG, Olson D, Cairns K. Xenobiotic metabolism enzyme gene expression in human bronchial epithelial and alveolar macrophage cells. Am J Respir Cell Mol Biol 1996; 14:262–271.
17. Tam YK. Individual variation in first-pass metabolism. Clin Pharmacokinet 1993; 25:300–328.
18. Hukkanen J, Pelkonen O, Hakkola J, Raunio H. Expression and regulation of xenobiotic-metabolizing cytochrome (P450 CYP) enzymes in human lung. Crit Rev Toxicol 2002.
19. Plopper CG, Buckpitt A, Evans M, Van Winkle L, Fanucchi M, Smiley-Jewell S, Lakritz J, West J, Lawson G, Paige R, Miller L, Hyde D. Factors modulating the epithelial response to toxicants in tracheobronchial airways. Toxicology 2001; 160:173–180.
20. Reddy SPM, Adiseshaiah P, Shapiro P, Vuong H. BMK1 (ERK5) regulates squamous differentiation marker SPRR1B transcription in Clara-like H441 cells. Am J Respir Cell Mol Biol 2002; 27:64–70.
21. Macé K, Bowman ED, Vautravers P, Shields PG, Harris CC, Pfeifer AMA. Characterisation of xenobiotic-metabolising enzyme expression in human bronchial mucosa and peripheral lung tissues. Eur J Cancer 1998; 34: 914–920.
22. Adams DR, Jones AM, Plopper CG, Serabjit-Singh CJ, Philpot RM. Distribution of cytochrome P-450 monooxygenase enzymes in the nasal mucosa of hamster and rat. Am J Anat 1991.
23. Reed CJ, Robinson DA, Lock EA. Antioxidant status of the rat nasal cavity. Free Radic Biol Med 2003; 34:607–615.

24. Rengasamy A, Barger MW, Kane E, Ma JK, Castranova V, Ma JY. Diesel exhaust particle-induced alterations of pulmonary phase I and phase II enzymes of rats. J Toxicol Environ Health 2003; 66:153–167.

25. Shelby MK, Cherrington NJ, Vansell NR, Klaassen CD. Tissue mRNA expression of the rat UDP-glucuronosyltransferase gene family. Am Soc Pharmacol Exp Ther 2003; 31:326–333.

26. Rahman Q, Abidi P, Afaq F, Schiffmann D, Mossman BT, Kamp DW, Athar M. Glutathione redox system in oxidative lung injury. Crit Rev Toxicol 1999; 29: 543–568.

27. Fanucchi MV, Buckpitt AR, Murphy ME, Storms DH, Hammock BD, Plopper CG. Development of phase II xenobiotic metabolizing enzymes in differentiating murine Clara cells. Toxicol Appl Pharmacol 2000; 168: 253–267.

28. Bond JA. Metabolism and elimination of inhaled drugs and airborne chemicals from the lungs. Pharmacol Toxicol 1993.

29. Campbell L, Abedel-Nasser G, Abulrob, Lana E, Kandalaft, Plummer S, Hollins AJ, Gibbs A, Gumbleton M. Constitutive expression of P-glycoprotein in normal lung alveolar epithelium and functionality in primary alveolar epithelial cultures. J Pharmacol Exp Ther 2003; 304:441–452.

30. Otto WR. Lung epithelial stem cells. J Pathol 2002; 197:527–535.

31. Marei HE, Abd el-Gawad M. Differentiation of ciliated cells in the terminal bronchioles of neonatal calves. Eur J Morphol 2001; 39:269–276.

32. Falk R, Philipson K, Svartengren M, Bergmann R, Hofmann W, Jarvis N, Bailey M, Camner P. Assessment of long-term bronchiolar clearance of particles from measurements of lung retention and theoretical estimates of regional deposition. Exp Lung Res 1999; 25:495–516.

33. Warheit DB, Hansen JF, Yuen IS, Kelly DP, Snajdr SI, Hartsky MA. Inhalation of high concentrations of low toxicity dusts in rats results in impaired pulmonary clearance mechanisms and persistent inflammation. Toxicol Appl Pharmacol 1997; 145:10–22.

34. Brown JS, Zeman KL, Bennett WD. Ultrafine particle deposition and clearance in the healthy and obstructed lung. Am J Respir Crit Care Med 2002; 166:1240–1247.

35. Svartengren K, Ericsson CH, Svartengren M, Mossberg B, Philipson K, Camner P. Deposition and clearance in large and small airways in chronic bronchitis. Exp Lung Res 1996; 22:555–576.

36. Hofmann W, Asgharian B. The effect of lung structure on mucociliary clearance and particle retention in human and rat lungs. Toxicol Schi 2003; 73:448–456.

37. Lay JC, Berry CR, Kim CS, Bennett WD. Retention of insoluble particles after local intrabronchial deposition in dogs. J Appl Physiol 1995:1921–1929.

38. Wagner EM, Foster WM. The role of the bronchial vasculature in soluble particle clearance. Environ Health Perspect 2001; 109:563–565.

39. Kreyling WG, Blanchard JD, Godleski JJ, Haeussermann J, Heyder J, Hutzler P, Schulz H, Sweeney TD, Takenaka S, Ziesenis A. Anatomic localization of 24- and 96-h particle retention in canine airways. Am Physiol Soc 1999: 269–284.

40. Clary-Meinesz C, Mouroux J, Huitorel P, Cosson J, Schoevaert D, Blaive B. Ciliary beat frequency in human bronchi and bronchioles. Chest 1997; 111:692–697.

41. Blouquit S, Morel H, Hinnrasky J, Naline E, Puchelle E, Chinet T. Characterization of ion and fluid transport in human bronchioles. Am J Respir Cell Mol Biol 2002; 27:503–510.

42. Foster WM. Mucociliary transport and cough in humans. Pulm Pharmacol Ther 2002; 15:277–282.

43. West MR, Ferguson DJ, Hart VJ, Sanjar S, Man Y. Maintenance of the epithelial barrier in a bronchial epithelial cell line is dependent on functional E-cadherin local to the tight junctions. Cell Commun Adhes 2002; 9:29–44.

44. Michelson PH, Tigue M, Jones JC. Human bronchial epithelial cells secrete laminin 5, express hemidesmosomal proteins, and assemble hemidesmosomes. J Histochem Cytochem 2000; 48:535–544.

45. Burleson GR. Models of respiratory immunotoxicology and host resistance. Immunopharmacology 2000; 48:315–318.

46. Hogg JC, Pare PD, Boucher RC. Bronchial mucosal permeability. Fed Proc 1979; 38:197–201.

47. Richardson JB, Ferguson CC. Neuromuscular structure and function in the airways. Fed Proc 1974; 38:202–208.

48. Lamb JP, Sparrow MP. Three-dimensional mapping of sensory innervation with substance P in porcine bronchial mucosa: comparison with human airways. Am J Respir Crit Care Med 2002; 166:1269–1281.

49. Brouns I, Van Genechten J, Hayashi H, Gajda M, Gomi T, Burnstock G, Timmermans JP, Adriaensen D. Dual sensory innervation of pulmonary neuroepithelial bodies. Am J Respir Cell Mol Biol 2003; 28:275–285.

50. Myers AC, Kajekar R, Undem BJ. Allergic inflammation-induced neuropeptide production in rapidly adapting afferent nerves in guinea pig airways. Am J Physiol Lung Cell Mol Physiol 2002; 282:L775–L781.

51. Tobin MJ. Chronic obstructive pulmonary disease, pollution, pulmonary vascular disease, transplantation, pleural disease, and lung cancer in AJRCCM 2000. Am J Respir Crit Care Med 2001; 164:1789–1804.

52. Desqueyroux H, Pujet JC, Prosper M, Le Moullec Y, Momas I. Effects of air pollution on adults with chronic obstructive pulmonary disease. Arch Environ Health 2002; 57:554–560.

53. March TH, Barr EB, Finch GL, Hahn FF, Hobbs CH, Menache MG, Nikula KJ. Cigarette smoke exposure produces more evidence of emphysema in B6C3F1 mice than in F344 rats. Toxicol Sci 1999; 51:289–299.

54. Hnizdo E, Vallyathan V. Chronic obstructive pulmonary disease due to occupational exposure to silica dust: a review of epidemiological and pathological evidence. Occup Environ Med 2003; 60:237–243.

55. Mio T, Romberger DJ, Thompson AB, Robbins RA, Heires A, Rennard SI. Cigarette smoke induces interleukin-8 release from human bronchial epithelial cells. Am J Respir Crit Care Med 1997; 155:1770–1776.

56. March TH, Barr EB, Finch GL, Nikula KJ, Seagrave JC. Effects of concurrent ozone exposure on the pathogenesis of cigarette smoke-induced emphysema in B6C3F1 mice. Inhal Toxicol 2002; 14:1187–1213.

57. Li XY, Gilmour PS, Donaldson K, MacNee W. Free radical activity and pro-inflammatory effects of particulate air pollution (PM10) in vivo and in vitro. Thorax 1996; 51:1216–1222.

58. MacNee W. Acute exacerbations of COPD. Swiss Med Wkly 2003; 133: 247–257.

59. MacNee W, Donaldson K. Mechanism of lung injury caused by PM10 and ultrafine particles with special reference to COPD. Eur Respir J Suppl 2003; 40:47s–51s.

60. Gilmour PS, Rahman I, Hayashi S, Hogg JC, Donaldson K, MacNee W. Adenoviral E1A primes alveolar epithelial cells to PM(10)-induced transcription of interleukin-8. Am J Physiol Lung Cell Mol Physiol 2001; 281: L598–L606.

61. Mauderly JL, Bice DE, Cheng YS, Gillett NA, Griffith WC, Henderson RF, Pickrell JA, Wolff RK. Influence of preexisting pulmonary emphysema on susceptibility of rats to inhaled diesel exhaust. Am Rev Respir Dis 1990; 141:1333–1341.

62. Barth PJ, Muller B, Wagner U, Bittinger A. Quantitative analysis of parenchymal and vascular alterations in NO_2-induced lung injury in rats. Eur Respir J 1995; 8:1115–1121.

63. Blank J, Glasgow JE, Pietra GG, Burdette L, Weinbaum G. Nitrogen-dioxide-induced emphysema in rats. Lack of worsening by beta-aminopropionitrile treatment. Am Rev Respir Dis 1988; 137:376–379.

64. Glasgow JE, Pietra GG, Abrams WR, Blank J, Oppenheim DM, Weinbaum G. Neutrophil recruitment and degranulation during induction of emphysema in the rat by nitrogen dioxide. Am Rev Respir Dis 1987; 135:1129–1136.

65. Stavert DM, Archuleta DC, Holland LM, Lehnert BE. Nitrogen dioxide exposure and development of pulmonary emphysema. J Toxicol Environ Health 1986; 17:249–267.

66. Lafuma C, Harf A, Lange F, Bozzi L, Poncy JL, Bignon J. Effect of low-level NO_2 chronic exposure on elastase-induced emphysema. Environ Res 1987; (43):75–84.

67. Mauderly JL, Bice DE, Cheng YS, Gillett NA, Henderson RF, Pickrell JA, Wolff RK. Influence of experimental pulmonary emphysema on the toxicological effects from inhaled nitrogen dioxide and diesel exhaust. Res Rep Health Eff Inst 1989; (30):1–47.

68. Kato A, Nagai A, Kagawa J. Morphological changes in rat lung after long-term exposure to diesel emissions. Inhal Toxicol 2000; 12:469–490.

69. Kleinerman J. Some effects of nitrogen dioxide on the lung. Fed Proc 1977; 36:1714–1718.

70. Juhos LT, Green DP, Furiosi NJ, Freeman G. A quantitative study of stenosis in the respiratory bronchiole of the rat in NO_2-induced emphysema. Am Rev Respir Dis 1980; 121:541–549.

71. Yao W, Wang G, Zhu H, Sun Y, Zhao M. Effect of ipratropium bromide on airway and pulmonary muscarinic receptors in a rat model of chronic obstructive pulmonary disease. Chin Med J (Engl) 2001; 114:80–83.

72. Smith LG, Busch RH, Buschbom RL, Cannon WC, Loscutoff SM, Morris JE. Effects of sulfur dioxide or ammonium sulfate exposure, alone or

combined, for 4 or 8 months on normal and elastase-impaired rats. Environ Res 1989; 49:60–78.

73. Xu J, Zhao M, Liao S. Establishment and pathological study of models of chronic obstructive pulmonary disease by SO$_2$ inhalation method. Chin Med J (Engl) 2000; 113:213–216.

74. Harkema JR, Wagner JG. Non-allergic models of mucous cell metaplasia and mucus hypersecretion in rat nasal and pulmonary airways. Novartis Found Symp 2002; 248:181–197.

75. Kodavanti UP, Mebane R, Ledbetter A, Krantz T, McGee J, Jackson MC, et al. Variable pulmonary responses from exposure to concentrated ambient air particles in a rat model of bronchitis. Toxicol Sci 2000; 54:441–451.

76. Saetta M, Turato G, Baraldo S, Zanin A, Braccioni F, Mapp CE, Maestrelli P, Cavallesco G, Papi A, Fabbri LM. Goblet cell hyperplasia and epithelial inflammation in peripheral airways of smokers with both symptoms of chronic bronchitis and chronic airflow limitation. Am J Respir Crit Care Med 2000; 161:1016–1021.

77. Cotran RS, Kumar V, Collins T, Robbins SL. Robbins Pathologic Basis of Disease. 6th ed. Philadelphia: Saunders, 1999.

78. Karakatsani A, Andreadaki S, Katsouyanni K, Dimitroulis I, Trichopoulos D, Benetou V, et al. Air pollution in relation to manifestations of chronic pulmonary disease: a nested case–control study in Athens, Greece. Eur J Epidemiol 2003; 18(1):45–53.

79. Nikula KJ, Green FH. Animal models of chronic bronchitis and their relevance to studies of particle-induced disease. Inhal Toxicol 2000; 12(suppl 4):123–153.

80. Harkema JR, Hotchkiss JA. Ozone- and endotoxin-induced mucous cell metaplasias in rat airway epithelium: novel animal models to study toxicant-induced epithelial transformation in airways. Toxicol Lett 1993; 68(1–2): 251–263.

81. Donaldson K, Brown GM, Brown DM, Slight J, Cullen RT, Love RG, et al. Inflammation in the lungs of rats after deposition of dust collected from the air of wool mills: the role of epithelial injury and complement activation. Br J Ind Med 1990; 47:231–238.

82. Wang H, Li J, Zhao Y. Autopsies of coal workers with chronic bronchitis [in Chinese]. Zhonghua Yu Fang Yi Xue Za Zhi 1998; 32:231–234.

83. Koike E, Hirano S, Shimojo N, Kobayashi T. cDNA microarray analysis of gene expression in rat alveolar macrophages in response to organic extract of diesel exhaust particles. Toxicol Sci 2002; 67:241–246.

84. Clarke RW, Catalano PJ, Koutrakis P, Murthy GG, Sioutas C, Paulauskis J, et al. Urban air particulate inhalation alters pulmonary function and induces pulmonary inflammation in a rodent model of chronic bronchitis. Inhal Toxicol 1999; 11:637–656.

85. Gordon T, Harkema JR. Cotton dust produces an increase in intraepithelial mucosubstances in rat airways. Am J Respir Crit Care Med 1995; 151: 1981–1988.

86. Hayashi M, Sornberger GC, Huber GL. Differential response in the male and female tracheal epithelium following exposure to tobacco smoke. Chest 1978; 73:515–518.

87. Scanlon PD, Seltzer J, Ingram RH Jr, Reid L, Drazen JM. Chronic exposure to sulfur dioxide. Physiologic and histologic evaluation of dogs exposed to 50 or 15 ppm. Am Rev Respir Dis 1987; 135:831–839.

88. Seltzer J, Scanlon PD, Drazen JM, Ingram RH Jr, Reid L. Morphologic correlation of physiologic changes caused by SO_2-induced bronchitis in dogs. The role of inflammation. Am Rev Respir Dis 1984; 129:790–797.

89. Morgenroth K. Morphological alterations to the bronchial mucosa in high-dosage long-term exposure to sulfur dioxide. Respiration 1980; 39:39–48.

90. Oda Y, Isohama Y, Kai H, Okano Y, Takahama K, Miyata T. Increased production and/or secretion of pulmonary surfactant in rats by long term sulfur dioxide exposure. J Pharmacobiodyn 1989; 12:726–730.

91. Schneider T, van Velzen D, Moqbel R, Issekutz AC. Kinetics and quantitation of eosinophil and neutrophil recruitment to allergic lung inflammation in a Brown Norway rat model. Am J Respir Cell Mol Biol 1997; 17:702–712.

92. Salmon M, Walsh DA, Koto H, Barnes PJ, Chung KF. Repeated allergen exposure of sensitized Brown-Norway rats induces airway cell DNA synthesis and remodelling. Eur Respir J 1999; 14:633–641.

93. Hamada K, Goldsmith CA, Goldman A, Kobzik L. Resistance of very young mice to inhaled allergen sensitization is overcome by coexposure to an air-pollutant aerosol. Am J Respir Crit Care Med 2000; 161:1285–1293.

94. Lambert A, Dong W, Winsett DW, Selgrade MK, Gilmour MI. Residual oil fly ash exposure enhances allergic sensitization to house dust mite. Toxicol Appl Pharmacol 1999; 158:269–277.

95. Jalaludin BB, O'Toole BI, Leeder SR. Acute effects of urban ambient air pollution on respiratory symptoms, asthma medication use, and doctor visits for asthma in a cohort of Australian children. Environ Res 2004; 95:32–42.

96. Vagaggini B, Taccola M, Cianchetti S, Carnevali S, Bartoli ML, Bacci E, Dente FL, Di Franco A, Giannini D, Paggiaro PL. Ozone exposure increases eosinophilic airway response induced by previous allergen challenge. Am J Respir Crit Care Med 2002; 166:1073–1077.

97. Scannell C, Chen L, Aris RM, Tager I, Christian D, Ferrando R, Welch B, Kelly T, Balmes JR. Greater ozone-induced inflammatory responses in subjects with asthma. Am J Respir Crit Care Med 1996; 154:24–29.

98. Balmes JR, Aris RM, Chen LL, Scannell C, Tager IB, Finkbeiner W, Christian D, Kelly T, Hearne PQ, Ferrando R, Welch B. Effects of ozone on normal and potentially sensitive human subjects. Part I: airway inflammation and responsiveness to ozone in normal and asthmatic subjects. Res Rep Health Eff Inst 1997; (78):1–37.

99. Holz O, Jorres RA, Timm P, Mucke M, Richter K, Koschyk S, Magnussen H. Ozone-induced airway inflammatory changes differ between individuals and are reproducible. Am J Respir Crit Care Med 1999; 159:776–784.

100. Vagaggini B, Carnevali S, Macchioni P, Taccola M, Fornai E, Bacci E, ML, Cianchetti S, Dente FL, Di Franco A, Giannini D, Paggiaro PL. Airway inflammatory response to ozone in subjects with different asthma severity. Eur Respir J 1999; 13:274–280.

101. Hiltermann TJ, de Bruijne CR, Stolk J, Zwinderman AH, Spieksma FT, Roemer W, Steerenberg PA, Fischer PH, van Bree L, Hiemstra PS. Effects

of photochemical air pollution and allergen exposure on upper respiratory tract inflammation in asthmatics. Am J Respir Crit Care Med 1997; 156: 1765–1772.

102. Depuydt PO, Lambrecht BN, Joos GF, Pauwels RA. Effect of ozone exposure on allergic sensitization and airway inflammation induced by dendritic cells. Clin Exp Allergy 2002; 32:391–396.

103. Stenfors N, Pourazar J, Blomberg A, Krishna MT, Mudway I, Helleday R, Kelly FJ, Frew AJ, Sandstrom T. Effect of ozone on bronchial mucosal inflammation in asthmatic and healthy subjects. Respir Med 2002; 96:352–358.

104. Bayram H, Sapsford RJ, Abdelaziz MM, Khair OA. Effect of ozone and nitrogen dioxide on the release of proinflammatory mediators from bronchial epithelial cells of nonatopic nonasthmatic subjects and atopic asthmatic patients in vitro. J Allergy Clin Immunol 2001; 107:287–294.

105. Peden DB, Boehlecke B, Horstman D, Devlin R. Prolonged acute exposure to 0.16 ppm ozone induces eosinophilic airway inflammation in asthmatic subjects with allergies. J Allergy Clin Immunol 1997; 100:802–808.

106. Bosson J, Stenfors N, Bucht A, Helleday R, Pourazar J, Holgate ST, Kelly FJ, Sandstrom T, Wilson S, Frew AJ, Blomberg A. Ozone-induced bronchial epithelial cytokine expression differs between healthy and asthmatic subjects. Clin Exp Allergy 2003; 33:777–782.

107. Hiltermann TJ, Stolk J, Hiemstra PS, Fokkens PH, Rombout PJ, Sont JK, Sterk PJ, Dijkman JH. Effect of ozone exposure on maximal airway narrowing in non-asthmatic and asthmatic subjects. Clin Sci (Lond) 1995; 89:619–624.

108. Mudway IS, Kelly FJ. Ozone and the lung: a sensitive issue. Mol Aspects Med 2000; 21:1–48.

109. Coulson FR, Fryer AD. Muscarinic acetylcholine receptors and airway diseases. Pharmacol Ther 2003; 98:59–69.

110. Ito T, Ikemi Y, Ohmori K, Kitamura H, Kanisawa M. Airway epithelial cell changes in rats exposed to 0.25 ppm ozone for 20 months. Exp Toxicol Pathol 1994; 46:1–6.

111. Oberdorster G. Pulmonary effects of inhaled ultrafine particles. Int Arch Occup Environ Health 2001; 74:1–8.

112. Sydbom A, Blomberg A, Parnia S, Stenfors N, Sandstrom T, Dahlen SE. Health effects of diesel exhaust emissions. Eur Respir J 2001; 17:733–746.

113. Okeson CD, Riley MR, Fernandez A, Wendt JO. Impact of the composition of combustion generated fine particles on epithelial cell toxicity: influences of metals on metabolism. Chemosphere 2003; 51:1121–1128.

114. Peden DB. Air pollution in asthma: effect of pollutants on airway inflammation. Ann Allergy Asthma Immunol 2001; 87:12–17.

115. Hashimoto S, Gon Y, Takeshita I, Matsumoto K, Jibiki I, Takizawa H, Kudoh S, Horie T. Diesel exhaust particles activate p38 MAP kinase to produce interleukin 8 and RANTES by human bronchial epithelial cells and *N*-acetylcysteine attenuates p38 MAP kinase activation. Am J Respir Crit Care Med 2000; 161:280–285.

116. Pandya RJ, Solomon G, Kinner A, Balmes JR. Diesel exhaust and asthma: hypotheses and molecular mechanisms of action. Environ Health Perspect 2002; 110(suppl 1):103–112.

117. Goldsmith CA, Ning Y, Qin G, Imrich A, Lawrence J, Murthy GG, Catalano PJ, Kobzik L. Combined air pollution particle and ozone exposure increases airway responsiveness in mice. Inhal Toxicol 2002; 14:325–347.

118. Churg A, Brauer M, Carmen Avila-Casado M, Fortoul TI, Wright JL. Chronic exposure to high levels of particulate air pollution and small airway remodeling. Environ Health Perspect 2003; 111:714–718.

119. Verones B, Oortgiesen M. Neurogenic inflammation and particulate matter (PM) air pollutants. Neurotoxicology 2001; 22:795–810.

120. Persinger RL, Poynter ME, Ckless K, Janssen-Heininger YM. Molecular mechanisms of nitrogen dioxide induced epithelial injury in the lung. Mol Cell Biochem 2002; 234–235:71–80.

121. Rombout PJ, Dormans JA, Marra M, van Esch GJ. Influence of exposure regimen on nitrogen dioxide-induced morphological changes in the rat lung. Environ Res 1986; 41:466–480.

122. Barck C, Sandstrom T, Lundahl J, Hallden G, Svartengren M, Strand V, Rak S, Bylin G. Ambient level of NO_2 augments the inflammatory response to inhaled allergen in asthmatics. Respir Med 2002; 96:907–917.

123. Siegel PD, Al Humadi NH, Nelson ER, Lewis DM, Hubbs AF. Adjuvant effect of respiratory irritation on pulmonary allergic sensitization: time and site dependency. Toxicol Appl Pharmacol 1997; 144:356–362.

124. Peden DB. Mechanisms of pollution-induced airway disease: in vivo studies. Allergy 1997; 52:37–44.

125. Sheppard D, Saisho A, Nadel JA, Boushey HA. Exercise increases sulfur dioxide-induced bronchoconstriction in asthmatic subjects. Am Rev Respir Dis 1981; 123:486–491.

126. American Thoracic Society/European Respiratory Society International Multidisciplinary Consensus Classification of the Idiopathic Interstitial Pneumonias. Am J Respir Crit Care Med 2002; 165:277–304. (This joint statement of the American Thoracic Society (ATS) and the European Respiratory Society (ERS) was adopted by the ATS board of directors, June 2001 and by the ERS Executive Committee, June 2001.)

127. Schenker M. Exposures and health effects from inorganic agricultural dusts. Environ Health Perspect 2000; 108:661–664.

128. Hubbard R, Venn A, Lewis S, Britton J. Lung cancer and cryptogenic fibrosing alveolitis. Am J Respir Crit Care Med 1999; 161:5–8.

129. Desai SR, Ryan SM, Colby TV. Smoking-related interstitial lung diseases: histopathological and imaging perspectives. Clin Radiol 2003; 58:259–268.

130. Pickrell JA, Hahn FF, Rebar AH, Horoda RA, Henderson RF. Changes in collagen metabolism and proteinolysis after repeated inhalation exposure to ozone. Exp Mol Pathol 1987; 46:159–167.

131. Last JA, Gelzleichter TR, Harkema J, Hawk S. Consequences of prolonged inhalation of ozone on Fischer-344/N rats: collaborative studies. Part I: content and cross-linking of lung collagen. Res Rep Health Eff Inst 1994:1–29.

132. Stockstill BL, Chang LY, Ménache MG, Mellick PW, Mercer RR, Crapo JD. Bronchiolarized metaplasia and interstitial fibrosis in rat lungs chronically exposed to high ambient levels of ozone. Toxicol Appl Pharmacol 1995; 134:251–263.

133. Christian D, Chen L, Scannell C, Ferrando R, Welch B, Balmes J. Ozone-induced inflammation is attenuated with multiday exposure. Am J Respir Crit Care Med 158:532–537.

134. Frank R, Liu M, Spannhake E, Mlynarek S, Macri K, Weinmann G. Repetitive ozone exposure of young adult. Evidence of persistent small airway dysfunction. Am J Respir Crit Care Med 164:1253–1260.

135. Jorres R, Holz O, Zachgo W, Timm P, Koschyk S, Muller B, Grimminger F, Seeger W, Kelly FJ, Dunster C, Frischer T, Lubec G, Waschewski M, Niendorf A, Magnussen H. The effect of repeated ozone exposures on inflammatory markers in bronchoalveolar lavage fluid mucosal biopsies. Am J Respir Crit Care Med 161:1855–1861.

136. Pinkerton KE, Dodge DE, Cederdahl-Demmler J, Wong VJ, Peake J, Haselton CJ, Mellick PW, Singh G, Plopper CG. Differentiated bronchiolar epithelium in alveolar ducts of rats exposed to ozone for 20 months. Am J Pathol 1993; 142:947–956.

137. Last JA, Gelzleichter TR, Pinkerton KE, Walker RM, Witschi H. A new model of progressive pulmonary fibrosis in rats. Am Rev Respir Dis 1993; 487–494.

138. Vetrano KM, Morris JB, Hubbard AK. Silica-induced pulmonary inflammation and fibrosis in mice is altered by acute exposure to nitrogen dioxide. J Toxicol Environ Health 1992; 37:425–442.

139. Churg A, Wright JL. Airway wall remodeling induced by occupational mineral dusts and air pollutant particles. Chest 2002.

140. Driscoll KE, Maurer JK, Lindenschmidt RC, Romberger D, Rennard SI, Crosby L. Respiratory tract responses to dust: relationships between dust burden, lung injury, alveolar macrophage fibronectin release, and the development of pulmonary fibrosis. Toxicol Appl Pharmacol 1990.

141. Fischbein A, Rohl AN, Suzuki Y, Bigman O. Interstitial pulmonary fibrosis in an automobile body shop worker. Toxicol Lett 1985.

142. Jederlinic PJ, Abraham JL, Churg A, Himmelstein JS, Epler GR, Gaensler EA. Pulmonary fibrosis in aluminum oxide workers. Investigation of nine workers, with pathologic examination and microanalysis in three of them. Am Rev Respir Dis 1990:1179–1184.

143. Dai J, Gilks B, Price K, Churg A. Mineral dusts directly induce epithelial and interstitial fibrogenic mediators and matrix components in the airway wall. Am J Respir Crit Care Med 1998; 158:1907–1913.

144. Schapira RM, Osornio-Vargas AR, Brody AR. Inorganic particles induce secretion of a macrophage homologue of platelet-derived growth factor in a density- and time-dependent manner in vitro. Exp Lung Res 1991; 17: 1011–1024.

145. Hyde DM, Plopper CG, Weir AJ, Murnane RD, Warren DL, Last JA, Pepelko WE. Peribronchiolar fibrosis in lungs of cats chronically exposed to diesel exhaust. Lab Invest 1985.

146. Kung VA. Morphological investigations of fibrogenic action of estonian oil shale dust. Environ Health Perspect 1979:153–155.

147. Schins RPF, Borm PJA. Mechanisms and mediators in coal dust induced toxicity: a review. Brit Occup Hyg Soc 1999; 43:7–33.

148. Yu IJ, Song KS, Chang HK, Han JH, Chung YH, Han KT, Chung KH, Chung HK. Recovery from manual metal arc-stainless steel welding-fume exposure induced lung fibrosis in Sprague–Dawley rats. Toxicol Lett 2003; 143:247–259.

149. Smyth A, O'Hea U, Williams G, Smyth R, Heaf D. Passive smoking and impaired lung function in cystic fibrosis. Arch Dis Child 1994; 71:353–354.

150. Rubin BK. Exposure of children with cystic fibrosis to environmental tobacco smoke. N Engl J Med 1990; 323:782–788.

151. Kovesi T, Corey M, Levison H. Passive smoking and lung function in cystic fibrosis. Am Rev Respir Dis 1993; 148:1266–1271.

152. Smyth A, O'Hea U, Feyerabend C, Lewis S, Smyth R. Trends in passive smoking in cystic fibrosis, 1993–1998. Pediatr Pulmonol 2001; 31:133–137.

153. Diamond G, Legarda D, Ryan LK. The innate immune response of the respiratory epithelium. Immunol Rev 2000; 173:27–38.

154. Houtmeyers E, Gosselink R, Gayan-Ramirez G, Decramer M. Regulation of mucociliary clearance in health and disease. Eur Respir J 1999; 13: 1177–1188.

155. Jakab GJ, Bassett DJ. Influenza virus infection, ozone exposure, and fibrogenesis. Am Rev Respir Dis 1990; 141:1307–1315.

156. Fusco D, Forastiere F, Michelozzi P, Spadea T, Ostro B, Arca M, Perucci CA. Air pollution and hospital admissions for respiratory conditions in Rome, Italy. Eur Respir J 2001; 17:1143–1150.

157. Harrod KS, Jaramillo RJ, Rosenberger CL, Wang SZ, Berger JA, McDonald JD, Reed MD. Increased susceptibility to RSV infection by exposure to inhaled diesel engine emissions. Am J Respir Cell Mol Biol 2003; 28:451–463.

158. Trimpe KL, Weiss H, Zwilling BS. The effect of SO_2 on the clearance of *Listeria* monocytogenes from the lungs of emphysematous hamsters. Environ Res 1986; 41:351–356.

159. Michel O, Duchateau J, Sergysels R. Effect of inhaled endotoxin on bronchial reactivity in asthmatic and normal subjects. J Appl Physiol 1989; 66: 1059–1064.

160. Witschi H. Tobacco smoke as a mouse lung carcinogen. Exp Lung Res 1998; 24:385–394.

161. Henry CJ, Kouri RE. Chronic inhalation studies in mice. II. Effects of long-term exposure to 2R1 cigarette smoke on (C57BL/Cum x C3H/AnfCum)F1 mice. J Natl Cancer Inst 1986; 77:203–212.

162. Finch GL, Nikula KJ, Belinsky SA, Barr EB, Stoner GD, Lechner JF. Failure of cigarette smoke to induce or promote lung cancer in the A/J mouse. Cancer Lett 1996; 99:161–167.

163. Last JA, Warren DL, Pecquet-Goad E, Witschi H. Modification by ozone of lung tumor development in mice. J Natl Cancer Inst 1987; 78:149–154.

164. Witschi H, Breider MA, Schuller HM. Failure of ozone and nitrogen dioxide to enhance lung tumor development in hamsters. Res Rep Health Eff Inst 1993; 60:1–25.

165. Sweet F, Kao MS, Lee SC, Hagar WL, Sweet WE. Ozone selectively inhibits growth of human cancer cells. Science 1980; 209:931–933.

166. Sills RC, Hong HL, Greenwell A, Herbert RA, Boorman GA, Devereux TR. Increased frequency of K-ras mutations in lung neoplasms from female B6C3F1 mice exposed to ozone for 24 or 30 months. Carcinogenesis 1995; 16:1623–1628.

167. Witschi H, Espiritu I, Pinkerton KE, Murphy K, Maronpot RR. Ozone carcinogenesis revisited. Toxicol Sci 1999; 52:162–167.

168. Kobayashi T, Todoroki T, Sato H. Enhancement of pulmonary metastasis of murine fibrosarcoma NR-FS by ozone exposure. J Toxicol Environ Health 1987; 20:135–145.

169. Richters A. Effects of nitrogen dioxide and ozone on blood-borne cancer cell colonization of the lungs. J Toxicol Environ Health 1988; 25:383–390.

170. Ichinose T, Sagai M. Combined exposure to NO_2, O_3 and H_2SO_4-aerosol and lung tumor formation in rats. Toxicology 1992; 74:173–184.

171. Pinkerton KE, Brody AR, Miller FJ, Crapo JD. Exposure to low levels of ozone results in enhanced pulmonary retention of inhaled asbestos fibers. Am Rev Respir Dis 1989; 140:1075–1081.

172. Heinrich U, Muhle H, Takenaka S, Ernst H, Fuhst R, Mohr U, Pott F, Stober W. Chronic effects on the respiratory tract of hamsters, mice and rats after long-term inhalation of high concentrations of filtered and unfiltered diesel engine emissions. J Appl Toxicol 1986; 6:383–395.

173. Iwai K, Higuchi K, Udagawa T, Ohtomo K, Kawabata Y. Lung tumor induced by long-term inhalation or intratracheal instillation of diesel exhaust particles. Exp Toxicol Pathol 1997; 49:393–401.

174. Hext PM. Current perspectives on particulate induced pulmonary tumours. Hum Exp Toxicol 1994; 13:700–715.

175. Ohyama K, Ito T, Kanisawa M. The roles of diesel exhaust particle extracts and the promotive effects of NO_2 and/or SO_2 exposure on rat lung tumorigenesis. Cancer Lett 1999; 139:189–197.

176. Heinrich U, Mohr U, Fuhst R, Brockmeyer C. Investigation of a potential cotumorigenic effect of the dioxides of nitrogen and sulfur, and of diesel-engine exhaust, on the respiratory tract of Syrian golden hamsters. Res Rep Health Eff Inst 1989; (26):1–27.

177. Richters A, Damji KS. The relationship between inhalation of nitrogen dioxide, the immune system, and progression of a spontaneously occurring lymphoma in AKR mice. J Environ Pathol Toxicol Oncol 1990; 10:225–230.

178. Richters A, Richters V. Nitrogen dioxide (NO_2) inhalation, formation of microthrombi in lungs and cancer metastasis. J Environ Pathol Toxicol Oncol 1989; 9:45–51.

179. Adkins B Jr, Van Stee EW, Simmons JE, Eustis SL. Oncogenic response of strain A/J mice to inhaled chemicals. J Toxicol Environ Health 1986; 17:311–322.

6

Irritant Agonists and Air Pollutants: Neurologically Mediated Respiratory and Cardiovascular Responses

STEPHEN H. GAVETT

National Health and Environmental Effects
Research Laboratory, U.S. Environmental
    Protection Agency, Research Triangle
Park, North Carolina, U.S.A.

**MARIAN KOLLARIK and BRADLEY
J. UNDEM**

Johns Hopkins University Asthma and
    Allergy Center, Baltimore,
Maryland, U.S.A.

I. Introduction

Situated within and just beneath the airway epithelium is a dense plexus of sensory nerves. These sensory (afferent) nerves serve as sentinels at the gateway between the organism and the inhaled air. This airway mucosal nerve plexus is present from the nose to the most peripheral airways. Irritants in the polluted air interact with these sensory nerves initiating a cascade of events that may lead to conscious sensations of irritation, subconscious changes in autonomic neural control, and/or defensive

---

This manuscript has been reviewed and approved for release by the National Health and Environmental Effects Research Laboratory, U.S. Environmental Protection Agency. Approval does not signify that the contents necessarily reflect the views and policies of the U.S. EPA, nor does mention of trade names or commercial products constitute endorsement or recommendation for use.

195

reflexes including cough and sneezing. Excessive afferent nerve irritation contributes to pathogenesis of cardio-respiratory diseases in susceptible individuals, or exacerbates preexisting diseases such as asthma and chronic obstructive lung disease. In this chapter, we will overview the basic neurobiology of the airways, with a special emphasis on the mucosal sensory innervation and the reflexes their activation engender. In addition, the literature that pertains specifically to airborne irritant mediated neuronal reflexes will be reviewed.

II. Sensory Innervation of the Airways
A. General Characterization of Sensory Nerves

Sensory nerves are characterized based on their activation profile, neurotransmitter chemistry, conduction velocity, and location of their cell bodies. The activation profile of airway sensory nerves typically falls into two general categories: mechanically sensitive (mechanosensors), and those that are activated by various chemicals. In the lower airways, many mechanosensors are sufficiently sensitive to lung distention that they are activated cyclically during eupneic breathing (1), for review see Ref. 2. This means that the central nervous system (CNS) is constantly receiving information (encoded in the form of action potentials) from the lungs. These lung distention (stretch)-sensitive nerves can be subcategorized based on their adaptation characteristics (3). Slowly adapting stretch receptors (SARs) discharge a sustained action potential train throughout a prolonged lung distention during inspiration. In contrast, rapidly adapting stretch receptors (RARs) discharge a short burst of action potentials during the dynamic phase of lung inflation and then abruptly adapt (4,5).

The sensory nerves in the plexus lining the epithelium of the airways do not respond to eupneic lung inflation (are not stretch receptors), but can be activated by various chemical substances associated with inflammation (e.g., bradykinin, ATP, serotonin) (6,7). These fibers form a diffuse lattice-like structure in the mucosa and are ideally situated to sense the inhaled air (8) (Fig. 1). It is likely that air pollutants that lead to irritation and/or reflex responses do so by first activating these chemosensitive nerves.

The velocity at which action potentials are conducted along the nerve fiber is another criterion used to characterize the nerve. The conduction velocity correlates with the diameter of the nerve fiber and the extent of its myelination. Medium-to-large diameter myelinated fibers that conduct action potentials at relatively high velocities ($5–50 \, m \, sec^{-1}$) are referred to as "A" fibers. On the other hand, small diameter unmyelinated fibers that conduct action potentials slowly ($<1 \, ms^{-1}$) are referred to as "C" fibers. The lung stretch-sensitive RARs and SARs are A-fibers, whereas most of the chemically sensitive sensory nerves in the airway mucosa are C-fibers (2).

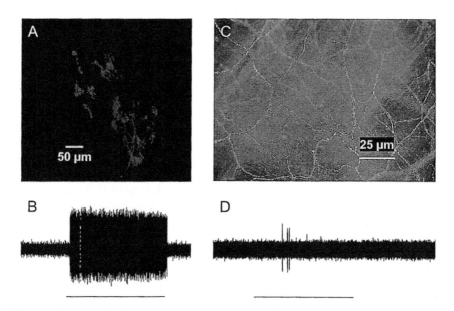

Figure 1 Two fundamental types of sensory nerves in the airways and lungs. (A) Structure of a low threshold mechanosensor located in the lung visualized by staining for the Na^+-K^+-ATPase α_3 subunit (courtesy of Jerry Yu, see also Ref. 187). Lung mechanosensors form specialized demarcated structures often closely juxtaposed to airway smooth muscle. Tracheal mechanosensors that mediate cough have similar structures. (B) Extracellular recording of lung mechanosensor activity shows a robust response to lung distention (denoted by horizontal bar). Mechanosensors have limited chemical sensitivity, but their activity can be modulated by irritants which affect airway smooth muscle or induce vascular effects. (C) Chemosensitive sensory nerves in the tracheal mucosa visualized by staining for substance P (courtesy of BJ Canning). Chemosensitive sensory nerves form dense diffuse plexuses and are in close contact with virtually all cell types in the tissue. They are relatively insensitive to mechanical stimuli (D, lung distention denoted by horizontal bar), but respond vigorously to a wide variety of chemical activators (not illustrated).

In C-fibers, neuropeptides often serve as central synaptic neurotransmitters. In addition, sensory neuropeptides could be released from the peripheral nerve ending and act locally in the innervated tissue (9). The available evidence suggests that stretch receptors (RARs and SARs) do not contain neuropeptides under normal conditions, whereas the chemosensitive nerves within epithelial plexus often contain neuropeptides such as neurokinins and calcitonin gene-related peptide (CGRP) (10). In human airways, the neuropeptides appear to be more richly expressed in the nerves within the nasal mucosa as compared to those in the lower airways.

The cell bodies of sensory nerves innervating the lower airways are situated in the vagal sensory ganglia and to a lesser extent in the dorsal root ganglia. Sensory neurons innervating nasal mucosa are situated in the trigeminal ganglia. The nerves originating in different ganglia project to different regions of CNS and appear to have distinct phenotypes (11).

B. Upper Airway Sensory Nerves

The olfactory epithelium is a major component of the nasal sensory inner-vation, but it will not be discussed in this chapter. The olfactory system comprises specialized epithelial cells that serve as odorant receptors in the inspired air (12). The epithelial cells transmit this information to the CNS via olfactory nerves. The activation of the olfactory pathways is believed not to directly trigger autonomic reflexes in man (12).

The sensory nerves to the nasal mucosa are provided by the branches of the trigeminal nerve (12). The maxillary branch gives rise to nasopalatine nerve, which supplies septum, palate, and posterior parts of the conchae. The anterior parts of the conchae are innervated by anterior ethmoidal nerve from the ophthalmic branch. The neurons supplying the nose are situ-ated in the ophthalmic and maxillary divisions of the trigeminal ganglia and are the source of nasal epithelial C-fibers (13,14). These C-fibers form a dense plexus in the nasal epithelium and many of them contain substance P and CGRP (15).

C. Lower Airways Sensory Nerves

The mucosa of the airways from the larynx to the peripheral bronchioles receives a relatively dense innervation. The majority of sensory nerves in the airway mucosa are thought to be highly branched unmyelinated C-fibers (16). The cell bodies of the airway sensory C-fibers are situated in the vagal sensory ganglia (nodose and jugular vagal ganglia) and the spinal thoracic dorsal root ganglia (17,18). The nerve fibers originating in the vagal ganglia are carried to the airways in the vagus nerve and its branches including superior and recurrent laryngeal nerves. The functional importance of spinal innervation is unknown and the current discussion will therefore focus on the vagal afferent nerve fibers.

The C-fibers in the lungs have been subcategorized based on their relative accessibility to chemical irritants administered via the pulmonary vs. bronchial circulation (6). The C-fibers with receptive fields more acces-sible from the pulmonary circulation are referred to as pulmonary C-fibers. The C-fibers that are more effectively activated by the chemical irritants in the bronchial circulation are referred to as bronchial C-fibers.

In addition to mucosal C-fibers, lungs receive low threshold mechan-osensitive A-fiber innervation. As mentioned above, these can be categor-ized, based on their adaptation rate to sustained lung inflation as either SARs or RARs (19). A subset of RARs has been termed "irritant" receptors, in as much as many respiratory irritants can lead to their activation (20).

Whether the "irritant" RARs are directly or indirectly activated by the irritants is difficult to assess in as much as many irritants can evoke bronchial smooth muscle contraction and vascular effects that in turn can lead to activation of mechanosensitive A-fibers. The precise location of the SARs and RARs has not yet been defined in detail, although at least some of the SARs are thought to be located within the bronchial smooth muscle layer (19).

The sensory network in the airways cannot be completely categorized based on the RAR, SAR, or C-fiber characterizations. For example, sensory nerve fibers in the guinea pig trachea have been identified that conduct action potentials faster than C-fibers, but much slower than RAR or SAR, fibers. Moreover the activation profile of these tracheal fibers is distinct from RAR, SAR, or C-fibers. These fibers are of interest in as much as their activation directly evokes cough reflexes in this species (21). In addition, neuroendocrine cells exist in mammalian airways that may also serve sensory functions. The pulmonary neuroendocrine system consists of specialized airway endocrine epithelial cells. The majority of these structures are intimately associated with vagal and/or spinal sensory nerve fibers (22). The pulmonary neuroendocrine cells (PNEC) can be solitary or clustered to form neuroepithelial bodies (NEB) (23). There is evidence that these cells serve as chemoreceptor sensory cells by detecting changes in oxygen content (23). Upon activation, these cells are thought to release a transmitter (e.g., 5-hydroxytryptamine or ATP) onto to the vagal or spinal afferent nerve thereby initiating central reflexes.

D. Mechanisms of Sensory Nerve Activation

There are numerous potential mechanisms by which inhaled pollutants could induce or increase airway afferent nerve activity (Fig. 2). The increase in nerve activity can be due to chemical interactions of the irritant at the nerve terminal or mediated indirectly via its action on non-neuronal cell types. Many mucosal sensory nerves are exquisitely sensitive to punctate mechanical perturbation of their receptive fields. Particles in the inhaled air could conceivably activate afferent nerve terminals via direct mechanical interaction. Inhaled pollutants may also activate the sensory nerves through mechanisms involving their physicochemical characteristics. Changes in the osmolarity of the fluid at the nerve terminal or changes in its pH can lead to action potential discharge in sensory C-fibers. In addition inhaled irritants may activate sensory nerves by direct interactions with certain ligand-gated ion channels.

The airway tissue consists of multiple cell types related through complex interactions. Thus, irritants may also activate airway sensory nerves indirectly via the action on other cell types. Irritants can activate and/or damage epithelial cells or other cell types resulting in the release of mediators such as ATP or eicosanoids that are capable of activating sensory nerves. Pollutants may initiate acute local inflammatory reactions leading

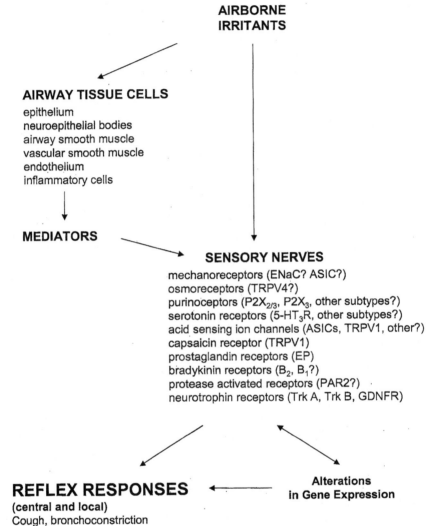

Figure 2 Mechanisms of sensory nerve activation by irritants. Inhaled irritants trigger respiratory and cardiovascular reflexes by acting directly on sensory nerve receptors, or indirectly by acting on other cell types which in turn activate sensory nerves. Direct acting irritants include acidic and aniso-osmotic solutions, some organic compounds such as alcohols and aldehydes, O_3, SO_2, certain types of particulate matter, and other air pollutants. Irritants also act on numerous cell types in the airways and lungs that can induce sensory nerve activation by mechanical effects (e.g., airway smooth muscle contraction) or by releasing chemical mediators, which interact with their specific receptors on the sensory nerves.

to recruitment of inflammatory cells. In addition to direct neuroexcitatory effects, the mediators released from the inflammatory cells exert vasoactive and smooth muscle constrictor effects which lead to sensory nerve activation mostly via mechanical means. Finally, in a more chronic setting, inhaled irritants may cause chronic inflammation that can induce long-term changes in the activity and excitability of sensory nerves.

Regardless of the direct or indirect mode of action, to activate the nerve terminal the inhaled pollutant must evoke a membrane depolarization (for review, see Ref. 24). The effective stimulus (physical or chemical) interacts with the nerve terminal in a manner that leads to opening and/or closing of specific ion channels resulting in membrane depolarization that is referred to as the generator potential. The generator potential is electrotonically conducted along the axon until it reaches the so-called active zone characterized by a high concentration of the voltage-gated sodium channels. If the membrane depolarization is of sufficient (threshold) magnitude in the active zone, a discharge of all-or-none action potentials is evoked. The frequency of action potential discharge increases with the magnitude of generator potential. Action potentials are then conducted to the first synapse in the central nervous system ultimately leading to sensations, and/or autonomic reflexes.

Some inhaled stimuli may affect the electrophysiological properties of the afferent nerve membrane without causing a generator potential and activating the nerve (24). Strictly speaking, these stimuli are not activators of the nerve, but rather are better characterized as modulators of the nerve excitability. The excitability of a nerve fiber may be increased by processes that lead to an increase in the amplitude of the generator potential, an increase in the efficiency of electronic conduction, or a decrease in action potential threshold. Some stimuli may act both as an activator (cause a generator potential) and as a modulator of neuronal excitability. In any event, an inhaled irritant may overtly activate sensory nerves leading to action potential discharge or increase the excitability of the nerves such that they are more sensitive to other activators.

Little is known about the mechanisms by which mechanical perturbation of airway afferent nerve terminals leads to the development of generator potentials. There are a wide variety of ion channels that are gated through mechanical forces, but as discussed elsewhere in more detail, how these participate in mechanical transduction in airway afferent nerves is unknown (25). Hyperosmolar solutions effectively lead to action potential discharge in airway mucosal afferent nerves (26,27). Again, the precise mechanism is unknown. Aniso-(unequal)-osmotic solutions could conceivably lead to mechanical deformation of the nerve terminal membrane causing activation of mechanically gated ion channels. Alternatively, epithelial cells could be stimulated by the aniso-osmotic solutions to release mediators such as lipoxygenase products that in turn activate the afferent nerves.

Instilling hyperosmolar solutions into a human nose causes immediate burning and itching sensations (28). The intensity of this sensory response is correlated with the amount of the lipoxygenase product 15-hydroxy-eicosatetraenoic (15-HETE) generated by the epithelial cells. The lipoxygenase products of arachidonic acid such as 15-HETE and 12-hydroperoxyeicosate-traenoic acid (12-HPETE) can activate directly sensory nerves via gating the vanilloid receptor TRPV1 (see below).

Ligand-gated ion channels expressed by the airway C-fibers include the ATP receptors (P2X channels), the 5-HT receptors (5-HT$_3$ receptor), the nicotine receptors, and certain TRP (Transient Receptor Potential) channels including the capsaicin-sensitive vanilloid receptor TRPV1 (7,21,29). Agonists of these channels lead to airway C-fibers activation. With few exceptions, air pollutants have not been shown to be high affinity agonists for these ligand-gated ion channels. The known exceptions are certain particulates, such as negatively charged carboxylate-modified polystyrene particles, which can directly activate TRPV1 (30), and, of course, nicotine in cigarette smoke, which acts on the nicotinic receptors.

Numerous organic compounds (alcohols, organic acids, aldehydes, ketones) when applied to the nasal mucosa evoke defensive reflexes (31–34). Often the concentration-dependency of these responses is indicative of a chemical–receptor interaction. A potential receptor class for these irritants is the TRP channels family (35). TRP channels are found on sensory C-fibers and evoke action potential discharge when activated. TRPV1 was discovered and defined based on its affinity for capsaicin and related vanilloids (formerly vanilloid receptor 1,VR1) (36). There are, however, endogenous activators of TRPV1 that include hydrogen ions (pH ~5.0), certain lipoxygenases products of arachidonic acid such as 12-HETE and 15-HETE, and certain endocannabinoids such as anadamide (36). Various alcohols can also activate TRPV1 (37). Interestingly, TRPV1, and perhaps other TRP channels, may be gated by electrostatic charges carried on inert particulate matter (PM) (30). Studies in cell culture systems and rodent models suggest that inflammatory and irritant effects of ambient air PM may be partially mediated by TRPV1 receptors (38–40). Another member of the TRP family named (designated) ANKTM1 has been localized to mammalian C-fiber neurons. Recent studies support the hypothesis that ANKTM1 can be gated by certain irritating isothiocyanates such as allylisothiocyante (mustard oil) and tetrahydorcannabinol (THC) (41).

Airborne irritants could lead to activation of other ligand-gated ion channels on mucosal sensory nerves by, for example inducing the release of ATP from epithelial cells or 5-HT from NEBs. Airborne irritants that evoke local inflammatory effects may lead to the production of various inflammatory mediators that act on G-protein-linked receptors on mucosal sensory nerves. Bradykinin directly evokes action potential discharge in airway C-fibers via the bradykinin B$_2$ receptor stimulation (42). Stimulation of other G-protein-coupled receptors such as the histamine H_1, certain protease activated receptors (PARs), and prostanoid receptors may act to increase excitability of airway sensory nerves (43,44).

III. CNS Integration

Activation of airway sensory nerves leads to action potential discharge that is conducted to the central terminal of the nerve where it evokes the release of central neurotransmitters. In the case of airway mucosal afferent nerves, the transmitters are thought to be typically excitatory amino acids such as glutamate. In addition, as mentioned above, the airway C-fiber afferent nerves use various neuropeptides as central neurotransmitters. The transmitter acts on receptors on the postsynaptic membrane causing depolarizing potentials in secondary neurons within the brainstem (for trigeminal and vagal afferents) or spinal cord (for spinal afferents). If the synaptic potential is of sufficient magnitude, action potential threshold is reached and neurotransmission continues to other areas in the CNS. Ultimately the information is transduced into conscious sensations (urge to sneeze or cough, chest tightness, etc) and/or reflexed out of the CNS via the autonomic nervous system.

The pattern of central projections of nasal mucosal trigeminal afferent nerves in the brainstem shown by neuronal tracing studies is in agreement with the hypothesis that the mucosal nerves are involved in nociception and defensive reflexes (45). More specifically, projections to the trigeminal brainstem nuclear complex were found in the superficial laminae of the subnucleus caudalis and in the subnucleus interpolaris, areas known to be involved in processing of nociceptive information. Labeling was also observed in the interstitial subnucleus of the nucleus tractus solitarius (nTS), which is involved in respiratory control (45). The vagal afferent nerves in the lower airways project primarily to the nTS in the brainstem. Inhalation of capsaicin or histamine has been shown to activate secondary neurons in the nTS secondary to glutamate and neurokinin neurotransmission (46).

When thinking about central integration of the information arising from the airways, it is important to keep in mind that mechanosensitive sensory nerves (but not most C-fibers) in the lungs are constantly being activated by cyclic changes in mechanical distension during breathing. It is likely that SAR and RAR mechanosensors as well as mucosal C-fibers synapse on their own distinct repertoires of secondary neurons in the CNS. In addition, however, the evidence favors the concept of convergence of inputs among the sensory nerve subtypes. Nasal afferents may converge with RAR and SAR input in the brainstem to affect respiratory control (47). Stimulation of laryngeal C-fibers can augment the increase in reflex parasympathetic output evoked by stimulation of RARs in the lungs (48).

Likewise, stimulation of C-fibers within the lungs can increase the sensitivity of the cough reflex evoked by activation of tracheal A-fibers (49). These effects are thought to be due to C-fiber activation releasing transmitters that increase the synaptic efficacy of A-fiber input. This can occur through a host of molecular mechanisms. Collectively, this process is referred to as "central sensitization" (50). Central sensitization is one possible mechanism whereby an inhaled pollutant stimulating sensory nerves in the nose or large airways leads to changes in reflexes evoked from distant sites such as the lower airways and cardiovascular system.

IV. Autonomic Nerves

The function of many cell types in the airways is regulated by autonomic nerves. Autonomic outflow is dependent on the activity of preganglionic neurons situated in the CNS. Preganglionic autonomic output can be profoundly up- or downregulated by the input from the airway sensory nerves. For example, activation of airway RAR and C-fibers can stimulate the activity of airway preganglionic parasympathetic nerves, whereas input from SAR nerves can inhibit preganglionic nerve activity (51). Preganglionic autonomic neurons project axons out of the CNS where they synapse on postganglionic neurons via nicotinic synaptic neurotransmission. The sympathetic postganglionic neurons innervating the airways are situated in the stellate and superior cervical ganglia. The cell bodies of postganglionic parasympathetic nerves innervating the nasal mucosa are situated in the sphenopalantine ganglia, whereas those innervating the lower airways are situated in small ganglia within the airways (52).

Stimulation of sympathetic nerves innervating the nose cause vasoconstriction, but has little effect on secretion (12). The vasoconstriction is thought to be due in large part to α-adrenergic receptor activation. Other sympathetic neurotransmitters such as neuropeptide Y have been identified in nasal nerves, but their contribution to sympathetic vascular control in the nose has not yet been clarified. The sympathetic nervous system is thought to be responsible for the so-called nasal cycle typified by periodic unilateral mucosal swelling and obstruction (12).

Stimulation of parasympathetic nerves in the nose leads to vasodilation and watery secretions. Blocking muscarinic cholinergic receptors inhibit both effects (53). As in the lower airways, there is evidence that noncholinergic parasympathetic nerves innervate the nasal mucosa. Both vasoactive intestinal peptide (VIP) and nitric oxide (NO) have been localized to nasal nerve fibers (12). These transmitters are effective vasodilators, but their role in human nasal physiology remains at present speculative.

The autonomic control of the lower airways has traditionally been viewed as a balance between the opposing actions of the sympathetic and parasympathetic systems. It was assumed that the actions of the parasympathetic nervous system were mediated by acetylcholine whereas the sympathetic nerves utilized noradrenaline to regulate airway function. In more recent times, it has become apparent that autonomic control is more complex than as simply described as the opposing actions of acetylcholine and noradrenaline. Multiple transmitters have been localized to the autonomic nerves innervating the airways. These transmitters have multiple effects on the end organs in the airways and their role as neurotransmitters and/or neuromodulators has been confirmed in many instances.

The parasympathetic nervous system provides both the contractile and relaxant innervation to bronchial smooth muscle. Parasympathetic nerve mediated bronchoconstriction is secondary to acetylcholine acting on muscarinic receptors. The only functional relaxant innervation of airway smooth muscle in many species including humans is also provided by the parasympathetic nervous system (54). Parasympathetic nerve-mediated relaxations of airway smooth muscle may be mediated by VIP and related peptides, as well as NO. These nonadrenergic, noncholinergic relaxant responses can be evoked in airways from the trachea to the small bronchi. It has been suggested that both constricting and relaxing transmitters are coreleased from the same postganglionic parasympathetic nerves. The evidence to date, however, favors the hypothesis that the relaxant and contractile nerves represent, two distinct parasympathetic pathways (55).

As with the bronchial smooth muscle, airway glands are regulated primarily by the parasympathetic nervous system. Acetylcholine is the primary neurotransmitter, but other peptide neurotransmitters may also play a role in regulating mucus secretion. In contrast, it has been shown that the neurotransmitters associated with sympathetic nerves have subtle if any direct effect on mucus secretion. However, these mediators may play a role in regulating parasympathetic nerve activity (56,57).

Both sympathetic and parasympathetic nerves regulate bronchial vascular tone (58–61). Sympathetic nerves mediate vasoconstriction through the actions of noradrenaline and neuropeptide Y, whereas parasympathetic nerves mediated vasodilatation through the actions of acetylcholine, nitric oxide, and perhaps peptides such as VIP. Reflex regulation of bronchial vascular tone is poorly defined, in large part due to the difficulty with which the bronchial vasculature is studied.

The release of acetylcholine is under the control of muscarinic autoreceptors (M_2) on postganglionic parasympathetic nerves (62,63). Acetylcholine binding to these receptors inhibits further release of acetylcholine from nerve terminals, serving as a mechanism to limit parasympathetically mediated bronchoconstriction. M_2-deficient mice exhibit enhanced bronchonstriction after methacholine challenge or vagal nerve stimulation (64). Disruption of neuronal M_2 receptor function occurs after allergic inflammation (65,66) and ozone exposure (67) resulting in airway hyperresponsiveness. Pilocarpine, an M_2 receptor-specific agonist, inhibits reflex bronchoconstriction induced by exposure to sulfur dioxide in normal, but not asthmatic subjects, suggesting this inhibitory mechanism is dysfunctional in asthmatic airways (68,69).

V. Airway and Cardiovascular Responses Initiated by Airway Mucosal Sensory Nerves

Irritants activate trigeminal, glossopharyngeal, or vagal nerves which evoke tingling, itching, stinging, burning, or otherwise painful sensations in the eyes or respiratory tract (70). Irritation of sensory nerves in the airway mucosa initiates reflexes that are often collectively referred to as defensive reflexes. These reflexes, which have been reviewed in considerable detail elsewhere, include changes in airway and cardiovascular function as well as changes in respiration which tend to prevent uptake of the irritant and prevent injury (6,29,71). Sensory nerve stimulation in the nose, trachea, and large bronchi may trigger conscious sensations of irritation as well as dyspnea. In the more peripheral airways, the afferent input is thought to lead primarily to reflex changes in autonomic tone and respiratory rhythm. Physiological responses to guard against exposure to irritants typically include bronchoconstriction and reductions in airflow, as measured by increased airway resistance (R) and decreased dynamic compliance (C_{dyn}). Increases in R reflect changes of airway diameter (which can be affected by airway smooth muscle constriction, mucus secretion, or edema), while decreases in C_{dyn} reflect reduced viscoelasticity, or distensibility, of the distal lung including the smallest airways.

Activation of airway mucosal sensory nerves leads to significant increases in parasympathetic outflow from the CNS. In the nose, this leads to rhinorrhea, and perhaps vasodilation (72). Indeed, in allergic individuals, the major component of nasal secretion evoked upon allergen application to the nasal septum can be antagonized by muscarinic receptor blockers (73). In the lower airways, the increased parasympathetic tone results in bronchoconstriction, increases in mucus secretion, and vasodilation (74).

Activation of airway sensory nerves can also evoke autonomic cardiovascular reflexes. Activation of mucosal C-fibers in the lower airways can lead to parasympathetic-mediated bradycardia and hypotension (vago-vagal reflexes) (29). Stimulation of nasal-pharyngeal afferent nerves can cause bradycardia often accompanied by hypertension (71). The bradycardia is most likely due to an increase in vagal parasympathetic activity, while hypertension is the consequence of increased sympathetic vasoconstrictor activity. In addition, nasal afferent activation may lead to an inhibition of baroreflex activity (75).

Activation of sensory nerves in the upper and lower airways influences respiratory rhythm (29,71). The most obvious defensive reflexes evoked by airway sensory nerve activation are the complex and highly coordinated cough and sneeze reflexes. The sensory nerves directly involved in the cough reflexes are mechanosensitive vagal A-fibers situated primarily in the larynx trachea and at bifurcations of large bronchi (21). Activation of mucosal C-fibers may also lead to irritating "itchy" airway sensations in the lower airways that provoke a cough response. Thus, inhalation of the C-fiber stimulant bradykinin or capsaicin consistently evokes cough in healthy humans (76,77). Relatively little is known about the specific nerve types subserving the sneeze reflexes, but as with cough, both mechanosensitive A-fibers as well as C-fibers are likely involved. In addition to cough and sneezing, vagal and trigeminal airway C-fiber stimulation can also lead to apneic or tachypneic reflexes.

A. Axon Reflexes

In addition to classically defined autonomic nerves, sensory C-fibers may subserve a local efferent function in the upper and lower airways (78). Many C-fibers are branched nerves that contain various neuropeptides (e.g., substance P, CGRP) in their peripheral terminals. Action potentials arising from the terminals may invade collateral branches causing the local release of sensory neuropeptides. This peripheral release of neurotransmitters from sensory nerve collaterals and the resulting end organ effects are referred to as an axon reflex. The released transmitters such as substance P, CGRP, and perhaps ATP, can cause numerous vascular effectors that have been collectively referred to as neurogenic inflammation (79). When administered exogenously, putative sensory neurotransmitters have profound effects in the airways including mucus secretion, vasodilatation, plasma exudation, and inflammatory cell recruitment (80). These observations naturally lead to the hypothesis that axonal reflexes contribute to the pathogenesis of inflammatory airways disease.

Axon reflexes have been well defined in the airways of rats and guinea pigs and evidence indicates that axon reflexes may regulate human upper airway responses to bradykinin and capsaicin (72,81). Moreover, the axon reflex may be amplified in the presence of ongoing inflammation in the nose (73,82). The role of axon reflexes in the lower airways is less clear. Morphological studies of the afferent innervation of the human airway mucosa reveal a dense plexus of afferent nerves innervating the epithelium, but a general sparseness of neuropeptide-containing nerve fibers.

VI. Neurologically Mediated Responses to Air Pollutants
A. Respiratory Responses to Sensory and Pulmonary Irritants

The biological effects of airborne irritants are typically determined by their water solubility, which controls the extent of penetration into the respiratory tract and corresponding characteristics of physiological responses (70). Sensory irritants, such as sulfur dioxide (SO_2), ammonia (NH_3), and formaldehyde (HCHO), are highly water-soluble agents which rapidly pass into the lining fluids of the eyes and upper respiratory tract, and elicit immediate painful or burning sensations. Bronchoconstriction, mucus secretion, and cough are typical responses to sensory irritants. At high concentrations, sensory irritants induce reflex inhibition of inspiration. Pulmonary irritants, such as ozone (O_3), nitrogen dioxide (NO_2), and phosgene ($COCl_2$), are less water-soluble chemicals which tend to deposit further down the respiratory tract, causing changes in breathing pattern and mechanics. Pulmonary irritants also deposit, to a lesser degree, in the nasopharynx and upper airways (83), which accounts for symptoms such as cough and painful breathing. As described previously, pulmonary irritant-induced changes in breathing pattern may be considered defensive reflexes which prevent injury by shifting the dose of the irritant to less susceptible tissues further up the respiratory tract. These reflex responses to inhaled irritants are typically characterized by rapid, shallow breathing (increased breath frequency and decreased tidal volume). However, these responses can also cause adverse consequences, especially in those individuals with respiratory or cardiac disease who are not able to maintain sufficient gas exchange. Healthy individuals who are able to maintain adequate gas exchange might respond to an irritant exposure with an insignificant or temporary alteration in respiratory function. An asthmatic might respond to the same exposure with an exaggerated bronchoconstriction reflex due to chronic airway inflammation, and may also be at increased risk due to diminished ventilatory reserve as a result of small airway damage and trapped air in the distal lung (84). Irritant responses have been assessed in experimental studies involving animals exposed to air pollutants, in clinical studies where healthy individuals and those with asthma or COPD are exposed to controlled low levels of air pollutants, and in epidemiologic studies of populations exposed to uncontrolled environmental air pollution.

B. Cardiovascular Responses

Inhaled irritants induce pulmonary reflexes which can result in responses in the heart as well as the lungs (85). As described above, activation of airway mucosal C-fibers often leads to parasympathetically mediated bradycardia and hypotension (6,29), although tachycardia with hypertension has also been demonstrated in humans after stimulation of the trachea (86). Although it is not clear whether C-fibers or RARs mediate these responses, it is clear that certain irritants may influence cardiovascular reflexes which alter the balance of parasympathetic and sympathetic activity in the heart. Recent studies have shown significant effects of air pollutants on cardiovascular function, especially with respect to the autonomic nervous system. An association between particulate air pollution and cardiac mortality has been proposed to be mediated by the autonomic nervous system (87). It is reasonable to assume then that cardiac effects of pollutants are mediated in part by stimulation of irritant receptors, which alters the balance of sympathetic and parasympathetic activity.

Three factors have been described which contribute to cardiovascular morbidity and mortality: the autonomic nervous system, the health of the myocardium, and its vulnerability to arrhythmogenic or ischemic conditions (88). Air pollutants may affect the function of all these components, especially in sensitive individuals such as patients with heart failure or chronic obstructive pulmonary disease (COPD), or the elderly. Since myocardial health and vulnerability to ischemia are not directly linked to neurological mechanisms, this section will only consider evidence for the direct role of the autonomic nervous system in response to air pollutants. The contribution of the autonomic nervous system to cardiovascular responses has been assessed by analysis of heart rate variability (HRV). Heart rate is continuously regulated by the opposing influences of parasympathetic and sympathetic activity. The parasympathetic effects, conducted through vagal nerves, slow the heart from its intrinsic rate of 100–120 beats per minute to a resting rate of 55–70 beats per minute (89). Various stressors stimulate sympathetic activity and increase heart rate from this resting level. Heart rate is measured in electrocardiogram (ECG) recordings as the interval between successive R peaks in the QRS complex, representing ventricular depolarizations. Only normal-to-normal (NN) beats originating in the sinus node (excluding atrial and ventricular ectopic beats) are used in the analysis of HRV. Studies using Holter monitors (ambulatory ECG devices) have become the standard method to obtain information about changes in HRV due to the effects of exposure to air pollutants in human volunteers (88). These recordings may be conducted for as little as 5–10 min, but usually for 24 hr to acquire the necessary data for full analysis of the periodicity of heart rate changes.

Heart rate variability is typically assessed using time domain or frequency domain indices. Time domain measures are derived from statistical analysis of the variability in NN intervals (Fig. 3). The most commonly used parameters include standard deviation of NN intervals (SDNN), root mean square of successive differences in NN intervals (rMSSD), and the percentage of successive NN intervals greater than 50 msec (pNN50). These parameters are highly correlated and reflect the influence of the parasympathetic system on the heart (88). Frequency domain measures are derived from power spectral analysis of NN intervals, which reveals periodic modulations of NN intervals (90). This periodicity can be expressed as the sum of a series of sine and cosine functions of varying amplitudes and frequencies (Fig. 4). Four components are present in humans: high frequency (HF; 0.15–0.4 Hz), low frequency (LF; 0.04–0.15 Hz), very low frequency (VLF; 0.003–0.04 Hz), and ultra-low frequency (ULF; < 0.003 Hz) power.

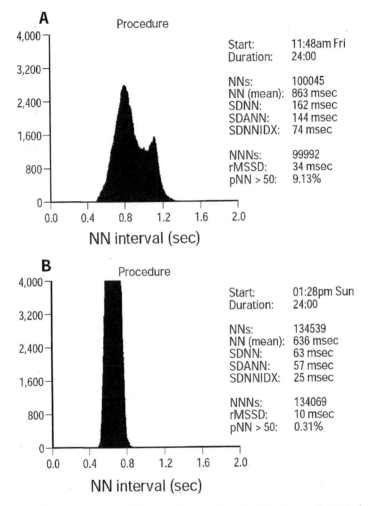

Figure 3 Time domain HRV analysis. (A) Distribution of NN intervals in healthy subject. (B) Distribution of NN intervals in patient with dilated cardiomyopathy. (Form Ref. 88.)

VLF and ULF power represent poorly understood long-term regulatory mechanisms, perhaps involving thermoregulation and the renin angiotensin system (88). HF power is almost entirely due to vagal parasympathetic modulation synchronous with respiration, while LF power largely reflects sympathetic tone and baroreflex sensitivity. Consequently the LF/HF ratio represents the overall balance of sympathetic and parasympathetic activity, referred to as sympathovagal tone (88). The total power (TP), measured as the sum of the four components, is equal to the heart period variance

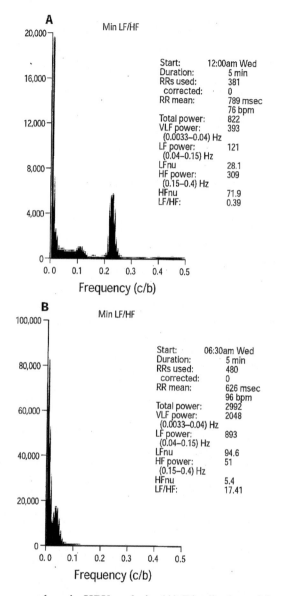

Figure 4 Frequency domain HRV analysis. (A) Distribution of frequencies (c/b, cycles/beat) in healthy subject. (B) Distribution of frequencies in patient after myocardial infarction. LFnu, low frequency content normalized for total power. HFnu, high frequency content normalized for total power. (From Ref. 88.)

(SDNN^2) and, along with SDNN, reflects the total HRV and the influence of the autonomic nervous system on the heart.

Heart rate variability decreases with age and with the presence of cardiopulmonary disease, indicating an imbalance in the autonomic control of cardiac function and increased susceptibility to cardiac events (88,90,91). Lower HRV is predictive of greater susceptibility to cardiovascular disease events, including angina pectoris, myocardial infarction, congestive heart failure, coronary heart disease, or death (91,92), and risk of mortality after myocardial infarction (93). Recent studies suggest a relationship between elevated levels of ambient air pollutants and effects on autonomic nervous system function, including effects on systemic arterial blood pressure (BP) and HRV.

C. Neurologically Mediated Cardiovascular Responses to Particulate Matter

Numerous studies have reported a role for respirable particulate matter in morbidity and mortality, especially in sensitive populations (94,95). These studies provide evidence that elevations in short-term ambient PM levels are associated with lung injury and inflammation, worsening of lung function, and hypoxia-related cardiovascular disease (96–99). The autonomic nervous system has been recognized as one of the important pathophysiological pathways leading to PM-associated cardiorespiratory health effects. These effects may occur in the absence of signs of hypoxia (100). Evidence indicating a role for neurological mechanisms in response to exposure to PM is mainly found in studies examining cardiac function in response to ambient or experimental exposures. Peters et al. (101) tested the hypothesis that air pollution episodes induce potentially life-threatening arrhythmias by monitoring patients with implanted cardioverter defibrillators. Frequency of defibrillation was significantly associated with increases in NO_2 and black carbon, and to a lesser extent with CO and PM_{10} (PM less than 10 μm aerodynamic diameter). These results suggest that air pollution is a risk factor for arrhythmic events.

The utility of this approach was demonstrated in studies of a January 1985 air pollution episode in central Europe, which resulted in elevated numbers of hospital admissions for cardiovascular diseases, attributed to acute coronary syndromes and arrhythmias (102). Retrospective analyses of these events showed increases in heart rate (103) and systolic blood pressure (104) associated with the air pollution episode days, as well as levels of total suspended particulates and sulfur dioxide, suggesting the effects could be related to changes in cardiovascular autonomic control.

The effects of exposure to ambient PM appear to depend on the health status of the individual. In recent studies of young healthy individuals, effects of $PM_{2.5}$ (PM less than 2.5 μm aerodynamic diameter) have been inconsistent. Devlin et al. (105) found no changes in HRV parameters in a panel of 11 young adults exposed to concentrated ambient air particles in the size range of 0.1–2.5 µm (CAPS; average 106 µg/m^3) in comparison to another panel of 11 young adults exposed to clean air. However, parameters of HRV decreased in 20 young healthy workers (106) and in 9 young adults (107) in association with ambient air PM$_{2.5}$, indicating a deleterious effect of ambient particles. In contrast, in a panel of 9 young adult male highway troopers, parameters of HRV were increased in association with ambient air PM$_{2.5}$ in their vehicles (average 24 µg/m^3), reflecting a presumed healthy physiologic response to PM, although some deleterious effects were noted, including increases in peripheral blood inflammation and coagulation markers and increased numbers of ectopic beats (108).

Associations of reduced HRV with levels of ambient fine PM have been consistently demonstrated in elderly populations. A study of 10 healthy elderly individuals exposed to a fairly low concentration of CAPS (average 41 µg/m^3) for 2 hr found significant decrements in several HRV parameters compared with measurements in the same individuals sham exposed to clean air (105). In a study of 21 elderly Boston residents monitored over several summer months (109), significantly lower HRV (as determined by SDNN and rMMSD) was associated with exposures to ambient PM$_{2.5}$ and ozone, suggesting that these pollutants decrease vagal tone, resulting in reduced HRV. A study of 56 elderly Baltimore residents also found associations between decreased HRV and elevations of ambient PM$_{2.5}$ measured one day previously (110). HRV parameters (SDNN, rMSSD, LF, HF) were also decreased in another panel study of 10 elderly subjects in relation to exposure to fine particles (107).

Autonomic control in relation to particle pollution has been studied in some animal models and in humans with cardiovascular disease. Dogs with experimentally induced coronary artery occlusion subsequently exposed to CAPS (average 286 µg/m^3) had enhanced ST segment elevation, indicative of worsened ischemia, in comparison with exposure to filtered air (111). Residual oil fly ash particles caused decreases in HRV in rats with left ventricular myocardial infarction, but not in sham-operated rats (112). A pilot study of seven mostly elderly subjects with cardiac disease found that PM$_{10}$ is associated with increased heart rate and decreased overall HRV as measured by SDNN, although rMSSD was increased (100). This study was consistent with that of a clinical study of 26 elderly subjects, where elevated levels of PM$_{2.5}$ were associated with decreased SDNN without any lag in effects, but only in the subgroup of 18 subjects with cardiovascular conditions (113). In a panel study of 131 adults with coronary artery disease, a small but significant decrease in blood pressure and heart rate were found in relation to particulate air pollution (114). These findings were opposite to those found in the earlier retrospective study of cardiovascular function after an air pollution episode, in which increases in blood pressure were found in the general population (104). Additionally, onset of myocardial infarction (MI) (115) and cardioverter defibrillator discharge (101) have been linked to increases in ambient PM. The increased risk of onset of MI was associated with PM levels in the 2 hr preceding the MI (115). The association of defibrillator events with PM was followed for 3 years in 100 heart patients with implanted defibrillators. Those with more than 10 defibrillator events had arrhythmias associated with exposures to NO_2, black carbon, CO, and $PM_{2.5}$, occurring 1–2 days after exposure to these pollutants (101). The strongest associations were found with NO_2, but associations were also found with $PM_{2.5}$ and PM_{10}. Finally, a study of 12 healthy and 12 asthmatic individuals found similar results (116,117): in the asthmatic group, systolic blood pressure modestly increased during filtered air exposure and decreased during CAPs exposure (average $106 \mu g/m^3$), whereas the pattern was reversed in healthy individuals (blood pressure increased during CAPS exposure).

The associations between PM exposure and autonomic control can also be found in instances of occupational exposures. A longitudinal study of 39 boilermakers and 1 pipefitter found decreased SDNN and increases in heart rate associated with occupational $PM_{2.5}$ exposure (118). These events were associated with long- and short-acting components, which were attributable to cytokine production and sympathetic activity, respectively. Further analysis of the elemental composition of the $PM_{2.5}$ was conducted in order to ascertain whether the observed effects could be associated with six commonly found metals in $PM_{2.5}$ (119). This analysis found a small increase in SDNN was associated with lead and vanadium in ambient $PM_{2.5}$. Other studies have not found significant cardiac effects with PM-associated metals. No effects on HR or HRV were observed after exposure of old dogs with preexisting cardiac abnormalities to metal compounds, including Mn, Ni, V, Fe, and Cu oxides or Ni and V sulfates at concentrations of $50 \mu g/m^3$(120).

D. Respiratory Responses to Ozone

Nitrogen dioxide formed from combustion processes and volatile organic compounds reacts with ultraviolet light and oxygen in a series of complex reactions to produce ozone (121), the primary oxidant pollutant of toxicological significance in ambient air. Ozone is less soluble in aqueous lining fluids of the respiratory tract than SO_2 but more soluble than oxygen—approximately half of inspired O_3 is taken up in the nasopharynx of rabbits, guinea pigs (122), and humans (83,123), whereas SO_2 is efficiently removed in this region (124). A significant fraction of inhaled O_3 penetrates to the deep lung where the thin alveolar epithelial–capillary endothelial barrier is particularly sensitive to ozone's oxidizing effects. Short-term exposures to elevated levels of O_3 induce lung inflammation and increased permeability of respiratory epithelium (125–127). Increases in lung epithelial permeability were noted 18–20 hours after exposure of healthy individuals to O_3 (0.15–0.35 ppm; 130 min) in the periphery, but not the base, of the lung (128). At this time, similar concentrations of O_3 also cause airway hyperresponsiveness to methacholine (129). At higher doses, O_3 induces an irritant response characterized by rapid, shallow breathing [increased frequency (f; tachypnea) and decreased tidal volume (V_T)] (130–133). These alterations in breathing pattern and mechanics effectively shift the deposited dose to the more proximal and less fragile tracheobronchial or nasopharyngeal regions. Central airway effects of O_3 are indicated by decreases in forced expiratory volume in 1 sec (FEV_1) and forced vital capacity (FVC), and at higher concentrations, increased airway resistance (134,135). Increased resistance may be caused by contraction of airway smooth muscle resulting in bronchoconstriction, submucosal edema, or mucus secretion. In addition, short-term exposures to ozone cause airway hyperresponsiveness to nonspecific contractile agonists such as histamine or methacholine (136).

The irritant response to ozone (rapid shallow breathing) and changes in spirometric measures of lung function such as FEV_1 and FVC adapt or attenuate after repeated exposures (137–139). Smaller airways may less readily adapt to repeated exposures compared with larger airways as indicated by persistent reductions in forced expiratory flow rate between 25% and 75% of FVC (FEF_{25-75}) compared with diminished responses in FEV_1 and FVC (139). Rapid shallow breathing in rats is attenuated upon repeated exposure to 0.35 or 0.5 ppm ozone, despite progressive lung damage (140). Adaptation is observed as early as 18 hr following an acute O_3 exposure and appears to precede the mobilization of antioxidants (141). The role of irritant pathways in the mechanisms responsible for adaptation is not well known.

Sensory C-fibers release a number of neuropeptide mediators which have important actions on respiratory function. Substance P and neurokinin A (NKA) are peptides cleaved from a common precursor termed preprotachykinin-1 (142). These and other tachykinin ligands bind to receptors termed NK1, NK2, and NK3. NK1 receptors have higher specificity for substance P than NKA, while the reverse is true for NK2 receptors. NK3 has a higher affinity for neurokinin B than NKA or substance P. NK1 receptors mediate hyperpermeability of endothelium and hypersecretion by airway epithelial goblet cells, while NK2 receptors mediate smooth muscle contraction resulting in bronchoconstriction (142,143). Neutral endopeptidase (NEP) and angiotensin-converting enzyme (ACE) both inactivate substance P by cleaving it to smaller peptides, while NEP also cleaves NKA.

There is a great deal of evidence indicating that bronchial sensory C-fibers mediate ozone-induced vagal reflex changes in breathing pattern (133). The reflex changes induced by bronchial C-fibers appear to protect against ozone-induced airway hyperresponsiveness (133,134). Substance

P and NKA may be involved in these responses, and ozone may increase their concentration due to loss of NEP activity (144). Pharmacologic inhibition of NEP function results in increased airway responsiveness to substance P in air-exposed, but not O_3-exposed guinea pigs since NEP levels are already reduced in this group (145). Treatment of neonatal rodents with capsaicin results in degeneration of C-fibers and permanent depletion of tachykinins from the lung (146). Studies which ablated the development of C-fibers using capsaicin in neonatal rats indicate that C-fibers protect against the development of ozone-induced airway hyperresponsiveness to methacholine (147) and lung injury and inflammation (148,149). In contrast, guinea pigs treated with capsaicin had reduced ozone-induced airway hyperresponsiveness (150). The difference in species response may lie in differing responsiveness to tachykinins substance P (SP) and neurokinin A (NKA), which are potent bronchoconstrictors in guinea pigs (151), but not rats (152).

Exposure of cultured human or canine bronchial epithelial cells to ozone causes injury as measured by decreases in transepithelial potential difference and increases in mannitol flux (153). NK1 and NK3 agonists and substance P inhibited ozone-induced injury, whereas the NK1 antagonist CP-96345 enhanced injury (153). These results suggest that tachykinins function to maintain bronchial epithelial barrier stability via NK1 receptor activation, and that C-fiber stimulation protects against irritant-induced lung injury. Combined treatment of rats with NK1 receptor antagonist CP-99994 and NK2 receptor antagonist SR-48968 or neonatal ablation of C-fibers with capsaicin caused enhanced neutrophilic response to ozone (1 ppm, 3 hr), but not enhanced airway hyperresponsiveness, suggesting that the tachykinin substance P and NKA both partially protect against ozone-induced lung inflammation (149). The enhanced inflammation in capsaicin-treated animals does not appear to be mediated by increased ventilation in comparison with untreated animals; in fact capsaicin treatment causes decreased ventilation in comparison to control rats (149) and guinea pigs (150). Consequently, increased inflammation in capsaicinized ozone-treated animals occurs despite a lower inhaled dose (149). In contrast to capsaicin-treated rats exposed to ozone which developed AHR (147), NK1 and NK2 receptor antagonism did not induce AHR in ozone-exposed rats (149). These results suggest that C-fibers inhibit the development of AHR, even though tachykinins are not involved. Other mediators such as CGRP and nitric oxide, which are colocalized in C-fibers, have bronchodilatory effects and their absence in capsaicin-treated animals may be responsible for AHR in this model (149). Nitric oxide may also be responsible for ozone-induced increases in vascular permeability (154). Substance P appears to protect lung epithelium from ozone-induced damage through increasing airway microvascular blood flow (155), helping to remove epithelial reactant products and reactive oxygen species from the airways. Mucus secretion is stimulated by substance P (156), which may reduce the dose of ozone reaching the epithelial layer. In addition, ozone may directly stimulate mucus transport through parasympathetic stimulation of tracheobronchial submucosal glands or alteration of epithelial permeability (157).

E. Responses to Sulfur Dioxide, Sulfuric Acid, and Nitrogen Dioxide

Sulfur dioxide is a common air pollutant which is highly water-soluble and therefore efficiently removed in the lining fluids of the upper respiratory tract (158). Healthy individuals are generally unresponsive to SO_2 concentrations less than $13.1 \, mg/m^3$ (5 ppm). In contrast, asthmatics respond to concentrations at least an order of magnitude lower (0.66–$1.3 \, mg/m^3$; 0.25–0.5 ppm) with an acute response characterized by bronchoconstriction, increases in airway resistance and decreases in expiratory flow rates, and symptoms of wheeze and shortness of breath (158). Effects can be observed at even lower concentrations when asthmatics are exposed to SO_2 during moderate exercise (159). Exposures of 0.05 ppm SO_2 caused increases in airway resistance in exercising asthmatics (160,161). These effects can be attributed to increased exposure due to enhanced ventilation and increased oral breathing (161).

In animal models, C-fibers appear to mediate different effects in response to SO_2 exposure, depending on intensity of exposure. In normal guinea pigs exposed to very high (500–2000 ppm) though brief (six breaths) exposures, SO_2 produced concentration-dependent increases in lung resistance and decreases in compliance (162). Intravenous administration of various receptor antagonists to guinea pigs prior to SO_2 exposure showed that the SO_2-induced increases in lung resistance are mainly mediated by NK2 receptors, and not by NK1 or muscarinic receptors (162). Neonatal capsaicin-treated rats exposed to very high concentrations of SO_2 gas (250 ppm, 5 hr/day, 5 days/week, 4 weeks) had increases in airway smooth muscle mass, lung inflammation and injury, lung resistance, and airway hyperresponsiveness to methacholine compared with control rats exposed to SO_2 (163). These results suggest that C-fibers limit the development of airway obstruction and airway hyperresponsiveness during induction of chronic bronchitis by SO_2 exposure, and that these effects are mediated by increases in smooth muscle mass.

Recent studies show that 0.2 ppm SO_2 causes changes in indices of autonomic nervous system function (164). SO_2 exposure caused increases in total power, HF and LF power in normal subjects and decreases in these indices in asthmatic subjects (164). In a retrospective study of cardiovascular function after air pollution, increases in systolic blood pressure were found with increasing levels of ambient SO_2 (104). In subgroups with high plasma viscosity levels and increased heart rates, systolic blood pressure was increased to a greater degree (104).

Sulfur oxides occur in the particulate phase as sulfuric acid (H_2SO_4) or its ammonia neutralization products letovicite [$(NH_4)_3H(SO4)_2$], ammonium bisulfate (NH_4HSO_4), and ammonium sulfate [$(NH_4)_2SO_4$] (158). The irritancy of these compounds appears to be related to acidity; studies in rabbits (165) and humans (166) show that H_2SO_4 induces a greater irritant response than NH_4HSO_4, which in turn is more irritant than $(NH_4)_2SO_4$. Ammonia produced in the nose and mouth neutralizes inhaled H_2SO_4 and reduces associated airway responses (167). Sulfuric acid is the most irritant of common ambient air acid species, including nitric acid (84). In healthy adults, no consistent effects of H_2SO_4 on pulmonary function or irritant symptoms have been reported at levels up to $1500\ \mu g/m^3$ for 1 hr, even with heavy exercise (168). However, some reports indicate exposures at levels less than $1000\ \mu g/m^3$ for several hours can result in airway hyperresponsiveness to cholinergic challenge without increasing airway inflammation (169). In contrast, asthmatic subjects are significantly more sensitive to H_2SO_4, with some reports indicating changes in pulmonary function at concentrations less than $100\ \mu g/m^3$ (170,171).

Oxides of nitrogen are emitted during combustion of a variety of fuels, especially from mobile sources. A small proportion of ambient nitrogen dioxide (NO_2) is emitted directly during combustion, although most is formed by the gradual oxidation of nitric oxide (NO) (172). Inhaled NO_2 is more water soluble than O_3, but less so than most sensory irritants, and consequently deposits primarily in the peripheral lung (84). Compared to O_3, NO_2 is less reactive and is only one-tenth as irritating (84). Further details of the effects of SO_2 as well as nitrogen oxides are examined in Chapter 5 (Air Pollutants, Epithelial Surfaces, and Lung Disease).

F. Responses to Volatile Organic Compounds

Various hydrocarbons and volatile organic compounds (VOCs) are present in JP-8 jet fuel. Repeated inhalation of aerosolized JP-8 induces physiological, biochemical, cellular, and morphological lung injury (173) as well as immunotoxic effects (174). Treatment of mice with an NK1 agonist prevented damage, while treatment with an NK1 antagonist exacerbated lung injury, expressed as increased lung permeability, alveolar macrophage toxicity, and bronchiolar epithelial injury (175). Similarly, immunotoxic effects were prevented and reversed by administration of substance P, which has highest affinity for the NK1 receptor (174,176). Neuropeptides also appear to be protective against injury induced by exposure to acrolein (177).

G. Responses to Mixtures of Air Pollutants

Mixtures of ambient air pollutants may result in the formation of secondary products with irritant properties. Recent studies indicate that unsaturated VOCs such as terpenes may react with oxidants (primarily ozone) to produce chemically reactive products which are sensory or pulmonary irritants. Mice exposed to combinations of isoprene and O_3, with or without NO_2, demonstrate a sensory irritant response (decreased f) (178). Similar reactions are observed with mixtures of O_3 with limonene (179) or α-pinene (180). Analysis of limonene/ozone reaction mixtures reveals the presence of irritants such as formaldehyde and acrolein (181), while methylvinyl ketone, methacrolein, and formaldehyde were detected in the isoprene/ozone reaction mixtures (178). The irritant effects of the identified reaction products and residual reactants could only partially explain the effects caused by the mixtures, suggesting that unknown highly irritant compounds are formed in these reactions.

Wood smoke, a complex mixture of gases and particles, stimulates both irritant RARs and C-fiber nerve endings in anesthetized rats (182). These effects appear to be mediated by the gas phase of the mixture, and hydroxyl radicals and cyclooxygenase enzyme products were found to stimulate these receptors (183,184). Interactions of O_3 with some types of PM, such as sulfuric acid-coated carbon particles, appear to prevent adaptation responses to repeated exposures to O_3 alone (185). The mechanisms responsible for prevention of these responses are not known, but these interactions indicate the importance of assessing the irritant and toxicologic properties of mixtures of urban air pollutants. Mixtures of pollutants designed to simulate urban air pollution were tested for their ability to affect respiratory function in rats exposed 4 hr/day, 3 days/week, for 4 weeks (186). Irritant respiratory responses, characterized by tachypnea and decreased tidal volume, were not observed in rats exposed to a low concentration of pollutants (0.15 ppm O_3, 0.1 ppm NO_2, 50 $\mu g/m^3$ NH_4HSO_4, 30 $\mu g/m^3$ carbon, 25 $\mu g/m^3$ HNO_3). Rats exposed to a medium concentration of pollutants (two-fold higher than the low concentration) exhibited irritant responses which were attenuated over time, indicative of adaptation to pollutant exposure. In contrast, high concentrations of pollutants (four-fold higher than the low concentration) caused progressive exacerbation of responses which correlated with other parameters of lung injury and cell proliferation (186). The concentrations, proportions, and components of air pollutant mixtures which cause enhanced irritancy or cardiopulmonary toxicity, as well as the mechanisms for these responses, remain to be determined.

VII. Summary

Lining the mucosa of all airways is a rich sensory innervation. In general, the sensory nerves comprise two major subtypes, the distention-sensitive mechanosensors (e.g., RAR and SAR) and the chemically sensitive nociceptors (e.g., nasal, bronchial, and pulmonary C-fibers). The consequence of activating airway sensory nerves depends on the nerve subtype, and their location within the airway. In the nose and large airways, sensory nerve activation can lead to various conscious sensations including irritation and pain. In all airways, activation of sensory nerves can affect patterns of respiration, and autonomic outflow leading to increases or decreases in parasympathetic and sympathetic tone.

Inhaling environmentally significant air pollutants can, in theory, result in activation of all types of sensory nerves either directly or through various indirect mechanisms. Activation of airway afferent nerves may explain how several classes of air pollutants induce neurologically mediated effects on the respiratory and cardiovascular systems. Very little is known, however, about the specific mechanisms underlying these processes. Pollutant-mediated neurological effects on the cardiovascular system are in particular poorly understood, being inferred largely from changes in heart rate variability, especially after exposures to elevated levels of ambient PM. The airway sensory innervation and accompanying reflexes they engender (cough, changes in autonomic outflow, etc.) may, in other cases, serve to protect the host from untoward effects of pollution. The specific role of C-fibers in protecting the respiratory system from injury induced by air pollutants has been convincingly demonstrated in animal models where these fibers have been ablated or the functions of specific sensory neuropeptides have been blocked by neuropeptide-specific antibodies.

References

1. Ho CY, Gu Q, Lin YS, Lee LY. Sensitivity of vagal afferent endings to chemical irritants in the rat lung. Respir Physiol 2001; 127(2–3):113–124.
2. Mazzone SB, Canning BJ, Widdicombe JG. Sensory pathways for the cough reflex. In: Chung F, Widdicombe JG, Boushey HA, eds. Cough: Causes, Mechanisms and Therapy. Oxford: Blackwell Publishing, 2003:161–172.
3. Knowlton GC, Larabee MG. A unitary analysis of pulmonary volume receptors. Am J Physiol 1946; 147:100–114.
4. Lee BP, Sant'Ambrogio G, Sant'Ambrogio FB. Afferent innervation and receptors of the canine extrathoracic trachea. Respir Physiol 1992; 90(1): 55–65.
5. McAlexander MA, Myers AC, Undem BJ. Adaptation of guinea-pig vagal airway afferent neurones to mechanical stimulation. J Physiol 1999; 521(Pt 1): 239–247.
6. Coleridge JC, Coleridge HM. Afferent vagal C fibre innervation of the lungs and airways and its functional significance. Rev Physiol Biochem Pharmacol 1984; 99:1–110.
7. Carr MJ, Undem BJ. Pharmacology of vagal afferent nerve activity in guinea pig airways. Pulm Pharmacol Ther 2003; 16(1):45–52.
8. Baluk P, Nadel JA, McDonald DM. Substance P-immunoreactive sensory axons in the rat respiratory tract: a quantitative study of their distribution and role in neurogenic inflammation. J Comp Neurol 1992; 319(4):586–598.

9. Mazzone SB. Targeting tachykinins for the treatment of obstructive airways disease. Treat Respir Med 2004; 3(4):201–216.

10. Hunter DD, Undem BJ. Identification and substance P content of vagal afferent neurons innervating the epithelium of the guinea pig trachea. Am J Respir Crit Care Med 1999; 159(6):1943–1948.

11. Riccio MM, Kummer W, Biglari B, Myers AC, Undem BJ. Interganglionic segregation of distinct vagal afferent fibre phenotypes in guinea-pig airways. J Physiol 1996; 496(Pt 2):521–530.

12. Eccles R. Anatomy and physiology of the nose and control of the nasal airflow. In: Adkinson NF, Yunginger JW, Busse WW, Bochner BS, Holgate ST, Simons FER, eds. Allergy. Philadelphia: Mosby, 2003:775–789.

13. Dinh QT, Groneberg DA, Mingomataj E, Peiser C, Heppt W, Dinh S, Arck PC, Klapp BF, Fischer A. Expression of substance P and vanilloid receptor (VR1) in trigeminal sensory neurons projecting to the mouse nasal mucosa. Neuropeptides 2003; 37(4):245–250.

14. Hunter DD, Dey RD. Identification and neuropeptide content of trigeminal neurons innervating the rat nasal epithelium. Neuroscience 1998; 83(2): 591–599.

15. Stjarne P, Lundblad L, Anggard A, Hokfelt T, Lundberg JM. Tachykinins and calcitonin gene-related peptide: co-existence in sensory nerves of the nasal mucosa and effects on blood flow. Cell Tissue Res 1989; 256(3):439–446.

16. Agostoni E, Chinnock JE, De Burgh Daly M, Murray JG. Functional and histological studies of the vagus nerve and its branches to the heart, lungs and abdominal viscera in the cat. J Physiol 1957; 135:182–205.

17. Kummer W, Fischer A, Kurkowski R, Heym C. The sensory and sympathetic innervation of guinea-pig lung and trachea as studied by retrograde neuronal tracing and double-labelling immunohistochemistry. Neuroscience 1992; 49(3):715–737.

18. Undem BJ, Chuaychoo B, Lee MG, Weinreich D, Myers AC, Kollarik M. Subtypes of vagal afferent C-fibers in guinea-pig lungs. J Physiol 2004; 556(3):905–917.

19. Widdicombe J. Airway receptors. Respir Physiol 2001; 125(1–2):3–15.

20. Mortola J, Sant'Ambrogio G, Clement MG. Localization of irritant receptors in the airways of the dog. Respir Physiol 1975; 24(1):107–114.

21. Canning BJ, Mazzone SB, Meeker SN, Mori N, Reynolds SM, Undem BJ. Identification of the tracheal and laryngeal afferent neurones mediating cough in anaesthetized guinea-pigs. J Physiol 2004; 557(2):543–558.

22. Brouns I, Van Genechten J, Hayashi H, Gajda M, Gomi T, Burnstock G, Timmermans JP, Adriaensen D. Dual sensory innervation of pulmonary neuroepithelial bodies. Am J Respir Cell Mol Biol 2003; 28(3):275–285.

23. Adriaensen D, Brouns I, Van Genechten J, Timmermans JP. Functional morphology of pulmonary neuroepithelial bodies: extremely complex airway receptors. Anat Rec 2003; 270A(1):25–40.

24. Fain GL. Molecular and Cellular Physiology of the Neurons. Cambridge: Harvard University Press, 1999.

25. Carr MJ, Undem BJ. Ion channels in airway afferent neurons. Respir Physiol 2001; 125(1–2):83–97.

26. Fox AJ, Barnes PJ, Dray A. Stimulation of guinea-pig tracheal afferent fibres by non-isosmotic and low-chloride stimuli and the effect of frusemide. J Physiol 1995; 482(Pt 1):179–187.

27. Pedersen KE, Meeker SN, Riccio MM, Undem BJ. Selective stimulation of jugular ganglion afferent neurons in guinea pig airways by hypertonic saline. J Appl Physiol 1998; 84(2):499–506.

28. Koskela H, Di Sciascio MB, Anderson SD, Andersson M, Chan HK, Gadalla S, Katelaris C. Nasal hyperosmolar challenge with a dry powder of mannitol in patients with allergic rhinitis. Evidence for epithelial cell involvement. Clin Exp Allergy 2000; 30(11):1627–1636.

29. Lee LY, Pisarri TE. Afferent properties and reflex functions of bronchopulmonary C-fibers. Respir Physiol 2001; 125(1–2):47–65.

30. Agopyan N, Li L, Yu S, Simon SA. Negatively charged 2- and 10-microm particles activate vanilloid receptors, increase cAMP, and induce cytokine release. Toxicol Appl Pharmacol 2003; 186(2):63–76.

31. Otto D, Molhave L, Rose G, Hudnell HK, House D. Neurobehavioral and sensory irritant effects of controlled exposure to a complex mixture of volatile organic compounds. Neurotoxicol Teratol 1990; 12(6):649–652.

32. Shusterman D. Toxicology of nasal irritants. Curr Allergy Asthma Rep 2003; 3(3):258–265.

33. Ekblom A, Flock A, Hansson P, Ottoson D. Ultrastructural and electrophysiological changes in the olfactory epithelium following exposure to organic solvents. Acta Otolaryngol 1984; 98(3–4):351–361.

34. van Thriel C, Seeber A, Kiesswetter E, Blaszkewicz M, Golka K, Wiesmuller GA. Physiological and psychological approaches to chemosensory effects of solvents. Toxicol Lett 2003; 140–141:261–271.

35. Vennekens R, Voets T, Bindels RJ, Droogmans G, Nilius B. Current understanding of mammalian TRP homologues. Cell Calcium 2002; 31(6):253–264.

36. Caterina MJ, Julius D. The vanilloid receptor: a molecular gateway to the pain pathway. Annu Rev Neurosci 2001; 24:487–517.

37. Trevisani M, Smart D, Gunthorpe MJ, Tognetto M, Barbieri M, Campi B, Amadesi S, Gray J, Jerman JC, Brough SJ, Owen D, Smith GD, Randall AD, Harrison S, Bianchi A, Davis JB, Geppetti P. Ethanol elicits and potentiates nociceptor responses via the vanilloid receptor-1. Nat Neurosci 2002; 5(6):546–551.

38. Veronesi B, Oortgiesen M. Neurogenic inflammation and particulate matter (PM) air pollutants. Neurotoxicology 2001; 22(6):795–810.

39. Veronesi B, Oortgiesen M, Roy J, Carter JD, Simon SA, Gavett SH. Vanilloid (capsaicin) receptors influence inflammatory sensitivity in response to particulate matter. Toxicol Appl Pharmacol 2000; 169(1):66–76.

40. Veronesi B, Wei G, Zeng JQ, Oortgiesen M. Electrostatic charge activates inflammatory vanilloid (VR1) receptors. Neurotoxicology 2003; 24(3):463–473.

41. Jordt SE, Bautista DM, Chuang HH, McKemy DD, Zygmunt PM, Hogestatt ED, Meng ID, Julius D. Mustard oils and cannabinoids excite sensory nerve fibres through the TRP channel ANKTM1. Nature 2004; 427(6971):260–265.

42. Fox AJ, Barnes PJ, Urban L, Dray A. An in vitro study of the properties of single vagal afferents innervating guinea-pig airways. J Physiol 1993; 469: 21–35.

43. Carr MJ, Schechter NM, Undem BJ. Trypsin-induced, neurokinin-mediated contraction of guinea pig bronchus. Am J Respir Crit Care Med 2000; 162(5):1662–1667.

44. Ho CY, Gu Q, Hong JL, Lee LY. Prostaglandin E(2) enhances chemical and mechanical sensitivities of pulmonary C fibers in the rat. Am J Respir Crit Care Med 2000; 162(2 Pt 1):528–533.

45. Anton F, Peppel P. Central projections of trigeminal primary afferents innervating the nasal mucosa: a horseradish peroxidase study in the rat. Neuroscience 1991; 41(2–3):617–628.

46. Haxhiu MA, Yamamoto B, Dreshaj IA, Bedol D, Ferguson DG. Involvement of glutamate in transmission of afferent constrictive inputs from the airways to the nucleus tractus solitarius in ferrets. J Auton Nerv Syst 2000; 80(1–2): 22–30.

47. Canning BJ, Reynolds SM, Mazzone SB. Multiple mechanisms of reflex bronchospasm in guinea pigs. J Appl Physiol 2001; 91(6):2642–2653.

48. Mazzone SB, Canning BJ. Synergistic interactions between airway afferent nerve subtypes mediating reflex bronchospasm in guinea pigs. Am J Physiol Regul Integr Comp Physiol 2002; 283(1):R86–R98.

49. Mazzone SB. Sensory regulation of the cough reflex. Pulm Pharmacol Ther 2004; 17(6):361–368.

50. Woolf CJ, Salter MW. Neuronal plasticity: increasing the gain in pain. Science 2000; 288(5472):1765–1769.

51. Widdicombe J, Lee LY. Airway reflexes, autonomic function, and cardiovascular responses. Environ Health Perspect 2001; 109(suppl 4):579–584.

52. Myers AC. Transmission in autonomic ganglia. Respir Physiol 2001; 125(1–2): 99–111.

53. Golding-Wood PH. Observations on petrosal and vidian neurectomy in chronic vasomotor rhinitis. J Laryngol Otol 1961; 75:232–247.

54. Ellis JL, Undem BJ. Pharmacology of non-adrenergic, non-cholinergic nerves in airway smooth muscle. Pulm Pharmacol 1994; 7(4):205–223.

55. Canning BJ, Undem BJ. Evidence that distinct neural pathways mediate parasympathetic contractions and relaxations of guinea-pig trachealis. J Physiol 1993; 471:25–40.

56. Davis B, Roberts AM, Coleridge HM, Coleridge JC. Reflex tracheal gland secretion evoked by stimulation of bronchial C-fibers in dogs. J Appl Physiol 1982; 53(4):985–991.

57. Rogers DF. Motor control of airway goblet cells and glands. Respir Physiol 2001; 125(1–2):129–144.

58. Haberberger R, Schemann M, Sann H, Kummer W. Innervation pattern of guinea pig pulmonary vasculature depends on vascular diameter. J Appl Physiol 1997; 82(2):426–434.

59. Zimmerman MP, Pisarri TE. Bronchial vasodilation evoked by increased lower airway osmolarity in dogs. J Appl Physiol 2000; 88(2):425–432.

60. Pisarri TE, Giesbrecht GG. Reflex tracheal smooth muscle contraction and bronchial vasodilation evoked by airway cooling in dogs. J Appl Physiol 1997; 82(5):1566–1572.

61. Widdicombe J. The tracheobronchial vasculature: a possible role in asthma. Microcirculation 1996; 3(2):129–141.

62. Fryer AD, Maclagan J. Muscarinic inhibitory receptors in pulmonary parasympathetic nerves in the guinea-pig. Br J Pharmacol 1984; 83(4):973–978.

63. Barnes PJ. Muscarinic receptors in airways: recent developments. J Appl Physiol 1990; 68(5):1777–1785.

64. Fisher JT, Vincent SG, Gomeza J, Yamada M, Wess J. Loss of vagally mediated bradycardia and bronchoconstriction in mice lacking M2 or M3 muscarinic acetylcholine receptors. Faseb J 2004; 18(6):711–713.

65. Elbon CL, Jacoby DB, Fryer AD. Pretreatment with an antibody to interleukin-5 prevents loss of pulmonary M2 muscarinic receptor function in antigen-challenged guinea pigs. Am J Respir Cell Mol Biol 1995; 12(3): 320–328.

66. Larsen GL, Fame TM, Renz H, Loader JE, Graves J, Hill M, Gelfand EW. Increased acetylcholine release in tracheas from allergen-exposed IgE-immune mice. Am J Physiol 1994; 266(3 Pt 1):L263–L270.

67. Schultheis AH, Bassett DJ, Fryer AD. Ozone-induced airway hyperresponsiveness and loss of neuronal M2 muscarinic receptor function. J Appl Physiol 1994; 76(3):1088–1097.

68. Fryer AD, Jacoby DB. Muscarinic receptors and control of airway smooth muscle. Am J Respir Crit Care Med 1998; 158(5 Pt 3):S154–160.

69. Minette PA, Lammers JW, Dixon CM, McCusker MT, Barnes PJ. A muscarinic agonist inhibits reflex bronchoconstriction in normal but not in asthmatic subjects. J Appl Physiol 1989; 67(6):2461–2465.

70. Alarie Y. Irritating properties of airborne materials to the upper respiratory tract. Arch Environ Health 1966; 13(4):433–449.

71. Canning BJ. Neurology of allergic inflammation and rhinitis. Curr Allergy Asthma Rep 2002; 2(3):210–215.

72. Tai CF, Baraniuk JN. Upper airway neurogenic mechanisms. Curr Opin Allergy Clin Immunol 2002; 2(1):11–19.

73. Sanico AM, Atsuta S, Proud D, Togias A. Plasma extravasation through neuronal stimulation in human nasal mucosa in the setting of allergic rhinitis. J Appl Physiol 1998; 84(2):537–543.

74. Mazzone SB, Canning BJ. Central nervous system control of the airways: pharmacological implications. Curr Opin Pharmacol 2002; 2(3):220–228.

75. Kobayashi M, Cheng ZB, Tanaka K, Nosaka S. Is the aortic depressor nerve involved in arterial chemoreflexes in rats? Nerv Syst 1999; 78(1):38–48.

76. Choudry NB, Fuller RW, Pride NB. Sensitivity of the human cough reflex: effect of inflammatory mediators prostaglandin E2, bradykinin, and histamine. Am Rev Respir Dis 1989; 140(1):137–141.

77. Fuller RW, Dixon CM, Cuss FM, Barnes PJ. Bradykinin-induced bronchoconstriction in humans. Mode of action. Am Rev Respir Dis 1987; 135(1): 176–180.

78. Widdicombe JG. Nasal pathophysiology. Respir Med 1990; 84(suppl A):3–9; discussion 9–10.
79. McDonald DM, Bowden JJ, Baluk P, Bunnett NW. Neurogenic inflammation. A model for studying efferent actions of sensory nerves. Adv Exp Med Biol 1996; 410:453–462.
80. Baluk P. Neurogenic inflammation in skin and airways. J Investig Dermatol Symp Proc 1997; 2(1):76–81.
81. Widdicombe JG. Neuroregulation of the nose and bronchi. Clin Exp Allergy 1996; 26(suppl 3):32–35.
82. Sanico AM, Philip G, Proud D, Naclerio RM, Togias A. Comparison of nasal mucosal responsiveness to neuronal stimulation in non-allergic and allergic rhinitis: effects of capsaicin nasal challenge. Clin Exp Allergy 1998; 28(1): 92–100.
83. Gerrity TR, Weaver RA, Berntsen J, House DE, O'Neil JJ. Extrathoracic and intrathoracic removal of O3 in tidal-breathing humans. J Appl Physiol 1988; 65(1):393–400.
84. Costa DL, Schelegle ES. Irritant air pollutants. In: Swift DL FW, ed. Air Pollutants and the Respiratory Tract. New York, NY: Marcel Dekker, 1999: 119–145.
85. Yeates DB, Mussatto DJ, Hameister WM, Daza A, Chandra T, Wong LB. Bronchial, alveolar, and vascular-induced anaphylaxis and irritant-induced cardiovascular and pulmonary responses. Environ Health Perspect 2001; 109(suppl 4):513–522.
86. Nishino T, Tagaito Y, Isono S. Cough and other reflexes on irritation of airway mucosa in man. Pulm Pharmacol 1996; 9(5–6):285–292.
87. Stone PH, Godleski JJ. First steps toward understanding the pathophysiologic link between air pollution and cardiac mortality. Am Heart J 1999; 138(5 Pt 1):804–807.
88. Zareba W, Nomura A, Couderc JP. Cardiovascular effects of air pollution: what to measure in ECG? Environ Health Perspect 2001; 109(suppl 4): 533–538.
89. Opthof T. The normal range and determinants of the intrinsic heart rate in man. Cardiovasc Res 2000; 45(1):177–184.
90. Malik M, Camm AJ, eds. Heart Rate Variability. New York: Blackwell Futura, 1995.
91. Tsuji H, Larson MG, Venditti FJ Jr, Manders ES, Evans JC, Feldman CL, Levy D. Impact of reduced heart rate variability on risk for cardiac events. The Framingham Heart Study. Circulation 1996; 94(11):2850–2855.
92. Liao D, Cai J, Rosamond WD, Barnes RW, Hutchinson RG, Whitsel EA, Rautaharju P, Heiss G. Cardiac autonomic function and incident coronary heart disease: a population-based case-cohort study. The ARIC Study. Atherosclerosis Risk in Communities Study. Am J Epidemiol 1997; 145(8): 696–706.
93. Vaishnav S, Stevenson R, Marchant B, Lagi K, Ranjadayalan K, Timmis AD. Relation between heart rate variability early after acute myocardial infarction and long-term mortality. Am J Cardiol 1994; 73(9):653–657.

94. Pope CA III, Dockery DW. Epidemiology of particle effects. In: Holgate ST, Samet JM, Koren HS, Maynard RL, eds. Air Pollution and Health. San Diego, CA: Academic Press, 1999:673–705.

95. U.S. Environmental Protection Agency. Air quality criteria for particulate matter EPA/600/P-95/001cF. Research Triangle Park, NC: U.S. Environmental Protection Agency, 1996.

96. Peters A, Wichmann HE, Tuch T, Heinrich J, Heyder J. Respiratory effects are associated with the number of ultrafine particles. Am J Respir Crit Care Med 1997; 155(4):1376–1383.

97. Pope CA III, Dockery DW. Acute health effects of PM10 pollution on symptomatic and asymptomatic children. Am Rev Respir Dis 1992; 145(5): 1123–1128.

98. Romieu I, Meneses F, Ruiz S, Sienra JJ, Huerta J, White MC, Etzel RA. Effects of air pollution on the respiratory health of asthmatic children living in Mexico City. Am J Respir Crit Care Med 1996; 154(2 Pt 1):300–307.

99. Vedal S, Petkau J, White R, Blair J. Acute effects of ambient inhalable particles in asthmatic and nonasthmatic children. Am J Respir Crit Care Med 1998; 157(4 Pt 1):1034–1043.

100. Pope CA III, Verrier RL, Lovett EG, Larson AC, Raizenne ME, Kanner RE, Schwartz J, Villegas GM, Gold DR, Dockery DW. Heart rate variability associated with particulate air pollution. Am Heart J 1999; 138(5 Pt 1):890–899.

101. Peters A, Liu E, Verrier RL, Schwartz J, Gold DR, Mittleman M, Baliff J, Oh JA, Allen G, Monahan K, Dockery DW. Air pollution and incidence of cardiac arrhythmia. Epidemiology 2000; 11(1):11–17.

102. Wichmann HE, Mueller W, Allhoff P, Beckmann M, Bocter N, Csicsaky MJ, Jung M, Molik B, Schoeneberg G. Health effects during a smog episode in West Germany in 1985. Environ Health Perspect 1989; 79:89–99.

103. Peters A, Perz S, Doring A, Stieber J, Koenig W, Wichmann HE. Increases in heart rate during an air pollution episode. Am J Epidemiol 1999; 150(10): 1094–1098.

104. Ibald-Mulli A, Stieber J, Wichmann HE, Koenig W, Peters A. Effects of air pollution on blood pressure: a population-based approach. Am J Public Health 2001; 91(4):571–577.

105. Devlin RB, Ghio AJ, Kehrl H, Sanders G, Cascio W. Elderly humans exposed to concentrated air pollution particles have decreased heart rate variability. Eur Respir J Suppl 2003; 40:76s–80s.

106. Magari SR, Schwartz J, Williams PL, Hauser R, Smith TJ, Christiani DC. The association between personal measurements of environmental exposure to particulates and heart rate variability. Epidemiology 2002; 13(3):305–310.

107. Chan CC, Chuang KJ, Shiao GM, Lin LY. Personal exposure to submicrometer particles and heart rate variability in human subjects. Environ Health Perspect 2004; 112:doi:10.1289/ehp.6897.

108. Riediker M, Cascio WE, Griggs TR, Herbst MC, Bromberg PA, Neas L, Williams RW, Devlin RB. Particulate matter exposure in cars is associated with cardiovascular effects in healthy young men. Am J Respir Crit Care Med 2004; 169(8):934–940.

109. Gold DR, Litonjua A, Schwartz J, Lovett E, Larson A, Nearing B, Allen G, Verrier M, Cherry R, Verrier R. Ambient pollution and heart rate variability. Circulation 2000; 101(11):1267–1273.
110. Creason J, Neas L, Walsh D, Williams R, Sheldon L, Liao D, Shy C. Particulate matter and heart rate variability among elderly retirees: the Baltimore 1998 PM study. J Expo Anal Environ Epidemiol 2001; 11(2):116–122.
111. Wellenius GA, Coull BA, Godleski JJ, Koutrakis P, Okabe K, Savage ST, Lawrence JE, Murthy GG, Verrier RL. Inhalation of concentrated ambient air particles exacerbates myocardial ischemia in conscious dogs. Environ Health Perspect 2003; 111(4):402–408.
112. Wellenius GA, Saldiva PH, Batalha JR, Krishna Murthy GG, Coull BA, Verrier RL, Godleski JJ. Electrocardiographic changes during exposure to residual oil fly ash (ROFA) particles in a rat model of myocardial infarction. Toxicol Sci 2002; 66(2):327–335.
113. Liao D, Creason J, Shy C, Williams R, Watts R, Zweidinger R. Daily variation of particulate air pollution and poor cardiac autonomic control in the elderly. Environ Health Perspect 1999; 107(7):521–525.
114. Ibald-Mulli A, Timonen KL, Peters A, Heinrich J, Wolke G, Lanki T, Buzorius G, Kreyling WG, de Hartog J, Hoek G, ten Brink HM, Pekkanen J. Effects of particulate air pollution on blood pressure and heart rate in subjects with cardiovascular disease: a multicenter approach. Environ Health Perspect 2004; 112(3):369–377.
115. Peters A, Dockery DW, Muller JE, Mittleman MA. Increased particulate air pollution and the triggering of myocardial infarction. Circulation 2001; 103(23):2810–2815.
116. Gong H Jr, Sioutas C, Linn WS. Controlled exposures of healthy and asthmatic volunteers to concentrated ambient particles in metropolitan Los Angeles. Res Rep Health Eff Inst 2003(118):1–36; discussion 37–47.
117. Gong H Jr, Linn WS, Sioutas C, Terrell SL, Clark KW, Anderson KR, Terrell LL. Controlled exposures of healthy and asthmatic volunteers to concentrated ambient fine particles in Los Angeles. Inhal Toxicol 2003; 15(4):305–325.
118. Magari SR, Hauser R, Schwartz J, Williams PL, Smith TJ, Christiani DC. Association of heart rate variability with occupational and environmental exposure to particulate air pollution. Circulation 2001; 104(9):986–991.
119. Magari SR, Schwartz J, Williams PL, Hauser R, Smith TJ, Christiani DC. The association of particulate air metal concentrations with heart rate variability. Environ Health Perspect 2002; 110(9):875–880.
120. Muggenburg BA, Benson JM, Barr EB, Kubatko J, Tilley LP. Short-term inhalation of particulate transition metals has little effect on the electrocardiograms of dogs having preexisting cardiac abnormalities. Inhal Toxicol 2003; 15(4):357–371.
121. Derwent RG. Atmospheric chemistry. In: Holgate S, Samet JM, Koren HS, Maynard RL, eds. Air Pollution and Health. San Diego, CA: Academic Press, 1999:51–62.

122. Miller FJ, McNeal CA, Kirtz JM, Gardner DE, Coffin DL, Menzel DB. Nasopharyngeal removal of ozone in rabbits and guinea pigs. Toxicology 1979; 14(3):273–281.

123. Hu SC, Ben-Jebria A, Ultman JS. Longitudinal distribution of ozone absorption in the lung: quiet respiration in healthy subjects. J Appl Physiol 1992; 73(4):1655–1661.

124. Kirkpatrick MB, Sheppard D, Nadel JA, Boushey HA. Effect of the oronasal breathing route on sulfur dioxide-induced bronchoconstriction in exercising asthmatic subjects. Am Rev Respir Dis 1982; 125(6):627–631.

125. Koren HS, Devlin RB, Graham DE, Mann R, McGee MP, Horstman DH, Kozumbo WJ, Becker S, House DE, McDonnell WF, Bromberg PA. Ozone-induced inflammation in the lower airways of human subjects. Am Rev Respir Dis 1989; 139(2):407–415.

126. Weinmann GG, Liu MC, Proud D, Weidenbach-Gerbase M, Hubbard W, Frank R. Ozone exposure in humans: inflammatory, small and peripheral airway responses. Am J Respir Crit Care Med 1995; 152(4 Pt 1):1175–1182.

127. Bhalla DK. Ozone-induced lung inflammation and mucosal barrier disruption: toxicology, mechanisms, and implications. J Toxicol Environ Health B Crit Rev 1999; 2(1):31–86.

128. Foster WM, Stetkiewicz PT. Regional clearance of solute from the respiratory epithelia: 18–20 h postexposure to ozone. J Appl Physiol 1996; 81(3): 1143–1149.

129. Foster WM, Brown RH, Macri K, Mitchell CS. Bronchial reactivity of healthy subjects: 18–20 h postexposure to ozone. J Appl Physiol 2000; 89(5): 1804–1810.

130. Mautz WJ, Bufalino C. Breathing pattern and metabolic rate responses of rats exposed to ozone. Respir Physiol 1989; 76(1):69–77.

131. Nielsen GD, Hougaard KS, Larsen ST, Hammer M, Wolkoff P, Clausen PA, Wilkins CK, Alarie Y. Acute airway effects of formaldehyde and ozone in BALB/c mice. Hum Exp Toxicol 1999; 18(6):400–409.

132. Folinsbee LJ, Silverman F, Shephard RJ. Exercise responses following ozone exposure. J Appl Physiol 1975; 38(6):996–1001.

133. Coleridge JC, Coleridge HM, Schelegle ES, Green JF. Acute inhalation of ozone stimulates bronchial C-fibers and rapidly adapting receptors in dogs. J Appl Physiol 1993; 74(5):2345–2352.

134. Schelegle ES, Carl ML, Coleridge HM, Coleridge JC, Green JF. Contribution of vagal afferents to respiratory reflexes evoked by acute inhalation of ozone in dogs. J Appl Physiol 1993; 74(5):2338–2344.

135. McDonnell WF, Horstman DH, Hazucha MJ, Seal E Jr, Haak ED, Salaam SA, House DE. Pulmonary effects of ozone exposure during exercise: dose–response characteristics. J Appl Physiol 1983; 54(5):1345–1352.

136. Golden JA, Nadel JA, Boushey HA. Bronchial hyperirritability in healthy subjects after exposure to ozone. Am Rev Respir Dis 1978; 118(2):287–294.

137. Hackney JD, Linn WS, Mohler JG, Collier CR. Adaptation to short-term respiratory effects of ozone in men exposed repeatedly. J Appl Physiol 1977; 43(1):82–85.

138. Folinsbee LJ, Bedi JF, Horvath SM. Respiratory responses in humans repeatedly exposed to low concentrations of ozone. Am Rev Respir Dis 1980; 121(3):431–439.

139. Frank R, Liu MC, Spannhake EW, Mlynarek S, Macri K, Weinmann GG. Repetitive ozone exposure of young adults: evidence of persistent small airway dysfunction. Am J Respir Crit Care Med 2001; 164(7):1253–1260.

140. Tepper JS, Costa DL, Lehmann JR, Weber MF, Hatch GE. Unattenuated structural and biochemical alterations in the rat lung during functional adaptation to ozone. Am Rev Respir Dis 1989; 140(2):493–501.

141. McKinney WJ, Jaskot RH, Richards JH, Costa DL, Dreher KL. Cytokine mediation of ozone-induced pulmonary adaptation. Am J Respir Cell Mol Biol 1998; 18(5):696–705.

142. Solway J, Leff AR. Sensory neuropeptides and airway function. J Appl Physiol 1991; 71(6):2077–2087.

143. Krause JE, Takeda Y, Hershey AD. Structure, functions, and mechanisms of substance P receptor action. J Invest Dermatol 1992; 98(6 suppl):2S–7S.

144. Hazbun ME, Hamilton R, Holian A, Eschenbacher WL. Ozone-induced increases in substance P and 8-epi-prostaglandin F2 alpha in the airways of human subjects. Am J Respir Cell Mol Biol 1993; 9(5):568–572.

145. Murlas CG, Lang Z, Williams GJ, Chodimella V. Aerosolized neutral endopeptidase reverses ozone-induced airway hyperreactivity to substance P. J Appl Physiol 1992; 72(3):1133–1141.

146. Nagy JI, Iversen LL, Goedert M, Chapman D, Hunt SP. Dose-dependent effects of capsaicin on primary sensory neurons in the neonatal rat. J Neurosci 1983; 3(2):399–406.

147. Jimba M, Skornik WA, Killingsworth CR, Long NC, Brain JD, Shore SA. Role of C fibers in physiological responses to ozone in rats. J Appl Physiol 1995; 78(5):1757–1763.

148. Sterner-Kock A, Vesely KR, Stovall MY, Schelegle ES, Green JF, Hyde DM. Neonatal capsaicin treatment increases the severity of ozone-induced lung injury. Am J Respir Crit Care Med 1996; 153(1):436–443.

149. Takebayashi T, Abraham J, Murthy GG, Lilly C, Rodger I, Shore SA. Role of tachykinins in airway responses to ozone in rats. J Appl Physiol 1998; 85(2):442–450.

150. Tepper JS, Costa DL, Fitzgerald S, Doerfler DL, Bromberg PA. Role of tachykinins in ozone-induced acute lung injury in guinea pigs. J Appl Physiol 1993; 75(3):1404–1411.

151. Lilly CM, Drazen JM, Shore SA. Peptidase modulation of airway effects of neuropeptides. Proc Soc Exp Biol Med 1993; 203(4):388–404.

152. Joos G, Kips J, Pauwels R, van der Straeten M. The effect of tachykinins on the conducting airways of the rat. Arch Int Pharmacodyn Ther 1986; 280(suppl 2):176–190.

153. Yu XY, Undem BJ, Spannhake EW. Protective effect of substance P on permeability of airway epithelial cells in culture. Am J Physiol 1996; 271(6 Pt 1): L889–L895.

154. Liu S, Kuo HP, Sheppard MN, Barnes PJ, Evans TW. Vagal stimulation induces increased pulmonary vascular permeability in guinea pig. Am J Respir Crit Care Med 1994; 149(3 Pt 1):744–750.

155. Piedimonte G, Hoffman JI, Husseini WK, Hiser WL, Nadel JA. Effect of neuropeptides released from sensory nerves on blood flow in the rat airway microcirculation. J Appl Physiol 1992; 72(4):1563–1570.

156. Wagner U, Fehmann HC, Bredenbroker D, Yu F, Barth PJ, von Wichert P. Galanin and somatostatin inhibition of substance P-induced airway mucus secretion in the rat. Neuropeptides 1995; 28(1):59–64.

157. Foster WM, Costa DL, Langenback EG. Ozone exposure alters tracheobronchial mucociliary function in humans. J Appl Physiol 1987; 63(3):996–1002.

158. Schlesinger RB. Toxicology of sulfur oxides. In: Holgate ST, Samet JM, Koren HS, Maynard RL, eds. Air Pollution and Health. San Diego, CA: Academic Press, 1999:585–602.

159. Linn WS, Avol EL, Peng RC, Shamoo DA, Hackney JD. Replicated dose–response study of sulfur dioxide effects in normal, atopic, and asthmatic volunteers. Am Rev Respir Dis 1987; 136(5):1127–1134.

160. Sheppard D, Saisho A, Nadel JA, Boushey HA. Exercise increases sulfur dioxide-induced bronchoconstriction in asthmatic subjects. Am Rev Respir Dis 1981; 123(5):486–491.

161. Bethel RA, Erle DJ, Epstein J, Sheppard D, Nadel JA, Boushey HA. Effect of exercise rate and route of inhalation on sulfur-dioxide-induced bronchoconstriction in asthmatic subjects. Am Rev Respir Dis 1983; 128(4):592–596.

162. Hajj AM, Burki NK, Lee LY. Role of tachykinins in sulfur dioxide-induced bronchoconstriction in anesthetized guinea pigs. J Appl Physiol 1996; 80(6):2044–2050.

163. Long NC, Martin JG, Pantano R, Shore SA. Airway hyperresponsiveness in a rat model of chronic bronchitis: role of C fibers. Am J Respir Crit Care Med 1997; 155(4):1222–1229.

164. Tunnicliffe WS, Hilton MF, Harrison RM, Ayres JG. The effect of sulphur dioxide exposure on indices of heart rate variability in normal and asthmatic adults. Eur Respir J 2001; 17(4):604–608.

165. Schlesinger RB. Comparative irritant potency of inhaled sulfate aerosols—effects on bronchial mucociliary clearance. Environ Res 1984; 34(2):268–279.

166. Utell MJ, Morrow PE, Hyde RW. Airway reactivity to sulfate and sulfuric acid aerosols in normal and asthmatic subjects. J Air Pollut Control Assoc 1984; 34(9):931–935.

167. Utell MJ, Mariglio JA, Morrow PE, Gibb FR, Spears DM. Effects of inhaled acid aerosols on respiratory function: the role of endogenous ammonia. J Aerosol Med 1989; 2:141–147.

168. Avol EL, Linn WS, Whynot JD, Anderson KR, Shamoo DA, Valencia LM, Little DE, Hackney JD. Respiratory dose–response study of normal and asthmatic volunteers exposed to sulfuric acid aerosol in the sub-micrometer size range. Toxicol Ind Health 1988; 4(2):173–184.

169. Frampton MW, Voter KZ, Morrow PE, Roberts NJ Jr, Culp DJ, Cox C, Utell MJ. Sulfuric acid aerosol exposure in humans assessed by bronchoalveolar lavage. Am Rev Respir Dis 1992; 146(3):626–632.

170. Koenig JQ, Covert DS, Larson TV, Pierson WE. The effect of duration of exposure on sulfuric acid-induced pulmonary function changes in asthmatic adolescent subjects: a dose–response study. Toxicol Ind Health 1992; 8(5): 285–296.

171. Hanley QS, Koenig JQ, Larson TV, Anderson TL, van Belle G, Rebolledo V, Covert DS, Pierson WE. Response of young asthmatic patients to inhaled sulfuric acid. Am Rev Respir Dis 1992; 145(2 Pt 1):326–331.

172. Ackermann-Liebrich U, Rapp R. Epidemiological effects of oxides of nitrogen, especially NO_2. In: Holgate ST, Samet JM, Koren HS, Maynard RL, eds. Air Pollution and Health. San Diego, CA: Academic Press, 1999: 561–584.

173. Robledo RF, Young RS, Lantz RC, Witten ML. Short-term pulmonary response to inhaled JP-8 jet fuel aerosol in mice. Toxicol Pathol 2000; 28(5):656–663.

174. Harris DT, Sakiestewa D, Robledo RF, Witten M. Protection from JP-8 jet fuel induced immunotoxicity by administration of aerosolized substance P. Toxicol Ind Health 1997; 13(5):571–588.

175. Robledo RF, Witten ML. NK1-receptor activation prevents hydrocarbon-induced lung injury in mice. Am J Physiol 1999; 276(2 Pt 1):L229–L238.

176. Harris DT, Sakiestewa D, Titone D, Robledo RF, Young RS, Witten M. Substance P as prophylaxis for JP-8 jet fuel-induced immunotoxicity. Toxicol Ind Health 2001; 16(7–8):253–259.

177. Turner CR, Stow RB, Talerico SD, Christian EP, Williams JC. Protective role for neuropeptides in acute pulmonary response to acrolein in guinea pigs. J Appl Physiol 1993; 75(6):2456–2465.

178. Wilkins CK, Clausen PA, Wolkoff P, Larsen ST, Hammer M, Larsen K, Hansen V, Nielsen GD. Formation of strong airway irritants in mixtures of isoprene/ozone and isoprene/ozone/nitrogen dioxide. Environ Health Perspect 2001; 109(9):937–941.

179. Wilkins CK, Wolkoff P, Clausen PA, Hammer M, Nielsen GD. Upper airway irritation of terpene/ozone oxidation products (TOPS). Dependence on reaction time, relative humidity and initial ozone concentration. Toxicol Lett 2003; 143(2):109–114.

180. Wolkoff P, Clausen PA, Wilkins CK, Hougaard KS, Nielsen GD. Formation of strong airway irritants in a model mixture of (+)-alpha-pinene/ozone. Atmos Environ 1999; 33(5):693–698.

181. Clausen PA, Wilkins CK, Wolkoff P, Nielsen GD. Chemical and biological evaluation of a reaction mixture of R-(+)-limonene/ozone: formation of strong airway irritants. Environ Int 2001; 26(7–8):511–522.

182. Kou YR, Wang CY, Lai CJ. Role of vagal afferents in the acute ventilatory responses to inhaled wood smoke in rats. J Appl Physiol 1995; 78(6): 2070–2078.

183. Kou YR, Lai CJ, Hsu TH, Lin YS. Involvement of hydroxyl radical in the immediate ventilatory responses to inhaled wood smoke in rats. Respir Physiol 1997; 107(1):1–13.

184. Lai CJ, Kou YR. Stimulation of vagal pulmonary C fibers by inhaled wood smoke in rats. J Appl Physiol 1998; 84(1):30–36.

185. Kleinman MT, Mautz WJ, Bjarnason S. Adaptive and non-adaptive responses in rats exposed to ozone, alone and in mixtures, with acidic aerosols. Inhal Toxicol 1999; 11(3):249–264.

186. Mautz WJ, Kleinman MT, Bhalla DK, Phalen RF. Respiratory tract responses to repeated inhalation of an oxidant and acid gas-particle air pollutant mixture. Toxicol Sci 2001; 61(2):331–341.

187. Yu J, Wang YF, Zhang JW. Structure of slowly adapting pulmonary stretch receptors in the lung periphery. J Appl Physiol 2003; 95(1):385–393.

7

Signal Transduction and Cytokine Expression in Particulate Matter (PM)-Induced Airway Remodeling

DIANNE M. WALTERS and JAMES C. BONNER

National Institute of Environmental Health Sciences, and
   CIIT Centers for Health Research, Research Triangle Park,
North Carolina, U.S.A.

I. Introduction

The inhalation of air pollution particulate matter (PM) has been associated with increased morbidity and mortality principally due to the physiologic impact of PM on the pulmonary and cardiovascular systems (1,2). Adverse respiratory effects in exposed human populations include increased asthmatic episodes and an increase in the prevalence of chronic bronchitis (3). Moreover, PM exposure could contribute to the increasing prevalence of chronic obstructive pulmonary disease (COPD) (4). Numerous studies with experimental animals have documented the effect of PM on various features of airway remodeling that occur during the pathogenesis of asthma and bronchitis, including inflammation, mucous cell metaplasia, airway smooth muscle thickening, and peribronchiolar fibrosis. These features of airway remodeling are illustrated in Fig. 1. However, the underlying cellular and molecular mechanisms that mediate PM-induced toxicity leading to these aspects of airway remodeling are poorly understood.

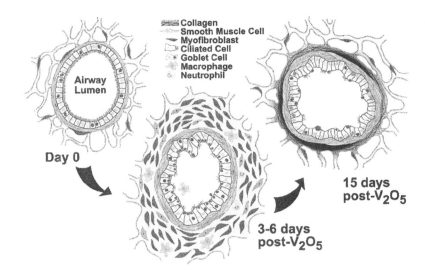

Figure 1   Airway remodeling following vanadium-induced lung injury. A single intra tracheal instillation of vanadium pentoxide (V_2O_5) in rats has been used to study cellular changes that occur during the pathogenesis of chronic airway diseases including bronchitis, asthma, and COPD (see Ref. 59). Vanadium-induced airway remodeling features mucous cell metaplasia, airway smooth muscle cell thickening, and peribronchiolar fibrosis.

In vitro mechanistic studies have proven invaluable in elucidating the mode of action of PM-induced toxicity at the cellular and molecular level. A variety of human and animal lung cell types have been utilized in studies with PM. Most of these investigations have focused on alveolar macrophages and airway epithelial cells, as these are the first cell types within the lung to encounter inhaled PM. Macrophages can be obtained with relative ease from human subjects through bronchoalveolar lavage, yet these cells must be used within a few hours after collection as they are terminally differentiated and cannot be grown in culture. Moreover, macrophages avidly engulf PM via phagocytosis and release a plethora of inflammatory mediators that are important in airway disease.

Human bronchial epithelial cells, usually obtained during lung transplant or at autopsy, have perhaps become the most intensely studied lung cell type. These cells can be stimulated to proliferate and can be maintained in a fully, differentiated state in an air–liquid interface system. A variety of immortalized human lung epithelial cell lines are also used in PM studies, such as BEAS-2B and H292 cells, and are valuable because they are easy to maintain and possess a high proliferative potential. However, a caveat is that these cell lines may not always accurately mimic the biological response of primary passage, differentiated human airway epithelial cells.

Finally, studies using mesenchymal cell types (fibroblasts and smooth muscle cells) are adding new information to our understanding of how PM affects airway smooth muscle thickening and airway fibrogenesis, respectively.

Despite the essential value of utilizing in vitro models, exposing cells in a dish to PM has some limitations. For example, one has to consider that the concentration of PM added to cells may not accurately reflect the dose of PM that accumulates within the airway during an in vivo exposure. Most in vitro studies use PM in suspension so that it can be distributed evenly within the cell culture system, whereas inhaled particles deposit directly on the surface of airway epithelial cells. Moreover, most in vitro experiments utilize a monolayer of a particular cell type. The complex interplay between pulmonary cell types that takes place within the lung cannot be adequately reproduced in such a simplistic and artificial setting. Nevertheless, much can be learned in these isolated systems in terms of how PM exerts its effects on cellular physiology, and this information can then be tested in the context of whole animal and ultimately human exposure studies.

A mixture of organic and inorganic agents contribute to the composition of PM, including transition metals released during the burning of petrochemicals (5,6), polycyclic aromatic hydrocarbons derived from diesel exhaust (7,8), and endotoxins from bacterial sources (9,10). Many of these constituents are known to stimulate a variety of intracellular signaling pathways that mediate cellular stress responses leading to the diversity of biological outcomes mentioned above that characterize airway remodeling. A major challenge to investigators in the field of PM research is to understand which signal transduction pathways lead to the gene expression profiles that mediate responses such as inflammation, cell proliferation, differentiation, and apoptosis. Cytokines and growth factors produced by a variety of airway cell types mediate many of these cellular responses. Understanding the intracellular signaling mechanisms that regulate cytokine expression after PM exposure is central to understanding airway remodeling.

The field of PM research is complicated by the heterogeneous nature of samples collected from various geographic sites and the possible interactive effects of PM-derived constituents. Many studies that have shed light on the cellular and molecular mechanisms through which PM exerts its pathophysiologic effects have come from studies aimed at the individual components of PM, such as transition metals, polycyclic aromatic hydrocarbons (PAH), and bacterial endotoxins. In this chapter, we will overview studies that have focused on the effects of PM on signal transduction and cytokine expression in a variety of airway cell types in order to address the issue of particle composition in mediating cytokine and growth factor expression associated with the pathology of airway disease.

II. Reactive Oxygen and Nitrogen Spcecies in Particle-Induced Lung Disease

A central principal to emerge from in vitro studies of PM is that reactive oxygen species (ROS) mediate many, if not all, of the biological effects of a variety of different particle types. The oxidative potential of PM is generally attributed to transition metals which can induce generation of ROS either via Fenton-like reactions, or by stimulating an oxidative burst in cells that have taken up PM. Particulate matter from a number of sources has been shown to induce oxidant generation that is associated with metal content of the sample. A number of studies have shown that residual oil fly ash (ROFA), a PM source rich in metal content, induces oxidant generation in alveolar macrophages and epithelial cells (11–13). In addition to resident cells of the lung, recruited inflammatory cells (i.e., neutrophils, macrophages, and eosinophils) have oxidant-generating capacity. Water-soluble metals appear to be particularly potent in inducing oxidant production (12). Likewise, diesel exhaust particles (DEP) and lipopolysaccharide (LPS) from gram negative bacteria have also been shown to stimulate the generation of ROS in alveolar macrophages. Phagocytosis of DEP by AM induces rapid oxidant generation leading to activation of apoptotic pathways (13). The organic constituents of DEP are likely responsible for these effects as extraction of PAHs and quinines abrogates ROS generation and apoptosis. Recently, stable radicals have been detected in $PM_{2.5}$ samples. These semiquinone radicals, derived from combustion of organic compounds such as tobacco or diesel fuel, can participate in redox cycling leading to sustained production of ROS (14). Thus, a variety of organic and inorganic constituents have the potential to cause ROS generation, either directly via redox chemistry or through stimulating pulmonary cells to increase ROS production.

Reactive oxygen species generated by PM exposure can act as signaling intermediates to activate intracellular signaling targets, including receptor tyrosine kinases, mitogen-activated protein (MAP) kinases, and transcription factors that in turn lead to transcriptional activation and the expression of genes involved in inflammation and airway remodeling. Inflammation following tissue injury is associated with increased generation of reactive oxygen species, such as superoxide anion ($O_2^{\bullet-}$) and hydrogen peroxide (H_2O_2) (15). Moreover, nitric oxide ($NO^{\bullet}$), which is synthesized by inflammatory cells, has the potential to react with $O_2^{\bullet-}$ via a nearly diffusion-limited reaction to form peroxynitrite ($ONOO^-$) (16). Reactive oxygen species and reactive nitrogen species (RNS) may serve physiological or pathophysiological functions. In the case of PM exposure, increased ROS and RNS production favors the latter outcome. For example, $NO^{\bullet}$ is thought to play a major role in host defense but is also presumed to contribute to tissue injury (17). Hydrogen peroxide and $O_2^{\bullet-}$-released into the extracellular environment by mononuclear cells during an oxidative burst may also play a role in immune defense, but can also mediate oxidant-induced cell injury and death (14). $ONOO^-$ is a potent cytotoxic species that has been proposed to contribute to the pathophysiology of a wide variety of inflammatory diseases. $ONOO^-$ principally causes the nitration of tyrosine residues on proteins and thereby modifies protein function, but also may induce oxidative reaction products through modifications of cysteine, methionine, and tryptophan. Nitrated proteins have been identified in lung tissue following exposure to particles and fibers (15,18), suggesting that $ONOO^-$ generation and subsequent tyrosine nitration leading to protein dysfunction could be a major factor in PM-induced airway disease.

Increasing evidence supports the idea that oxidants serve as signaling intermediates required for receptor tyrosine kinase function and downstream activation of MAP kinases. In particular, H_2O_2 generated intracellularly following the binding of platelet-derived growth factor (PDGF) or epidermal growth factor (EGF) to their respective receptors appears to reversibly inhibit protein tyrosine phosphatase activity which is required for phosphorylation of receptor tyrosine kinases (19,20). Inasmuch, low levels of oxidants serve as essential mediators of normal cell physiologic function, including proliferation, migration, and differentiation. For example, resting lung fibroblasts in culture generate micromolar levels of H_2O_2 that likely maintain their proliferative potential when stimulated with growth factors (21). This endogenously produced pool of H_2O_2 could also play an important role in mediating PM-induced gene expression and cytotoxic effects. In particular, vanadium that are associated with certain PM react with cell-derived H_2O_2 to form the potent protein tyrosine phosphatase (PTP) inhibitor, peroxovanadate. The PTP inhibition by agents such as H_2O_2 is reversible and necessary for normal cell function. However, PTP inhibition by peroxovanadate is irreversible and causes prolonged MAP kinase activation and cellular stress. Therefore, the timing of phosphorylation and dephosphorylation reactions within a cell is critical to normal cell function. Particulate matter and its metal constituents cause prolonged phosphorylation, leading to the increased production of proinflammatory mediators and ultimately causing cellular stress and apoptosis.

III. Inflammation and Induction of Proinflammatory Mediators
A. Cytokine Production

Various sources of PM cause airway inflammation and this early inflammatory response has been linked to the exacerbation of asthma and other adverse respiratory symptoms in exposed individuals. Numerous studies have focused on the ability of PM to induce the expression of proinflammatory cytokines and growth factors (Table 1). Particulate matter initially stimulates the airway epithelium and resident alveolar macrophages to release cytokines involved in the acute inflammatory response, such as

Table 1 Expression of PM-stimulated Cytokines by Lung Cells in Vitro and PM-Derived Agents Implicated in Cytokine Expression

PM sample	Cytokine	Agents	Cell type	Reference
ROFA	IL-6, MIP-2	V	Epithelial (RTE)	22,37
	IL-8, IL-6, TNF-α	—	Epithelial (NHBE)	27
	MIP-2, TNF-α	V	Macrophage (RAW264.7)	12
Utah Valley	IL-8	Cu	Epithelial (BEAS-2B)	23
	IL-8	Zn, V, Cu, Fe, Ni	Epithelial (NHBE)	46
Mexico city	TNF-α, IL-6	LPS, Cu, Zn, Ni	Monocyte (J774A.1)	24
UAP[a]	TNF-α, IL-6	LPS	Macrophage (human AM)	9,39
DEP	IL-8, GM-CSF, IL-1β	PAH	Epithelial (HBE)	25
	IL-8	PAH	Epithelial (HNEC)	26

[a]UAP-urban air particulates from St. Louis; Washington, D.C.; Ottawa; and Dusseldorff.

IL-1β, TNF-α, IL-6, and IL-8. These cytokines stimulate a variety of biologic responses. For example, IL-8 released by the airway epithelium is a potent chemokine that mediates neutrophil recruitment into the lung to resolve inflammation. Other cytokines, such as TNF-α and interleukin-13 (IL-13), stimulate airway mesenchymal cells (myofibroblasts and airway smooth muscle cells) to produce growth factors such as TGF-β and PDGF, which play a role in the development of airway fibrosis. Some of interactions between these cytokines and growth factors are illustrated in Fig. 2.

Many studies have focused on a specific constituent of PM that mediates cytokine production. For example, the transition metals such as vanadium and copper were found to mediate cytokine gene expression induced by ROFA and Utah Valley PM, respectively (22,23). In contrast, cytokine expression induced by Mexico City PM and urban air particulates from several other major cities was driven by LPS (9,24). Polycyclic aromatic hydrocarbons (PAH) caused cytokine production induced by DEP

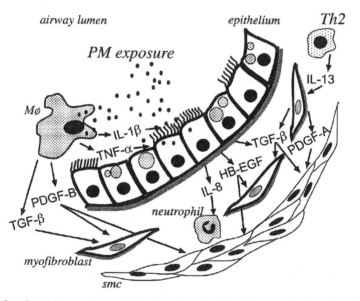

Figure 2 Cytokine and growth factors involved in airway cell signaling interactions following PM exposure. Particulate matter exposure first targets alveolar macrophages and airway epithelial cells and stimulates the expression of a variety of cytokines and growth factors that signal mesenchymal cells (myofibroblasts, smooth muscle cells) and inflammatory cells (neutrophils, Th2 lymphocytes) in the surrounding airway tissue. Some cytokines that are upregulated during acute inflammation (TNF-α, IL-1β, IL-13) appear to be important in stimulating the release of growth factors involved in chronic airway remodeling and fibrosis (TGF-β, PDGF).

(25,26). Airway epithelial cells and lung macrophages are the first to encounter inhaled particles. In particular, the airway epithelial cells serve not only as a physical barrier, but also function as an effector cell in the inflammatory process. Therefore, many investigators have utilized cultured lung epithelial cell lines or primary cultures to study the effects of PM on the expression of proinflammatory mediators. Epithelial cells have been shown to express several proinflammatory cytokines in response to various PM sources. For example, ROFA induces expression of IL-1β, IL-6, IL-8, and TNF-α in epithelial cells in vitro (Table 1). Each of these proinflammatory cytokines induce cellular responses that are linked to airway repair or remodeling. For example, IL-8 is a chemoattractant for neutrophils and PM-induced lung inflammation is characterized by neutrophilic and monocytic infiltration (27). IL-1β, TNF-α, and IL-6 stimulate the production of a variety of factors, including lipid mediators, proteinases, adhesion molecules, and other proinflammatory cytokines. The TNF-α appears to be critical for the development of fibrotic reactions, as it stimulates the production of TGF-β1 (28). TGF-β1 is a principal factor that increases collagen deposition by myofibroblasts adjacent to airways in the lung. Therefore, many of the proinflammatory cytokines that are upregulated early (i.e., within hours) by PM exposure mediate downstream events that culminate in the production of other cytokines and growth factors. These mediators, in turn, stimulate connective tissue cell growth and extracellular matrix deposition that alter airway wall structure.

Increasing evidence indicates that the inhalation of PMs increases symptom severity in allergic asthmatics (29). Asthma is characterized mainly as an immune response that features the recruitment of eosinophils and the subsequent production of Th2 type cytokines, including IL-13 and IL-4 (30). The majority of PM studies in rodent models have utilized a single exposure strategy that does not result in increased Th2 cytokines. However, a growing number of studies have demonstrated that under the appropriate experimental conditions in animals pre-exposed to a sensitizing agent PM has the ability to increase the expression of Th2 type cytokines. For example, Gavett et al. (31) showed that oil fly ash enhances Th2 cytokine production, eosinophil recruitment, and airway hyper-responsiveness in mice that were previously sensitized to ovalbumin. Diaz-Sanchez et al. (32) showed that DEP ehanced the production of Th2 cytokines in individuals exposed to ragweed allergen. These studies suggest that PM exacerbates allergic asthma at least in part by enhancing Th2 cytokine production.

B. Intracellular Signaling Pathways

A variety of agents associated with PM have the potential to stimulate cytokine production. Transition metals such as vanadium, zinc, copper, and arsenic have been reported to induce gene expression and secretion of a

Table 2 Transition Metals Associated with PM Mediating Cytokine Expression in Vitro and Implicated Intracellular Signaling Molecules

Constituent	Cytokine	Signaling molecule(s)	Cell type	Reference
Vanadium	TNF-α, IL-8	NF-κB	Epithelial (BEAS-2B)	27
	HB-EGF	EGFR, p38, ERK	Epithelial (NHBE)	45
	HB-EGF	EGFR, p38	Fibroblast (HLF)	47
Zinc	IL-8	EGFR	Epithelial (NHBE)	46
Copper	IL-8	NF-κB	Epithelial (BEAS-2B)	23
Arsenic	IL-8	NF-κB	Epithelial (NHBE)	36

variety of cytokines through the activation of several well-characterized signal transduction pathways (Table 2). Some of the signal transduction pathways targeted by PM that result in the expression of cytokine genes are illustrated in Fig. 3. For the most part, these metals act via oxidant-dependent mechanisms wherein free radicals (hydroxl radical and super-oxide) or hydrogen peroxide are generated (33,34). Jaspers et al. (35,36) have demonstrated that ROS generated from metals such as vanadium and arsenic are capable of activating transcription factors such as nuclear factor-κB (NF-κB), which is a major signaling molecule that mediates proin-flammatory cytokine production. Quay et al. (37) demonstrated that ROFA particles induced IL-6 expression through NF-κB activation in the BEAS-2B epithelial cell, line, and IL-6 expression was blocked by the free radical scavenger *N*-acetyl-L-cysteine and by the metal chelator deferoxamine (37). The mechanism through which ROS activate NF-κB is not clearly understood. However, NF-kB is a redox-sensitive transcription factor and therefore free radicals could play a role in its activation (38). Alternatively, some sources of PM also contain LPS, which binds to membrane CD14 and activates the toll-like receptor termed TLR4 to activate NF-κB and stimulate cytokine production (39,40).

Transition metals also stimulate cytokine and growth factor produc-tion via NF-κB-independent mechanisms. For example, the epidermal growth factor receptor (EGFR) is a central target of metal-induced oxida-tive stress (41). Reactive oxygen species reversibly inhibit PTPs associated with the intracellular domain of the EGFR. Inactivation of PTPs leads to EGFR phosphorylation and downstream activation of MAP kinase path-ways (42). The precise mechanisms through which the EGFR is activated likely depend on the particular metals in question. For example, vanadium is capable of generating H_2O_2 and forms peroxovanadate, which is struc-turally similar to the phosphate molecule and acts as a potent irreversible PTP inhibitor (43). Through PTP inhibiton, vanadium is capable of acti-vating the EGFR via a ligand-independent mechanism. However, metals

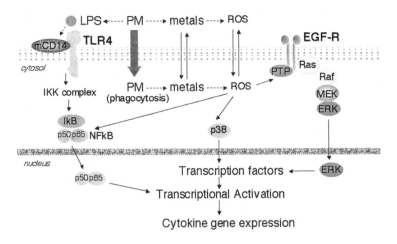

Figure 3 Activation of intracellular signaling pathways and cytokine gene expression by air pollution PM. Particulate matter-associated agents such as LPS or transition metals stimulate transcriptional activation via different mechanisms. Lipopolysaccharide binds membrane CD14 (mCD14) to activate the toll-receptor (TLR4) and thereby stimulate the NF-kB pathway. Transition metals such as V and Zn activate the EGFR signaling pathway leading to downstream phosphorylation of ERK via the generation of ROS. The ROS are also capable of activating p38 MAP kinase and NF-κB.

may also cause the release of cell-associated EGFR ligands to bind and activate the EGFR through ligand-dependent (i.e., ligand–receptor binding) mechanisms. Both zinc and vanadium have been shown to activate the EGFR in human bronchial epithelial cells at least in part by cleavage of the membrane-tethered EGFR ligand, HB-EGF (44,45).

Wu et al. (46) showed that PM collected from the Utah Valley containing Zn, Fe, Mn, Cu, V, Ni, and Pb activates the EGFR signaling pathway. In this study, the EGFR signaling pathway was shown to mediate IL-8 expression. However, whether EGFR activation was mediated by a specific metal in the mixture or an interaction between metals remains unclear. Individual metal components have been demonstrated to activate the EGFR signaling pathway. For example, vanadium alone can activate EGFR in human lung fibroblasts, leading to HB-EGF expression (47). V or Zn activates EGFR in human bronchial epithelial cells which result in Ras-dependent activation of MEK and ERK (48,49). It has also been reported that Src-dependent phosphorylation of EGFR is required for Zn-induced Ras activation (50). Thus, much is known regarding the mechanisms through which individual metals activate the EGFR signaling pathway, yet little is known regarding possible interactive or synergistic effects of metals within the PM mixture.

Mitogen-activated protein kinases are pivotal intracellular signaling proteins that function in cell growth, development, and differentiation (51). There are three major classes of MAP kinases: extracellular signal-regulated kinases (ERKs), c-Jun-N-terminal kinases (JNKs), and p38 MAP kinases. All of these MAP kinases are targets of oxidative stress, making them prime targets for PM-induced cytokine expression and apoptosis (52,53). Several components of PM are known to activate all three classes of MAP kinases, including metals, LPS, and ROS generated from these constituents. In particular, the coactivation of ERKs and p38 MAP kinase are required to cause the production of several cytokines and growth factors. Carter et al. (54) reported that LPS-induced TNF-α production by human alveolar macrophages required p38 MAP kinase and ERK activation. Similarly, these same two MAP kinases were found to be required for vanadium-induced stimulation of HB-EGF production by human bronchial epithelial cells and human lung fibroblasts (45,47).

The intracellular signaling pathways that are activated by PM are complex due to the diversity of agents associated with particles. A plethora of information exists on the cell signaling pathways that are activated (or deactivated) by ROS, LPS, and a variety of purified transition metals associated with various PM samples. However, little is known regarding the interactive effects of these PM-derived constituents. PM-derived constituents likely have a multitude of interactive effects on cell signaling pathways and their associate biological responses. For example, Wagner et al. (55) demonstrated that endotoxin enhances ozone-induced mucous cell metaplasia in rat nasal epithelium. Imrich et al. (56) demonstrated that LPS priming of lung macrophages enhanced production of TNF-α following exposure to ambient PM. The signaling mechanisms that account for this enhanced biologic response after the combination of LPS and oxidative stress are not well understood. However, it is likely that cross-talk between LPS- and ROS-induced intracellular signaling pathways plays a significant role in the amplification of a biologic response to PM. For example, it is possible that LPS-induced signaling through TLR4 and ROS signaling through EGFR could converge to cause a biological response that is enhanced in magnitude compared to the activation of either TLR4 or EGFR alone. This concept emphasizes the potential importance of understanding how particle composition dictates the overall magnitude of biologic response to PM exposure.

IV. PM-Induced Airway Fibrotic Reactions
A. Vanadium as a Model of PM-Induced Chronic Bronchitis and COPD

Exposure to air pollution particulates has not been associated with progressive, lethal fibrotic reactions in the lung parenchyma as has been documented for other fibrotic agents such as asbestos fibers (57). However, airway remodeling in asthma, chronic bronchitis, and COPD features more subtle fibrotic lesions surrounding the small airways of the lung, basement membrane thickening and peribronchiolar fibrosis, that contribute to airway narrowing and loss of compliance (58). These observations have sparked a considerable focus on epithelial–fibroblast interactions in mediating the pathogenesis of airway fibrosis. Like parenchymal fibrosis, airway fibrosis involves the proliferation of myofibroblasts surrounding the airways and subsequent collagen deposition by these cells (59). Additionally, PM-induced airway fibrosis includes thickening of the subepithelial basement lamina and increased collagen deposition in the peribronchiolar region that surrounds the airway smooth muscle. Many of these changes are consistent with the pathology of chronic bronchitis and COPD. Vanadium pentoxide, a transition metal found in many sources of PM, causes airway remodeling reminiscent of chronic bronchitis and COPD and could serve as a useful model for these PM-associated diseases (59). The cellular changes observed during the progression of airway disease in rodents are illustrated in Fig. 1.

In vivo studies with vanadium pentoxide show similar airway pathology to that of ROFA-induced lesions, including peribronchiolar fibrosis and mucous cell metaplasia (59–61). Numerous studies with vanadium in vitro have demonstrated that this transition metal causes the activation of MAP kinases and a variety of transcription factors including NF-κB, AP-1, NFAT, p53, and STAT-1 (62–65). The activation of these transcription factors is dependent on the upstream activation of kinases. For example, Jaspers and coworkers reported that vanadium-induced NF-κB-dependent transcription depends on the activation of p38 MAP kinase in airway epithelial cells (35). Zhang et al. (45) showed that human bronchial epithelial cells exposed to vanadium-induced oxidative stress released HB-EGF, and this EGFR ligand was found to be a major mitogen for human lung myofibroblasts in culture. Moreover, this same investigation revealed that HB-EGF-induced mitogenesis of myofibroblasts was due in part to the autocrine release of FGF-2. The cytokine signaling between airway epithelial cells and myofibroblasts involving HB-EGF, along with other profibrotic growth factors such as TGF-β and PDGF, is illustrated in Fig. 2. Animal models of fibrosis also support a role for the EGFR and its ligands. Rice et al. (66) reported that a tyrphostin inhibitor of EGFR tyrosine kinase reduced vanadium-induced pulmonary fibrosis in rats. These studies indicate that HB-EGF and perhaps other EGFR ligands contribute to airway epithelial cell and fibroblast proliferation after exposure to vanadium-containing PM.

Certain particles contain negligible amounts of vanadium, but are rich in other transition metals. For example, Adamson et al. (67) investigated a PM sample collected from Ottawa, Ontario and reported that epithelial cell proliferation and fibrosis was due to zinc present in the PM sample. Particulate matter collected from Utah Valley was found to be rich in zinc and copper, and the presence of these metals correlated with PM-induced IL-8 production (23,48). These investigators subsequently found that zinc mediates the cleavage of HB-EGF from the cell membrane of the airway epithelium, which then activates the EGFR to cause epithelial cell proliferation (46). Therefore, HB-EGF may also be an important mediator of airway fibrosis and remodeling after exposure to PMs that are rich in zinc. Thus, while different metals mediate the toxic effects of various PM sources, some of these transition metals exert their toxic effects through common signaling pathways.

B. Profibrotic Cytokines and Growth Factors

Fibrosis is characterized by the proliferation of lung myofibroblasts and the excessive production of collagen and other extracellular matrix proteins by these cells. A variety of growth factors and cytokines have been implicated in the pathogenesis of fibrosis. Many of these profibrotic peptides are expressed days after exposure to a fibrotic agent. Most studies with PM have addressed the acute response of pulmonary inflammation, while relatively little attention has been paid to chronic airway remodeling. However, cytokines that are elevated during acute inflammation could play a role in the development of airway fibrosis. For example, many PM samples that are rich in metals or contain LPS stimulate the release of IL-1β and TNF-α. These cytokines are elevated within hours after PM exposure and do not directly promote myofibroblast growth or the deposition of extracellular matrix proteins. Instead, these early proinflammatory cytokines stimulate a variety of different biological effects, including the increased expression of profibrotic growth factors and their receptors. For example, TNF-α stimulates the production of TGF-β1, a major stimulator of collagen deposition (28). IL-1β increases the expression of PDGF-AA and its receptor on lung myofibroblasts (68,69).

The increased expression of PDGF α-receptor (PDGF-Rα) by IL-1β has been implicated in the progression of PM- and metal-induced airway fibrosis. Lindroos et al. (69) reported that PDGF-Rα is up-regulated in vivo following the intratracheal instillation of ROFA in rats. Upregulation of the PDGF-Rα is also strongly induced in the lungs of rats exposed to vanadium pentoxide (70). In these studies, it was demonstrated that vanadium or ROS generated by vanadium did not directly stimulate upregulation of growth factor receptors. Instead, vanadium-induced oxidative stress first caused IL-1β release by alveolar macrophages, which then served as the major stimulus for PDGF-Rα expression. Particulate matter from Mexico city has been reported to induce expression of the PDGF-Rα and this is mainly mediated through LPS adsorbed to the particles (10). Moreover, purified *Escherichia Coli* LPS has been reported as a potent inducer of the PDGF-Rα (71). Therefore, bacterial agents associated with PM as well as IL-1β

produced by PM-stimulated cells are capable of increasing PDGF-Rα expression.

The PDGF ligands are also upregulated by a variety of different particles and fibers. Particle-stimulated alveolar macrophages primarily secrete PDGF-B chain isoforms (PDGF-AB and PDGF-BB), whereas lung fibroblasts produce only the PDGF-AA isoform (72,73). Yamashita et al. (74) showed that PDGF-B chain isoforms are also involved in the augmentation of airway responsiveness through remodeling of airways in diesel exhaust PM-treated mice. Therefore, the coordinated upregulation of the PDGF isoforms and the PDGF-Rα could be important in mediating airway fibrosis following exposure to a variety of different types of PM.

Diesel exhaust particles have been reported to stimulate the release of IL-1β and TNF-α (75), and the role of these cytokines in promoting the induction of profibrotic growth factors has been discussed above. The DEP can also cause a Th2 type response when combined with allergen challenge. Diaz-Sanchez et al. (32) reported that Th2 cytokines, such as IL-13, are also increased in vivo in rodents following exposure to DEP. IL-13 is a key mediator that has been linked to the pathogenesis of asthma (30). Moreover, the overexpression of IL-13 in transgenic mice causes airway fibrosis, goblet cell hyperplasia, and eosinophilic inflammation (76). Little is known regarding the mechanisms through which DEP mediates airway remodeling and fibrosis. However, since IL-13 is upregulated by DEP, it is likely that this cytokine contributes to the pathogenesis of DEP-induced airway disease. IL-13 also stimulates the release of profibrotic growth factors. Lee et al. (77) have reported that IL-13 stimulates the expression of TGF-β1, a potent stimulator of collagen deposition. Ingram et al. (78) recently reported that IL-13 induced the secretion of PDGF-AA in lung fibroblasts. These observations suggest that DEP could stimulate IL-13 to signal the autocrine or paracrine release of growth factors that mediate airway fibrogenesis.

As mentioned above, TGF-β1 is a central mediator of collagen deposition during the progression of fibrosis. The overexpression of TGF-β1 in mice by adenoviral vectors causes massive fibrotic reactions (79). Moreover, the overexpression of either TNF-α or IL-13 causes similar fibrotic reactions and this has been attributed to TGF-β1 expression (28,80). Therefore, TGF-β1 is downstream of TNF-α and IL-13, and these cytokines upregulate collagen production via TGF-β1. Moreover, TGF-β1 causes the production of another profibrotic cytokine termed connective tissue growth factor (CTGF) that has been implicated in the progression of pulmonary fibrosis (81). It is likely that PM exposure activates numerous cytokine/growth factor cascades that lead to airway remodeling and fibrosis in chronically exposed individuals.

V. PM-Induced Airway Epithelial Cell Growth and Differentiation

A. EGFR and Mucous Cell Metaplasia

Airway epithelial cell growth and differentiation are central features of remodeling during chronic inflammatory disease processes such as asthma and bronchitis. In particular, mucous cell metaplasia and the formation of mucus-producing goblet cells contribute to the pathology of these diseases. Particulate matter-induced oxidative stress has been shown to stimulate the differentiation of airway epithelial cells to a mucin-producing, secretory cell phenotype (82,83). A major target of PM-induced toxicity that could mediate airway epithelial cell differentiation and mucin production is the EGFR.

The EGFR and its ligands are elevated during the pathogenesis of asthma in humans, and induction of this system correlates with goblet cell hyperplasia in the airways of asthmatics (84,85). Understanding the mechanisms that regulate the EGFR and its ligands in mediating mucous hypersecretion by airway epithelial cells has become an active area of research in attempts to understand airway remodeling in asthma. The role of EGFR and its ligands in orchestrating epithelial growth, repair, and differentiation during airway remodeling following PM exposure is complex and involves: (1) the cleavage and release of membrane-bound EGFR ligands (TGF-α, HB-EGF) from the cell membrane by a variety of endogenous mediators that activate metalloproteinases, (2) inflammatory cytokines (e.g., TNF-α) and proteinases (e.g., neutrophil elastase) produced by leukocytes that have the potential to induce EGFR expression, and (3) the ligand-independent activation of EGFR by ROS generated by leukocytes or by inhaled pollutants.

The mechanisms through which PM causes mucin production are not clearly understood and direct evidence is lacking. However, there is clear evidence that PM and PM-derived metals can activate the EGFR and the activation of this receptor has been tied to mucin hypersecretion. Takeyama et al. (86) first identified the EGFR system as a regulatory axis for mucin production in airways. Prior to this work, it had been reported that neutrophils mediated goblet cell degranulation, and this was associated with increased elastase activity (87). Moreover, neutrophil elastase has been shown to increase the mRNA stability of MUC5AC (a major respiratory mucin) and increased production of MUC5AC glycoprotein via the generation of ROS (88). Recently, Kohri et al. (89) demonstrated that neutrophil elastase triggers cleavage of membrane-tethered TGF-α to bind and phosphorylate EGFR in an autocrine manner, resulting in downstream signaling pathways that culminate in the expression of MUC5AC. It is presently unclear whether neutrophil elastase mediates the activation of the EGFR after the inhalation of PM. It is reasonable to speculate that elastase may play a role as neutrophilic infiltration is a feature of PM-induced airway inflammation. However, PM has been shown to activate the EGFR via elastase-independent-mechanisms. Metals associated with certain PM samples, including vanadium and zinc, have been reported to activate the EGFR either through ligand-independent mechanisms or by stimulating the autocrine shedding of the membrane-tethered EGFR ligand, HB-EGF (44,45).

B. EGFR and Epithelial Cell Proliferation

Other cytokines that are upregulated during PM-induced airway remodeling may also exert their biologic effects via the EGFR system. Interleukin-13, a Th2 cytokine, plays a critical role in the pathogenesis of asthma and recent reports have linked IL-13-induced airway epithelial cell proliferation and mucin production to EGFR activation. Booth et al. (90) reported that IL-13 stimulated the release of TGF-α from the membranes of human bronchial epithelial cells, which then bound to the EGFR and initiated proliferation. Shim et al. (91) demonstrated that the intratracheal instillation of IL-13 into the lungs of rats caused goblet cell metaplasia and increased mucin production via a complex mechanism wherein IL-13 induced the production of IL-8, thereby causing neutrophil recruitment. In that study, the authors proposed that TNF-α secreted by recruited neutrophils induced EGFR expression in the airway epithelium. Recently, these investigators reported that IL-13 stimulates EGFR activation and mucin production by activating TNFα-converting enzyme, TACE (92).

Inhaled pollutants that cause airway inflammation and remodeling also have the capacity to trigger EGFR phosphorylation through ligand-independent mechanisms. Ligand-independent receptor activation is a mechanism wherein exogenous stressors (e.g., ROS, metals) enter the cells and by-pass the extracellular, ligand-binding domain of the EGFR to activate the intracellular domain of the receptor (93,94). This concept is illustrated in Fig. 3, where PM-induced metals generate H_2O_2, which then activates the EGFR and downstream signaling pathway leading to transcriptional activation and biological responses such as increased cytokine production. A variety of environmental agents that generate oxidative stress can activate EGFR via ligand-independent activation, and this is most likely achieved through inhibition of phosphatase activity associated with the kinase domain of the EGFR (43). For example, metals associated with air pollution particulates such a vanadium are potent EGFR activators in bronchial epithelial cells and pulmonary myofibroblasts (48,93). These studies identify the EGFR as a common target of pollutant-induced oxidative stress that mediates airway epithelial cell proliferation and/or mucin production.

Particulate matter-induced EGFR activation may also mediate inflammatory responses. As mentioned above, the activation of EGFR by Utah Valley PMs resulted in increased IL-8 release (46). IL-8 causes a neutrophilic infiltration that in many cases results in the resolution of an inflammatory response. It is therefore possible in some instances that the induction of proinflammatory mediators could serve to resolve an inflammatory response to favor tissue repair rather than a fibrotic outcome. Another example is the induction of COX-2 through activation of the EGFR (95). It is well known that PM activates the EGFR via a ligand-independent mechanisms wherein ROS generated from the PM or certain transition metals such as vanadium associated with the PM cause phosphatase inhibition that results in phosphorylation of tyrosine residues within the intracellular domain of the EGFR. While EGFR activation results in the expression of many proinflammatory and profibrotic mediators, the activation of this receptor also induces COX-2, which is the principal enzyme that metabolizes arachidonic acid to PGE_2. The PGE_2 released by lung cells binds to specific cell-surface EP receptors (96) and serves to suppress airway fibrogenesis in a number of ways, including suppression of fibroblast growth and chemotaxis, inhibition of collagen synthesis, and downregulation of growth factors such as CTGF (Fig. 4). Residual oil fly ash, which contains abundant vanadium, has also been shown to induce COX-2 (97). Moreover, COX-2 deficient mice have been shown to be

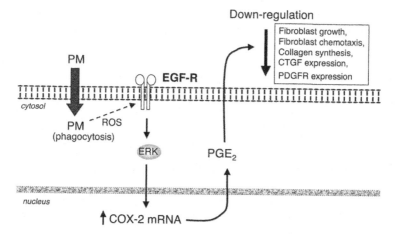

Figure 4   Induction of COX-2 expression by PM via the EGFR signaling cascade. Air pollution PM activates the EGFR via ROS-dependent mechanisms to signal MAP kinase activation and thereby increases COX-2 mRNA and protein. The COX-2 converts arachidonic acid to a variety of prostanoids, including PGE_2, which has an inhibitory effect on a variety of profibrotic outcomes, including fibroblast growth and collagen deposition.

susceptible to vanadium-induced lung fibrosis (98). One possible mechanism may involve the increased production of TNF-α in the COX-2 deficient mice. Another possibility is that PGE$_2$, which is generated by COX-2, serves to inhibit lung myofibroblast growth and this is mediated in part through downregulation of PDGF-Rα (99). These findings suggest that COX-2-derived mediators, particularly PGE$_2$, could be important antifibrotic mediators and that COX-2 plays a protective role against PM-induced airway fibrogenesis.

VI. Summary

Abundant evidence indicates that PM exposure causes adverse respiratory effects and represents the greatest risk to individuals with pre-existing respiratory diseases, such as asthma and chronic bronchitis. It is clear that PM from a number of different geographic locations causes inflammatory responses and remodeling of airway structure through the release of a variety of proinflammatory mediators, including cytokines, growth factors, proteinases, and lipid mediators. Our understanding of the mechanisms of PM-induced lung disease is complicated by the heterogeneous nature of PM samples and our lack of knowledge on the interactive effects of organic and inorganic PM-associated constituents. Nevertheless, considerable progress has been made toward understanding the cellular and molecular mechanisms through which PM exerts its toxic effects in the lung and in vitro models have proven extremely useful in this regard.

It is clear that oxidative stress is an underlying factor that contributes to the biological effects of PM. The ROS generated by both organic and inorganic constituents of PM enter cells through phagocytosis or diffusion across the cell membrane to target cell signaling proteins, including phosphatases, kinases, and redox-sensitive transcription factors. The EGFR has emerged as a central target for PM-induced toxicity in epithelial cells and fibroblasts. For example, in airway epithelial cells, it now appears that PM can cause a diversity of biological effects through activation of the EGFR, including mucin production, cell proliferation, and the production of numerous cytokines and growth factors. Therefore, air pollution PM acts as a cellular stressor that disrupts normal cell signaling pathways to promote or exacerbate airway diseases. TLR4 also appears to be a central target of PM that is activated by particle-associated endotoxins or perhaps by oxidative stress. TLR4 is linked to the NF-κB signaling pathway and this pathway is extremely important to proinflammatory cytokine expression during an inflammatory response.

Future endeavors should focus on cell systems that will allow a better understanding of cell–cell interactions during PM-induced airway disease. Epithelial–fibroblast interactions appear critical to the development of airway fibrosis and co-culture models may prove invaluable in this regard. A functional genomics and proteomics approach could be exceedingly important in establishing toxicogenomic profiles of different PM samples from urban areas. In general, a better understanding of the cellular and molecular mechanisms through which PM disrupts intracellular signaling pathways will allow us to more precisely regulate PM that contains constituents known to cause the greatest risk to human health.

References

1. Schwartz J. Particulate air pollution and chronic respiratory disease. Environ Res 1993; 62:7–17.
2. Dockery DW, Pope CA, Xu X, Spengler JD, Ware JH, Fay ME, Ferris BG, Speizer FE. An association between air pollution and mortality in six U.S. cities. N Engl J Med 1993; 329:1753–1759.
3. Pope CA III, Dockery DW, Schwartz J. Review of epidemiological evidence of health effects of particulate air pollution. Inhal Toxicol 1995; 7:1–18.
4. Anderson HR, Spix C, Medina S, Schouten JP, Castellsaque J, Rossi G, Zmirou D, Touloumi G, Wojtyniak B, Ponka A, Bacharova L, Schwartz J, Katsouyanni K. Air pollution and daily admissions for chronic obstructive pulmonary disease in 6 European cities: results from the APHEA project. Eur Respir J 1998; 10:1064–1071.
5. Kodavanti UP, Hauser R, Christiani DC, Meng ZH, McGee J, Ledbetter A, Richards J, Costa DL. Pulmonary responses to oil fly ash particles in the rat differ by virtue of their specific soluble metals. Toxicol Sci 1998; 43:204–212.
6. Dreher KL, Jaskot RH, Lehmann JR, Richards JH, McGee JK, Ghio AJ, Costa DL. Soluble transition metals mediate residual oil fly ash induced acute lung injury. J Toxicol Environ Health 1997; 50:285–305.
7. Diaz-Sanchez D, Jyrala M, Ng D, Nel A, Saxon A. In vivo nasal challenge with diesel exhaust particles enhances expression of the CC chemokines Rantes, MIP-1a, and MCP-3 in humans. Clin Immunol 2000; 97:140–145.
8. Nightingale JA, Maggs R, Cullinan P, Donnelly LE, Rogers DF, Kinnersley R, Fan Chung K, Barnes PJ, Ashmore M, Newman-Taylor A. Airway inflammation after controlled exposure to diesel exhaust particulates. Am J Respir Crit Care Med 2000; 162:161–166.
9. Becker S, Soukup JM, Gilmour MI, Devlin RB. Stimulation of human and rat alveolar macrophages by urban air particulates: effects of oxidant radical generation and cytokine production. Toxicol Appl Pharmacol 1996; 141:637–648.
10. Bonner JC, Rice AB, Lindroos PM, O'Brien PO, Dreher KL, Rosas I, Alfaro-Moreno E, Osornio-Vargas AR. Induction of the lung myofibroblast PDGF receptor system by urban ambient particles from Mexico city. Am J Respir Cell Mol Biol 1998; 19:672–680.
11. Kadiiska MB, Mason RP, Dreher KL, Costa DL, Ghio AJ. In vivo evidence of free radical formation in the rat lung after exposure to an emission source air pollution particle. Chem Res Toxicol 1997; 10:1104–1108.

12. Goldsmith CA, Imrich A, Danaee H, Ning YY, Kobzik L. Analysis of air pollution particulate-mediated oxidant stress in alveolar macrophages. J Toxicol Environ Health 1998; 54:529–545.

13. Hiura TS, Kaszubowski MP, Li N, Nel AE. Chemicals in diesel exhaust particles generate reactive oxygen radicals and induce apoptosis in macrophages. J Immunol 1999; 163:5582–5591.

14. Squadrito GL, Cueto R, Dellinger B, Pryor WA. Quinoid redox cycling as a mechanism for sustained free radical generation by inhaled airborne particulate matter. Free Rad Biol Med 2001; 31(9):1132–1138.

15. Rosen GM, Pou S, Ramos CL, Cohen MS, Britigan BE. Free radicals and phagocytic cells. FASEB J 1995; 9:200–209.

16. Pryor WA, Squadrito GL. The chemistry of peroxynitrite: a product from the reaction of nitric oxide with superoxide. Am J Physiol 1995; 268:L699–L722.

17. Carreras MC, Pargament GA, Catz SD, Poderoso JJ, Boveris A. Kinetics of nitric oxide and hydrogen peroxide production and formation of peroxynitrite during the respiratory burst of human neutrophils. FEBS Lett 1994; 34:65–68.

18. Zhu S, Manuel M, Tanaka S, Choe N, Kagan E, Matalon S. Contribution of reactive oxygen and nitrogen species to particulate-induced lung injury. Environ Health Perspect 1998; 106:1157–1163.

19. Sundaresan M, Yu ZX, Ferrans VJ, Irani K, Finkel T. Requirement for generation of H_2O_2 for platelet-derived growth factor signal transduction. Science 1995; 270:296–299.

20. Bae YS, Kang SW, Seo MS, Baines IC, Tekle E, Chock PB, Rhee SG. Epidermal growth factor (EGF)-induced generation of hydrogen peroxide. Role in EGF receptor-mediated tyrosine phosphorylation. J Biol Chem 1997; 272: 217–221.

21. Wang Y-Z, Ingram JL, Walters DM, Rice AB, Santos JH, Van Houten B, Bonner JC. Vanadium-induced STAT-1 activation in lung myofibroblasts requires H_2O_2 and p38 MAP kinase. Free Rad Biol Med 2003; 35:845–855.

22. Dye JA, Adler KB, Richards JH, Dreher KL. Role of soluble metals in oil fly ash-induced airway epithelial injury and cytokine gene expression. Am J Physiol 1999; 277:L498–L510.

23. Kennedy T, Ghio AJ, Reed W, Samet J, Zagorski J, Quay J, Carter J, Dailey L, Hoidal JR, Devlin RB. Copper-dependent inflammation and nuclear factor-κB activation by particulate air pollution. Am J Respir Cell Mol Biol 1998; 19: 366–378.

24. Osornio-Vargas AR, Bonner JC, Alfaro-Moreno E, Martinez L, Garcia-Cuellar C, Ponce-de-Leon Rosales S, Miranda J, Rosas I. Proinflammatory and cytotoxic effects of Mexico city air pollution particulate matter in vitro are dependent on particle size and composition. Environ Health Perspect 2003; 111:1289–1293.

25. Boland S, Baeza-Squiban A, Fournier T, Houcine O, Gendron MC, Chevrier M, Jouvenot G, Coste A, Aubier M, Marano F. Diesel exhaust particles are taken up by human airway epithelial cells in vitro and alter cytokine production. Am J Physiol 1999; 276:L604–L613.

26. Terada N, Hamano N, Maesako KI, Hiruma K, Hohki G, Suzuki K, Ishikawa K, Konno A. Diesel exhaust particulates upregulate histamine receptor mRNA

and increase histamine-induced IL-8 and GM-CSF production in nasal epithelial cells and endothelial cells. Clin Exp Allergy 1999; 29:52–59.

27. Carter JD, Ghio AJ, Samet JM, Devlin RB. Cytokine production by human airway epithelial cells after exposure to an air pollution particle is metal-dependent. Toxicol Appl Pharmacol 1997; 146:180–188.

28. Sime PJ, Marr RA, Gauldie D, Xing Z, Hewlett BR, Graham FL, Gauldie J. Transfer of tumor necrosis factor-α to rat lung induces severe pulmonary inflammation and patchy interstitial fibrogenesis with induction of transforming growth factor-β1 and myofibroblasts. Am J Pathol 1998; 153:825–832.

29. Salvi S, Holgate ST. Mechanisms of particulate matter toxicity. Clin Exp Allergy 1999; 29:1187–1194.

30. Wills-Karp M, Luyimbazi J, Xu X, Schofield B, Neben TY, Karp CL, Donaldson DD. Interleukin-13: central mediator of allergic asthma. Science 1998; 282:2258–2260.

31. Gavett S, Madison S, Stevens M, Costa D. Residual oil fly ash amplifies allergic cytokines, airway hyperresponsiveness, and inflammation in mice. Am J Respir Crit Care Med 1999; 160:1897–1904.

32. Diaz-Sanchez D, Tsien A, Fleming J, Saxon A. Combined diesel exhaust particulate and ragweed allergen challenge markedly enhance human in vivo nasal ragweed specific IgE and skew cytokine production to a Th2 type phenotype. J Immunol 1997; 158:2406–2413.

33. Pritchard RJ, Ghio AJ, Lehmann JR, Winsett DW, Tepper JS, Park P, Gilmour MI, Dreher KL, Costa DL. Oxidant generation and lung injury after particulate air pollutant exposure increase with the concentrations of associated metals. Inhal Toxicol 1996; 8:457–477.

34. Ghio AJ, Stonehuerner J, Pritchard RJ, Piantadosi CA, Quigley DR, Dreher KL, Costa DL. Humic-like substances in air pollution particulates correlate with concentrations of transition metals and oxidant generation. Inhal Toxicol 1996; 8:479–494.

35. Jaspers I, Samet JM, Erzurum S, Reed W. Vanadium-induced κB-dependent transcription depends upon peroxide induced activation of the p38 mitogen-activated protein kinase. Am J Respir Cell Mol Biol 2000; 23:95–102.

36. Jaspers I, Samet JM, Reed W. Arsenite exposure of cultured airway epithelial cells activates κB-dependent interleukin-8 gene expression in the absence of nuclear factor-κB nuclear translocation. J Biol Chem 1999; 274:31025–31033.

37. Quay JL, Reed W, Samet J, Devlin RB. Air pollution particles induced IL-6 gene expression in human airway epithelial cells via NF-kappaB activation. Am J Respir Cell Mol Biol 1998; 19:98–106.

38. Bowie A, O'Neill LA. Oxidative stress and nuclear factor-kappaB activation: a reassessment of the evidence in the light of recent discoveries. Biochem Pharmacol 2000; 59:13–23.

39. Soukup JM, Becker S. Human alveolar macrophage responses to air pollution particulates are associated with insoluble components of course material, including particulate endotoxin. Toxicol Appl Pharmacol 2001; 171:20–26.

40. Bowie A, O'Neill LA. The interleukin-1 receptor/Toll-like superfamily: signal generators for pro-inflammatory interleukins and microbial products. J Leukoc Biol 2000; 67:508–514.

41. Bonner JC. The epidermal growth factor receptor at the crossroads of airway remodeling. Am J Physiol 2002; 283:L528–L530.
42. Guyton KZ, Liu Y, Gorospe M, Xu Q, Holbrook ML. Activation of mitogen-activated protein kinase by H_2O_2. Role in cell survival following oxidant injury. J Biol Chem 1996; 271:4138–4142.
43. Samet JM, Stonehuerner J, Reed W, Devlin RB, Dailey LA, Kennedy TP, Bromberg PA, Ghio AJ. Disruption of protein tyrosine phosphate homeostasis in bronchial epithelial cells exposed to oil fly ash. Am J Physiol 1997; 272: L426–L432.
44. Wu W, Samet JM, Silbajoris R, Dailey LA, Sheppard D, Bromberg PA, Graves LM. Heparin-binding EGF cleavage mediates zinc-induced EGF receptor phosphorylation. Am J Respir Cell Mol Biol 2004; 30:540–547.
45. Zhang L, Rice AB, Adler K, Sannes P, Martin L, Gladwell W, Koo JS, Gray TE, Bonner JC. Vanadium stimulates human bronchial epithelial cells to produce heparin- binding epidermal growth factor-like growth factor: a mitogen for lung fibroblasts. Am J Respir Cell Mol Biol 2001; 24:123–131.
46. Wu W, Samet JM, Ghio AJ, Devlin RB. Activation of the EGF receptor signaling pathway in airway epithelial cells exposed to Utah Valley PM. Am J Physiol 2001; 281:L483–L489.
47. Ingram JL, Rice AB, Santos J, Van Houten B, Bonner JC. Vanadium-induced HB-EGF expression in human lung fibroblasts is oxidant dependent and requires MAP kinases. Am J Physiol 2003; 284:L774–L782.
48. Wu W, Graves LM, Jaspers I, Devlin RB, Reed W, Samet JM. Activation of the EGF receptor signaling pathway in human airway epithelial cells exposed to metals. Am J Physiol 1999; 277:L924–L931.
49. Wu W, Jaspers I, Zhang W, Graves LM, Samet JM. Role of Ras in metal-induced EGF receptor signaling and NF-κB activation in human airway epithelial cells. Am J Physiol 2002; 282:L1040–L1048.
50. Wu W, Graves LM, Gill GN, Parsons SJ, Samet JM. Src-dependent phosphorylation of the epidermal growth factor receptor on tyrosine 845 is required for zinc-induced Ras activation. J Biol Chem 2002; 277:24252–24257.
51. Davis RJ. Transcriptional regulation by MAP kinases. Mol Reprod Devel 1995; 42:459–467.
52. Martindale JL, Holbrook NJ. Cellular response to oxidative stress: signaling for suicide and survival. J Cell Physiol 2002; 192:1–15.
53. Torres M. Mitogen-activated protein kinase pathways in redox signaling. Front Biosci 2003; 8:369–391.
54. Carter AB, Monick MM, Hunninghake GW. Both ERK and p38 kinases are necessary for cytokine gene transcription. Am J Respir Cell Mol Biol 1999; 20:751–758.
55. Wagner JG, Van Dyken SJ, Hotchkiss JA, Harkema JR. Endotoxin enhancement of ozone-induced mucous cell metaplasia is neutrophil-dependent in rat nasal epithelium. Tox Sci 2001; 60:338–347.
56. Imrich A, Ning YY, Koziel H, Coull B, Kobzik L. Lipopolysaccharide priming amplifies lung macrophage tumor necrosis factor production in response to air particles. Toxicol Appl Pharmacol 1999; 159:117–124.

57. Rom WN, Travis WD, Brody AR. Cellular and molecular basis of the asbestos-related diseases. Am Rev Respir Dis 1991; 143:403–422.
58. Brewster CEP, Howarth PH, Djukanovic R, Wilson J, Holgate ST, Roche WR. Myofibroblasts and subepithelial fibrosis in bronchial asthma. Am J Respir Cell Mol Biol 1990; 3:507–511.
59. Bonner JC, Rice AB, Moomaw CR, Morgan DL. Airway fibrosis in rats induced by vanadium pentoxide. Am J Physiol 2000; 278:L209–L216.
60. Kodavanti UP, Jaskot RH, Su WY, Costa DL, Ghio AJ, Dreher KL. Genetic variability in combustion particle-induced chronic lung injury. Am J Physiol 1997; 272:L521–L532.
61. Silbajoris R, Ghio AJ, Samet JM, Jaskot R, Dreher KL, Brighton LE. In vivo and in vitro correlation of pulmonary MAP kinase activation following metallic exposure. Inhal Toxicol 2000; 12:453–468.
62. Chen F, Demers LM, Vallyathan V, Ding M, Lu Y, Castranova V, Shi X. Vanadate induction of NF-κB involves IκB kinase b and SAPK/ERK kinase 1 in macrophages. J Biol Chem 1999; 29:20307–20312.
63. Ding M, Li JJ, Leonard SS, Ye J-P, Shi X, Colburn NH, Castranova V, Vallyathan V. Vanadate-induced activation of activator protein-1: role of reactive oxygen species. Carcinogenesis 1999; 20:663–668.
64. Huang C, Ding M, Li J, Leonard SS, Rojanasukul Y, Castranova V, Vallyathan V, Ju G, Shi X. Vanadium-induced nuclear factor of activated T cells activation through hydrogen peroxide. J Biol Chem 2001; 276:22397–22403.
65. Huang C, Zhang Z, Ding M, Li J, Ye J, Leonard SS, Shen H-M, Butterworth L, Lu Y, Costa M, Rojanasaku Y, Castranova V, Vallyathan V, Shi X. Vanadate induces p53 transactivation through hydrogen peroxide and causes apoptosis. J Biol Chem 2000; 275:32516–32522.
66. Rice AB, Moomaw CR, Morgan Dl, Bonner JC. Specific inhibitors of PDGF- or EGF-receptor tyrosine kinase reduce pulmonary fibrosis in rats. Am J Pathol 1999; 155:213–221.
67. Adamson IYR, Prieditis H, Hedgecock C, Vincent R. Zinc is the toxic factor in the lung response to an atmospheric particulate sample. Toxicol Appl Pharmacol 2000; 166:111–119.
68. Raines EW, Dower SK, Ross R. Interleukin-1 mitogenic activity for fibroblasts and smooth muscle cells is due to PDGF-AA. Science 1989; 243: 393–396.
69. Lindroos PM, Coin PG, Badgett A, Morgan DL, Bonner JC. Alveolar macrophages stimulated with titanium dioxide, chrysotile asbestos, and residual oil fly ash up-regulate the PDGF receptor-α on lung fibroblasts through an IL-1 β-dependent mechanism. Am J Respir Cell Mol Biol 1997; 16:283–292.
70. Bonner JC, Lindroos PM, Rice AB, Moomaw CR, Morgan DL. Induction of PDGF receptor-α in rat myofibroblasts during pulmonary fibrogenesis in vivo. Am J Physiol 1998; 274:L72–L80.
71. Coin PG, Lindroos PM, Osornio-Vargas AR, Roggli VL, Bonner JC. Lipopolysaccharide up-regulates platelet-derived growth factor (PDGF) a-receptor expression in rat lung myofibroblasts and enhances responses to all PDGF isoforms. J Immunol 1996; 156:4797–4806.

72. Bonner JC, Osornio-Vargas AR, Badgett A, Brody AR. Differential proliferation of rat lung fibroblasts induced by the platelet-derived growth factor (PDGF)-AA, -AB, -BB isoforms secreted by rat alveolar macrophages. Am J Respir Cell Mol Biol 1991; 5:539–547.

73. Lasky JA, Coin PG, Lindroos PM, Ostrowski LE, Brody AR, Bonner JC. Chrysotile asbestos stimulates gene expression and secretion of PDGF-AA by rat lung fibroblasts: evidence for an autocrine loop. Am J Respir Cell Mol Biol 1995; 12:162–170.

74. Yamashita N, Sekine K, Miyasaka T, Kawashima R, Nakajima Y, Nakano J, Yamamoto T, Horiuchi T, Hirai K, Ohta K. Platelet-derived growth factor is involved in the augmentation of airway responsiveness through remodeling of airways in diesel exhaust particulate-treated mice. J Allergy Clin Immunol 2001; 107:135–142.

75. Yang HM, Ma JYC, Castranova V, Ma JKH. Effects of diesel exhaust particles on the release of IL-1 and TNFα from rat alveolar macrophages. Exp Lung Res 1997; 23:269–284.

76. Zu Z, Homer RJ, Wang Z, Chen Q, Geba GP, Wang J, Zhang Y, Elias JA. Pulmonary expression of interleukin-13 causes inflammation, mucus hypersecretion, subepithelial fibrosis, physiologic abnormalities, and eotaxin production. J Clin Invest 1999; 103:779–785.

77. Lee CG, Homer RJ, Zhu Z, Lanone S, Wang X, Koteliansky V, Shipley JM, Gotwals P, Noble P, Chen Q, Senior RM, Elias JA. Interleukin-13 induces tissue fibrosis by selectively stimulating and activating transforming growth factor beta(1). J Exp Med 2001; 194:809–813.

78. Ingram JL, Rice AB, Geisenhoffer K, Madtes DK, Bonner JC. IL-13 and IL-1beta promote lung fibroblast growth through coordinated up-regulation of PDGF-AA and PDGF-Ralpha. FASEB J 2004; 18:1132–1134.

79. Gauldie J, Sime PJ, Xing Z, Marr B, Tremblay GM. Transforming growth factor- beta gene transfer to the lung induces myofibroblast presence and pulmonary fibrosis. Curr Top Pathol 1999; 93:35–45.

80. Lasky JA, Ortiz LA, Tonthat B, Hoyle GW, Corti M, Athas G, Lungarella G, Brody A, Friedman M. Connective tissue growth factor mRNA expression is upregulated in bleomycin-induced lung fibrosis. Am J Physiol 1998; 275: L365–L371.

81. Jiang N, Dreher KL, Dye JA, Li Y, Richards JH, Martin LD, Adler KB. Residual oil fly ash induces cytotoxicity and mucin secretion by guinea pig tracheal epithelial cells via an oxidant-dependent mechanism. Toxicol Appl Pharmacol 2000; 163:221–230.

82. Wright DT, Fischer BM, Li C, Rochelle LG, Akley NJ, Adler KB. Oxidant stress stimulates mucin secretion and PLC in airway epithelium via a nitric oxide-dependent mechanism. Am J Physiol (London) 1996; 271: L854–L861.

83. Amishima H, Munakata M, Nasuhara Y, Sato A, Takahashi T, Homma Y, Kawakami Y. Expression of epidermal growth factor and epidermal growth factor receptor immunoreactivity in the asthmatic airway. Am J Respir Crit Care Med 1998; 157:1907–1912.

84. Takeyama K, Fahy JV, Nadel JA. Relationship of epidermal growth factor receptors to goblet cell production in human bronchi. Am J Respir Crit Care Med 2001; 163:511–516.

85. Takeyama K, Dabbagh K, Lee HM, Agusti C, Lausier JA, Ueki IF, Gratan KM, Nadel JA. Epidermal growth factor system regulates mucin production in airways. Proc Natl Acad Sci USA 1999; 96:3081–3086.

86. Takeyama K, Dabbagh K, Shim JJ, Dao-Pick T, Ueki IF, Nadel JA. Oxidative stress causes mucin synthesis via transactivation of epidermal growth factor receptor: role of neutrophils. J Immunol 2000; 164:1546–1552.

87. Voynow JA, Young LR, Wang Y, Horger T, Rose MC, Fischer BM. Neutrophil elastase increases MUC5AC mRNA and protein expression in respiratory epithelial cells. Am J Physiol 1999; 276:L835–L843.

88. Fischer BM, Voynow JA. Neutrophil elastase induces MUC5AC gene expression in airway epithelium via a pathway involving reactive oxygen species. Am J Respir Cell Mol Biol 2002; 26:447–452.

89. Kohri K, Ueki IF, Nadel JA. Neutrophil elastase induces mucin production by ligand- dependent epidermal growth factor receptor activation. Am J Physiol 2002; 283:L531–L540.

90. Booth BW, Adler KB, Bonner JC, Tournier F, Martin LD. Interleukin-13 induces proliferation of human bronchial epithelial cells in vitro via a mechanism mediated by transforming growth factor-α. Am J Respir Cell Mol Biol 2001; 25:739–743.

91. Shim JJ, Dabbagh K, Ueki IF, Dao-Pick T, Burgel PR, Takeyama K, Tam DC, Nadel JA. IL-13 induces mucin production by stimulating epidermal growth factor receptors and by activating neutrophils. Am J Physiol 2001; 280: L134–L140.

92. Shao MX, Ueki IF, Nadel JA. Tumor necrosis factor α-converting enzyme mediates MUC5AC mucin expression in cultured human airway epithelial cells. PNAS 2003; 100:11618–11623.

93. Wang Y-Z, Bonner JC. Mechanism of extracellular signal-regulated kinase (ERK)-1 and ERK-2 activation by vanadium pentoxide in rat pulmonary myofibroblasts. Am J Respir Cell Mol Biol 2000; 22:590–596.

94. Zhang, P, Wang YZ, Kagan E, Bonner JC. Peroxynitrite targets the epidermal growth factor receptor, Raf-1, and MEK independently to activate MAPK. J Biol Chem 2000; 275:22479–22486.

95. Ashida M, Bito T, Budiyanto A, Ichihashi M, Ueda M. Involvement of EGF receptor activation in the induction of cyclooxygenase-2 in HaCaT keratinocytes after UVB. Exp Dermatol 2003; 12(4):445–452.

96. Nataraj C, Thomas DW, Tilley SL, Nguyen MT, Mannon R, Koller BH, Coffman TM. Receptors for prostaglandin E(2) that regulate cellular immune responses in the mouse. J Clin Invest 2001; 108:1229–1235.

97. Samet JM, Ghio AJ, Costa DL, Madden MC. Increased expression of COX-2 mediates oil fly ash-induced lung injury. Exp Lung Res 2000; 26:57–69.

98. Bonner JC, Rice AB, Ingram JL, Moomaw CR, Nyska A, Bradbury A, Sessoms AR, Chulada PC, Morgan DL, Zeldin DC, Langenbach R. Suscept-

ibility of cyclooxygenase-2-deficient mice to pulmonary fibrogenesis. Am J Pathol 2002; 161:459–470.

99. Boyle JE, Lindroos PM, Rice AB, Zhang L, Zeldin DC, Bonner JC. Prostaglandin-E_2 counteracts interleukin-1β-stimulated up-regulation of platelet-derived growth factor α-receptor on rat pulmonary myofibroblasts. Am J Respir Cell Mol Biol 1999; 20:433–440.

8

Chronic Exposure and Susceptibility to Oxidant Air Pollutants

IRA B. TAGER

Division of Epidemiology, School of Public Health, University of California, Berkeley, California, U.S.A.

I. Introduction

This chapter deals with the effects of chronic exposure to oxidant air pollutants on human health, hi the ambient environment, the principal oxidant pollutants are ozone (O_3), constituents of particulate matter (PM) (transition metals, organic compounds and their derivatives), and oxides of nitrogen, the most important of which is NO_2 (in terms of being studied in relation to human health effects). The chapter focuses broadly on the health effects that have been associated with the oxidant gases and PM, since most of the detailed data related to PM are covered in several other chapters. However, since oxidant gases occur in the presence of PM that contains oxidant organic compounds that can result in redox cycling (1,2), some discussion related to PM-associated health effects is unavoidable.

A. General Mechanism for Health Effects Related to Oxidant Air Pollutants

Oxidative stress is one major mechanism through which ambient air pollutants (PM and xidant gases) are thought to lead to acute and to chronic health outcomes. Ozone is a highly reactive molecule that produces its effects through the mediation of free radical reactions in the lining fluid of the pulmonary airways: (1) oxidation of biomolecules to yield free radical species that leads to inflammation and DNA damage; (2) driving radical-dependent production of toxic, nonradical species from organic compounds such as aldehydes through ozonolysis of cell membrane fatty acids (3–6); (3) oxidation of arachadonic acid in cell membranes that leads to proinflammatory metabolites of arachadonic acid; and (4) alteration of structural and functional proteins (discussed in Ref. 7). Current concepts of ozone interactions with the respiratory tract are summarized in Fig. 1 and by Mudway and Kelly (6).

NO$_2$ is a reactive species that, like O$_3$, reacts within the surface lining layer of the pulmonary airways to form free radical reaction products (8). In the ambient environment, NO$_2$ participates in a complex series of redox reactions that lead to the formation of free radicals and strong oxidants such as peroxyacyl nitrate (PAN) (9). While any of the reactive molecules produced by atmospheric transformation of NO$_2$ can contribute to the ambient oxidant burden, NO$_2$ transformations in the lung do not seem to

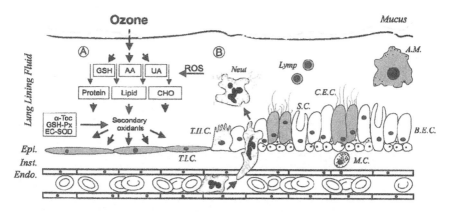

Figure 1   Ozone (O$_3$) is rapidly taken up in the surface lining fluid (SLF) of the airways, and relatively little O$_3$ reacts directly with underlying cells, except where the SLF is denuded. O$_3$ is highly reactive with antioxidants in the SLF (GSH—reduced glutathione, AA—ascorbic acid, UA—uric acid), which provide the first line of protection against O$_3$. Secondary anti—oxidants in the SLF are α tocopherol (α Toc), glutathione peroxidases (GSH-Px) and extracellular superoxide dismutase (EC-SOD). Reactions with proteins can lead to inactivation of enzymes; reactions with lipids leads to the formation of proinflammatory products, particularly of arachadonic acid. C.E.C—ciliated epithelial cell, T.I.C. and T.II.C—type I and II epithelial cells, AM—alveolar macrophage, B.E.C—bronchial epithelial cell, Epi—epithelium, Inst.—inrerstitium, Endo.—endothelium, Neut—neutrophil, lymph—lymphocyte, ROS—reactive oxygen species. (From Ref. 6.)

pose as great an oxidant stress as those for O_3, at least as measured by the ability of NO_2 to decxease the activity and levels of human epithelial lining fluid glutathione peroxidases (10) and in vitro ability to degrade lung elastin (7). Moreover, in controlled exposure studies, much higher concentrations than are encountered ordinarily in ambient environments are required to produce evidence of host responses to NO_2 (11). These artificial exposure conditions may not capture the full toxicological potential of oxides of nitrogen, which are converted to reactive nitrogen species in aqueous and gas phases in the presence of superoxide (12), the later being an important product of O_3 chemical reactions and the redox cycling of organic compounds found in PM.

A considerable body of recent research has established the importance of the generation of reactive oxygen metabolites (ROM) as a potentially important mechanism related to the health effects associated with particle air pollution. Figure 2 summarizes mechanisms proposed for reactive organic species derived from mobile sources. A similar general mechanism can be supported by the substantial body of data on the oxidant properties of transition metals (e.g., iron, nickel, vanadium, copper) found in ambient PM from fixed and mobile sources (13–18).

Data from several sources point to the potential consequences for human health of chronic exposure to the oxidizing potential of ambient air pollution. Repeated, cyclical exposure of monkeys to concentrations of O_3 at levels still observed in many parts of the world, leads to chronic inflammation and remodeling of small airways (19,20) of the type seen with exposure to tobacco smoke (21). In vitro evidence that O_3 (22,23) and PM (24–27) can lead to DNA damage in respiratory (nasal) epithelium is supported by population-based studies in highly polluted environments (28–30). Oxidation of low-density lipoproteins (LDL) is considered to be an integral part of the pathophysiology of atherosclerotic cardiovascular disease (31). The direct penetration of ultrafme PM into the circulation (32) raises the possibility of added oxidant stress either directly or through promotion of inflammation. Any process that contributes to inflammation and recruitment of inflammatory cells into the walls of atherosclerotic lesions will enhance the oxidative processes involved in atherosclerosis (33). Ambient PM has been shown to lead to the increased production and release of polymorphonuclear leukocytes into the circulation (34–37), which can be expected to increase underlying risk of acute cardiovascular events (38). Finally, repeated oxidative stress from variety of sources is seen as an important component of the pathophysiology of chronic obstructive lung disease (39). Increased deposition of particle aerosols in central and peripheral lung compartments has been observed in persons with Chronic obstructive lung disease (COPD) under controlled exposure conditions (mass median diameter 1 μm, geometric SD 1.2) (40). This increased deposition could be worsened in the presence in high ambient O_3 concentrations (41).

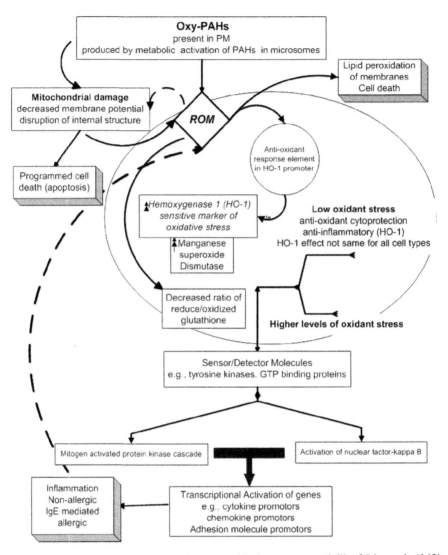

Figure 2 Basic elements of "stratified oxidative stress model" of Li, et al. (142) (area enclosed in gray circle) and consequences of ROM that are not controlled by antioxidant defenses. Solid arrows represent the pathways; dashed arrows identify feedback loops that perpetuate the adverse outcomes. ROM—reactive oxygen metabolites. (Adapted from Ref. 143.)

Further support for the pathophysiological importance, oxidant stress comes from controlled studies on antioxidant vitamin supplementation. Antioxidant supplementation has been observed to diminish decrements in lung function (volumes and flows) related to repeated exposures to 1 hr maximum ambient O_3 levels in adults and asthmatic children in Mexico City (42,43) and in amateur cyclists during exercise (44,45). Controlled exposure studies also have demonstrated a protective effect of antioxidant supplementation on postozone exposure bronchial reactivity to $SO2$ in young adults with asthma (46) and reductions in forced vital capacity (FVC) and forced expiratory volume in 1 sec (FEV_1) in health young adults (47).

B. Why a Focus on Health Effects Related to Chronic Exposure?

In its promulgation of the 1996 revision of the PM standard, EPA, based on its risk assessment, noted the relatively larger contribution of long-term compared to short-term exposure on mortality burden (48). Over the past few years, additional data have accumulated on the health effects of long-term exposure to PM (see Table 9–11 of Ref. 49). Careful review of the data that focused on PM effects indicates that similar effects are associated with long-term exposure to ambient O_3 during the summer season (see Fig. 5 ozone 1982–1998 3rd quarter in Ref. 50 and Fig. 12 in this text). New data from Children's Health Study (CHS) cohort in southern California indicate that: (1) chronic exposure to O_3 may be a cause of asthma amongst those highly exposed based on outdoor activity patterns (51); (2) average ambient levels of pollutants in a complex oxidant environment adversely affect lung function growth in children (52,53) and increase the presence of bronchitic symptoms in children with asthma (54). Data from the National Morbidity, Mortality and Air Pollution Study (NMMAPs) have demonstrated short-term mortality effects related to O_3. These data, when coupled with more recent data, indicate that so-called acute effects on mortality can persist for months (55–59) and, in part, may be related to cumulated exposures. Finally, an increasing body of pathological data in humans provides direct evidence of the tissue effects of chronic exposures to high oxidant environments (see above). A recent study examined the lungs of life-long female residents (mean age 66 ± 9 years) of Mexico City who had no evidence of chronic respiratory disease and who had never smoked or cooked with biomass fuels (60). Compared with lungs from Vancouver, Canada, a low pollutant environment, the Mexico City lungs demonstrated abnormalities in the membranous and respiratory bronchioles (increased muscle and fibrosis) (Fig. 3). Electron microscopy revealed chained carbonaceous and carbon/sulfur aggregates of ultrafine PM in the airway mucosa (60). Although the focus of this paper is on PM, the ambient air in Mexico City is a complex oxidant environment with high O_3 as well as high PM. This collective body of new data clearly points to the need to place increased emphasis on the potential for human health effects that are a consequence of cumulative effects of exposures to relatively high mean levels and/or repeated exposures to short-term increases in ambient oxidant pollutant levels (61).

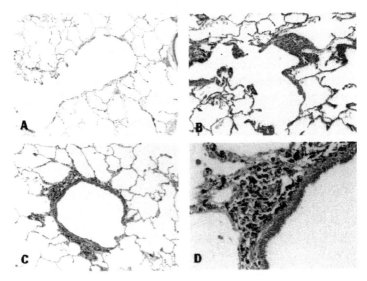

Figure 3 Respiratory bronchioles (RB) from lung from autopsies in Vancouver, Canada (A) and Mexico City (B–D). Relative to A, RB from BB has increased muscle. C and D show extensive deposition of dust in walls of RB. (From Ref. 60.)

II. Standards, Origin, and Sources
A. Standards

Table 1 presents a summary of the current ambient air quality standards for the United States, the State of California, and the World Health Organization for O_3, NO_2, and PM.

B. Origin of and Spatial Distribution of Oxidant Pollutants

This chapter focuses on the oxidant gases ozone and oxides of nitrogen. Sources and spatial distribution of PM are covered in Chapter 2, Particulate Dosimetry in the Respiratory Tract.

1. Ozone

Tropospheric[a] zone is a secondary pollutant that is formed from NO_x and volatile organic compounds in the presence of sunlight (photons $\sim$0.2 μm). Consequently, the highest concentrations are found during day-light hours, with peaks most likely to occur in the mid-afternoon hours. Principally,

[a] The troposphere extends from the earth's surface to an average of 14 km (actual height depends on latitude and season) (62).

Table 1 Summary of Air Quality Standards for Oxidant Air Pollutants[a]

Pollutant	Averaging time	United States	California	World Health Organization (1999)
Ozone	1 hr	0.120 ppm (235 µg/m³)	0.090 ppm (180 µg/m³)	Annual range: 10–100 µg/m³
	8 hr	0.080 ppm (157 µg/m³)	None	Guideline level: 120 µg/m³ (0.060 ppm)
Respirable PM (PM$_{10}$)	24 hr	150 µg/m³	50 µg/m³ (under review)	No guideline value recommended
	Annual mean (arithmetic)	50 µg/m³	20 µg/m³	
Fine PM (PM$_{2.5}$)	24 hr	65 µg/m³	None	No guideline value recommended
	Annual mean (arithmetic)	15 µg/m³	12 µg/m³	
Nitrogen dioxide	24 hr	None	None	Annual range: 10–150 µg/m³
	1 hr	None	0.250 ppm (470 µg/m³)	Guideline level 1 hr level: 200 µg/m³ (0.106 ppm)
	Annual mean (arithmetic)	0.053 ppm (100 µg/m³)	None	Annual mean: 40 µg/m³ (0.021 ppm)

[a] *Sources:* US: http://www.epa.gov/air/criteria.html; California: http://www.arb.ca.go v/research/aaq s/caaq s/caaqs.htm; WHO: http://www.who.int/environmentalinforma tion/Air/Guidelines/Chapter3.htm; Ref. 65.

O_3 is an outdoor pollutant, with indoor sources being rare in, residential dwellings. Ozone is produced by laser printers and photocopiers that can be found in large numbers in occupational settings (63). A complete review of the tropospheric photochemistry can be found in the 1996 Air Quality Criteria Document for Ozone and Related Photochemical Oxidants (62). The basic atmospheric chemistry is summarized in Fig. 4. Processes that lead to the production of nitrogen oxides (NO_x) have the potential to increase tropospheric O_3 concentrations. Mobile sources related to transportation and recreation and fossil fuel burning from power plants and industrial sources

Basic Photolysis Process
$$2NO + O_2 \rightarrow 2NO_2$$
$$NO_2 + h\nu \rightarrow NO + 0(^3P)$$
$$0(^3P) + O_2 + M \rightarrow O_3 + M$$
$$NO + O_3 \rightarrow NO_2 + O_2$$

Processes that Disturb Equilibrium State
Production of NO_2 without intermediate O_3

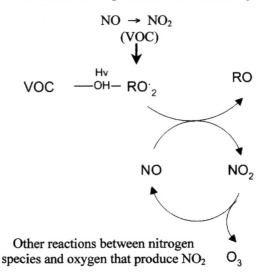

Figure 4 Simplified photolysis processes that lead to O_3 formations. The basic photolytic reaction is an equilibrium reaction. The presence of natural volatile organic compounds (VOCs) (e.g., from plants) contribute to the nonanthropogenic background O_3 concentrations. Volatile organic compounds derived from anthropogenic activities (e.g., motor vehicles, industrial processes) and additional reactions between nitrogen species with O_2 contribute to an expanded pool of oxides of nitrogen that can, in the presence of photons, lead to increased production of O_3 beyond the equilibrium state. RO•$_2$, alkyl-peroxy radical; OH, hydroxyl radical. (From Ref. 62.)

make the principal contribution to the NO_x inventory, while transportation and nonfuel burning industrial sources make up the bulk of the VOC inventory (Fig. 5) (64). As a consequence of these declines in NO_x and VOC emissions, the 1- and 8-hr average O_3 concentrations declined 22% and 14%,

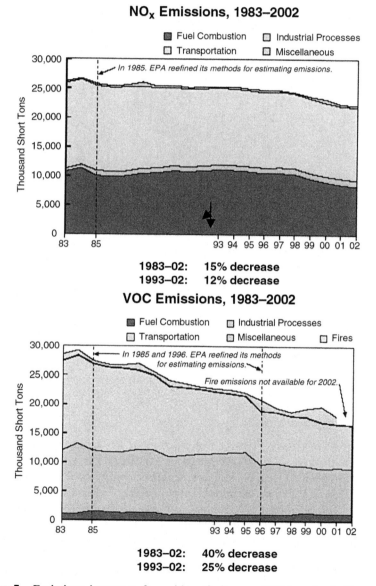

Figure 5 Emissions inventory for oxides of nitrogen (NO_x) and volatile organic compounds for 1983–2002. (From Ref. 64.)

Ozone Concentrations in the Easterm Regions of the U.S. and Canada
(Average Annual 4th Highest Daily Maximum) 8-hour Ozone, 1999-2001

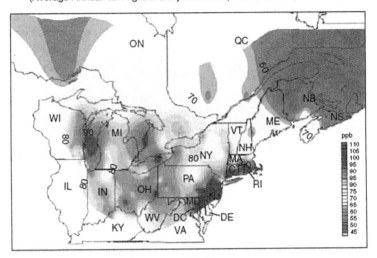

Figure 6 Illustration of the region character of the spatial distribution of O_3. Distribution of fourth highest day maximum O_3 concentration in the eastern United States and Canada, 1999–2001. (Available from http://www.epa.gov/ceiswebl/ceishome/atlas/nationalatlas/ozone.htm.)

respectively, over the period 1983–2002. Nonetheless, in 2002, 68.0 and 136.4 million people in the United States were living in areas that exceeded the 1- and 8-hr O_3 standards, respectively (64). Ozone tends to be a regional pollutant (Fig. 6), with concentrations increasing as air masses are transported away from primary sources of NO_x and undergo the photochemical process summarized in Fig. 4 continuing to lead to O_3 formation.

2. *Oxides of Nitrogen (NO_x) and Nitrogen Dioxide (NO_2)*

Oxides of nitrogen are primary pollutants that are emitted as a result of burning fossil fuels (Fig. 5). As noted in Fig. 4, NO is converted to NO_2 near the emission source. NO_x also consists of several other nitrogen oxide species (Table 2). These components participate in a variety of chemical reactions (Table 2), one of the most important of which is the formation of nitrates that make up an important component of $PM_{2.5}$, especially in the parts of western states in the United States, where there are abundant sources of ammonia. Currently, in the United States, there are no areas that are above the annual standard of 0.053 ppm (64), although in many parts of the world, the World Health Organization (WHO) annual mean of $40\,\mu g/m^3$ (0.021 ppm) is exceeded due to high concentrations of motor

Table 2 Components of NO_x and Summary of Chemical Reactions of Nitrogen Species in the Atmosphere

Component	Reaction process	Comment
Components of NO_x		
Nitrogen trioxide (NO_3)	$O_3 + NO_3$	Rapid photolysis-only important at night, very reactive with organic compounds
Dinitrogen trioxide (N_2O_3)	$NO + NO_2$—equilibrium reaction	Equilibrium concentrations 10^{-7}–10^{-9} ppm; reacts with water to for nitrous acid (HONO)
Dinitrogen tetroxide (N_2O_4)	$2NO_2$—equilibrium reaction	Equilibrium concentrations 10^{-6}–10^{-8}
Dinitrogen pentoxide (N_2O_5)	$NO_2 + NO_3 + M$—equilibrium reaction	Nighttime component; combines with liquid water to form nitric acid (HNO_3)
Nitrates, nitrites, and nitrogen acids		
Nitric acid (HNO_3)	$NO_2 + HO\bullet;\ N_2O_5 + H_2O$ (liquid)	Highly volatile; does not condense into aerosol at usual atmospheric concentrations; reacts with ammonia gas (NH_3) or aerosol that contains crustal material form nitrates
Nitrous acid (HONO)	$NO + OH + M$	Formed during daylight when hydroxyl radicals are present
Organic nitrates	$R–CH_2–O\bullet + NO_2 \rightarrow RCH–ONO_2$ (alkyl nitrate) $CH_3C(O)OO\bullet NO_2 \rightarrow CH_3C(O)OONO_{23}$ (peroxyacetyl nitrate—PAN)	PAN is best studied reaction. PAM thermally labile
Aerosal nitrates	$NH_3 + HNO_3$	Reversible reaction; equilibrium constant temperature- and humidity-dependent

Source: From Ref. 67.

vehicles (65). In 2002, approximately 50% of 125 sites that reported annual means to the USEPA database exceeded the WHO standard (64) (Fig. 7). However, no population estimates are available for these sites.

Transport of nitrogen species is dependent on both meteorological and chemical processes. As detailed in 1993 EPA Criteria Document for Oxides of Nitrogen (62), a typical scenario can be summarized as follows: NO_x emitted early in the morning will disperse vertically and move down wind. On sunny days, most NO_x is converted to PAN and HNO_3, and most of the HNO_3 is removed by depositional processes and conversion to nitrates as the air plume moves (Table 2). After sunset, dark phase chemistry proceeds and transport continues. As the plume moves, NO_x concentrations decrease as a result of dilution and chemical transformation. The typical daily urban pattern of NO_x and O_3 is given in Fig. 8 (66). Peaks of NO and NO_2 occur in the early morning and are followed by an ozone peak in the late morning to early afternoon, the height of the latter is determined not only by NO_x concentrations but by the concentrations of VOCs. At emission sources, O_3 concentrations may not build up due to scavenging by NO (Fig. 4).

Unlike O_3, there are important indoor sources of NO_x (9): gas appliances (stoves, dryers, water heaters), kerosene heaters, wood stoves, and tobacco products (particularly from side stream smoke). Levels in homes with a major NO_x source have been reported to be 0.025 ± 0.004 ppm compared to 0.009 ± 0.002 ppm in homes without such sources (67). Indoor:outdoor NO_2 ratios of 2.3 ± 1.9 and 1.2 ± 0.5 have been reported for homes with and without gas ranges, respectively (68). Ice skating rinks represent an important indoor source related to recreation, with mean levels as high as 0.206 ppm (69).

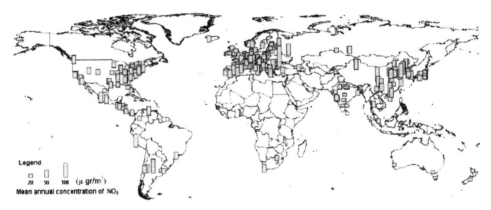

Figure 7 Distribution of NO_2 levels around the globe based on latest available data. Comparisons are made against the WHO annual mean standard of $40 \, \mu g/m^3$ (0.021 ppm). Areas with highest NO_2 levels are those with greatest concentrations of motor vehicles. (From Ref. 65.)

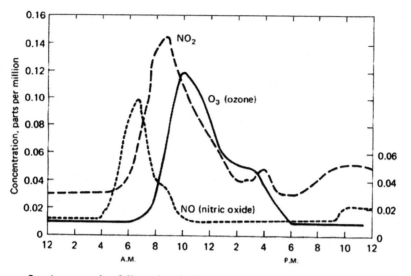

Figure 8 An example of diurnal variation of NO, NO_2 and O_3 in Los Angeles, CA, July 19, 1965. (From Ref. 66.)

III. Health Effects Related to Chronic Exposure to Oxidant Air Pollutants

To a great extent, data from epidemiological studies of acute exposure have served as the basis for current designations of susceptible populations. Frank and Tankersley (61) have offered a useful formulation that provides a unifying construct for susceptibility to adverse health outcomes related to chronic exposure to oxidant air pollutants. Briefly, these authors suggest that disruption of what they term the "deterministic chaos" (a complex interplay of systems that is characterized by stability around "set points," periodicity, and rapid response) can lead to responses to stress that are not sufficiently flexible to preserve homeostasis and/or may appear unrelated to the magnitude and duration of an environmental stress (such as have been seen with increases in daily mortality at relatively low levels of ambient air pollutants). Aging and chronic disease processes are the principal examples given by the authors, but, by extension, developmental immaturity as seen in the fetus and in infants likely is part of this process.

A considerable body of epidemiological data has established associations between prenatal exposure to relatively high levels of ambient air pollutants and a variety of adverse birth outcomes—intrauterine mortality (70), low birth weight (71–76), preterm delivery (74,77,78), small for gestational age (76,79) and neonatal mortality (80). Increased postnatal mortality also has been reported from several studies (81–84). While all of these studies have sought to ascribe these various effects to a specific pollutant(s), in studies where data for more than a single pollutant are presented, it is difficult to ignore the complex mixtures of PM and gases in which the outcomes were evaluated. A question arises as to whether the alterations in fetal development that are implied by the adverse birth outcomes have implications over the long term and thereby define "susceptibility" to ambient air pollutants. Asthma appears to be more common in children of low birth weight (85) and appears to be more related to growth retardation than to prematurity (85,86). Moreover, the observation that asthmatic children who were born either before 37 weeks gestations or of low birth weight (< 2500 g) had a substantially increased risk of symptoms and reduced lung function in responses to increases in daily levels of summertime air pollutants in the eastern one-half of the United States (characterized by high O_3 and PM dominated by sulfates) (87) indicates that alterations in fetal development related to exposure to ambient air pollution not only may increase the risk of chronic respiratory disease but also may confer ongoing susceptibility to the adverse health consequences of ambient oxidant pollutant environments. The extent to which such susceptibility actually contributes to long-term health risks is difficult to assess. Migration of children from "high" to low ambient pollutant environments has been associated with improvements in lung function and associated decrements in children who move to environments with higher ambient pollution levels (88). On the other hand, studies of birth cohorts have reported: (1) associations between birth weight and lung function in the eighth decade of life (89); and (2) associations between childhood exposures, which include air pollution, and respiratory symptoms and lung function at age 36 years, even after adjustment for exposures in adult life such as cigarette smoking (90).

Although most of the data that relate to "susceptible" populations have been derived from studies on health outcomes related to acute increases in ambient pollutants, we easily can make inferences to chronic exposures from these data. As noted in Fig. 2, oxidant stress, in the end, is a potent proinflammatory stimulus; and inflammation itself is a major source of oxidant stress (91) (and reviewed by Chow et al. (92). If oxidant stress is a major component of the pathophysiological effects of oxidant air pollutants on human health, then it stands to reason that any disease process for which inflammation is a major component (asthma (93), chronic obstructive lung disease and emphysema (94), atherosclerotic cardiovascular disease, respiratory infections (33) could be influenced adversely by long-term exposure to oxidant air pollutants exposure. Oxidative stress is thought to play an important role in normal aging (95), and highly oxidant environments can be expected to contribute to the overall burden of oxidant damage related to normal aging. Indeed, epidemiological data have identified the elderly and persons with chronic respiratory and cardiovascular diseases (and diseases that contribute to the risk of cardiovascular diseases such as diabetes mellitus) and malignancy to be at increased risk for adverse health outcomes related to ambient air pollution.

The genetic underpinnings for human susceptibility to long-term exposure to oxidant pollutant environments are emerging. Particular focus has been on the glutathione-*S*-transferase (GST) supergene family, the members of which play an important role in the protection of cells against oxidative stress through catalysis of reactions of glutathione with electrophiles, which thereby lead to a reduction in their reactivity with cellular macromolecules (96,97). Romieu et al. (99) studied the influence of the GSTM1-null genotype on the adverse effects of ambient O_3 and the protective effect of vitamin E (98). Percentage decrements in maximum mid-expiratory flow (MMEF, FEF_{25-74}) rate were greater in children with the null genotype, and the primary benefit of supplemental vitamin E on mitigation of lung function decrements was seen in the GSTM1-null children. The effects were greatest in children with moderate and severe asthma. An Italian study of healthy, nonsmoking cyclists who cycled on days with O_3 concentrations between 32 and 103 ppb demonstrated that participants who had wild-type NAD(P):quinine oxidoreductase (NQO1)[b] and the GSTM1-null genotype had greater declines in FEV_1 than subjects with all other combinations of these two genes (Fig. 9) and greater evidence of DNA damage as measured by formation of 8-hydroxy-2'-deoxyguanoside (8-OhdG) (101). A controlled O_3 exposure study (0.100 ppm for 2 hr of mild exercise) by the same authors observed greater evidence of oxidative stress (thiobarbituric acid reactive substances) and LTB-4 (neutrophil chemotactic mediator) production and 8-OhdG formation in subjects with the NQO1 wild-type and GSTM1-null genotype compared to all other combinations (102). Data from the CHS have found associations between the GSTM1-null and GSTP1 polymorphisms and deficits in growth of FEV_1 (103). The largest effects were observed for FEV_1 in non-Hispanic whites when the GSTM1-null and GSTP1 (val/val) genotypes were present together. Given the data from this study on the effects of oxidant pollutants on lung function growth (52,53), these data clearly point to important susceptible subgroups in the population. Finally, a very recent study has linked lowered levels of glutathione peroxidase I activity with increased risk of acute cardiovascular events (deaths and nonfatal heart attacks), an effect that was significantly increased in cigarette smokers (104).

---

[b]NQO1 detoxifies quinones, which are important components of PM, to their hydroquinones (HQs) without the production of intermediate, redox-cycling semiquinones (99). HQs are stable compounds that do not undergo redox cycling but can undergo further oxidation by O_2 and O_3 (100). Glutathione-*S*-transferases catalyze the metabolism of reactive species (e.g., peroxides) that are formed from these oxidative processes.

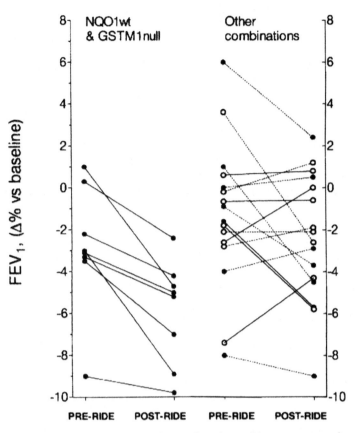

Figure 9   Response of FEV_1 to 2-hr cycling in ambient ozone environments. NQOlwt = NQO1 wild type. Under "other combinations," non-NQOlwt genotype and GSTMl-null (closed circles), non-NQOlwt genotype and GSTM1 + (open circles) (From Ref. 101.)

IV.   Exposure and Deposition as Susceptibility Factors for Health Effects Related to Chronic Exposures

The details related to deposition and clearance of particle pollutants are covered in detail in Chapter 2. Over longer periods of time, factors that affect exposure (ambient concentrations, location in indoor vs. outdoor environments) and deposition, for any given exposure (oral vs. nasal breathing, rate and depth of ventilation, presence of underlying respiratory tract disease), will vary greatly within individuals and across populations. The ability to integrate all of these factors over any length of time for large populations in whom health outcomes related to chronic exposures will be assessed is difficult, if not impossible, even in birth cohort studies. Attempts to incorporate "dose" [a function of exposure, ventilation (frequency and depth, oral, nasal) and deposition] into epidemiological studies are difficult. Accurate assessment of dose received for any given ambient exposure in free-living populations is not feasible at the present time. However, reliability for some estimates may be acceptable for epidemiological studies under certain circumstances. Künzli et al. (105) determined the variability of estimated measures of "effective life time exposure" to ozone in college freshmen in California (based on exposure based on a dense O_3 monitoring network, lifetime residential history and questionnaire-based patterns of outdoor activities). Variance components analysis indicated that between 25% and 45% of the variability between two estimates made 7 days apart was due to between assessment variability. Gonzales et al. (106) studied 18 college freshmen who wore passive ozone monitors and completed daily diaries during summer months in the San Fernando Valley of southern California; and 1 year later completed a questionnaire to assess their exposure to O_3 during the time the passive monitor were worn (106). Mean differences in the estimates between the measured exposures and those estimated from the questionnaire 1 year later (estimated minus measured) were 21.6 and 6.4 ppb when questions about home ventilation were and were not included in estimation of exposure. Collectively, these studies indicate the extent of the difficulties related to estimation of exposures over long periods of time in epidemiological studies, to say nothing of trying to translate these estimates into estimates of dose. Moreover, these studies do not take account of factors such as changing predominance of oral vs. nasal breathing during rest at different ages and the relative extent to which individuals switch to oral breathing during exercise. These factors may influence total uptake of O_3 (pages 8–9 to 8–30 USEPA/600P-93/004cF of Ref. 107) and clearly increase uptake of PM (108), adapted from Figs. 10–15 (see Chapter 2).

Several publications provide support for the use of measures of ambient concentrations of oxidants as surrogates for dose (in conjunction with some data on activity patterns) and chronic health effects. In the CHS, time spent outdoors and time spent in high ventilation activities, outdoors were associated with decreases in lung function growth (52) and increases in the occurrence of asthma (51), respectively. Künzli et al. (110) observed that estimates of lifetime exposure to ambient concentration of ozone in college freshman was associated with decreased levels of small airways function (109) as would have been predicted by studies in primates (19,20). However, none of these studies account fully for the complexity of the ambient pollutant mixture to which individuals are exposed each day and over time.

If oxidant damage is a common pathway through which acute, subacute, and chronic exposures to ambient air pollutants lead to adverse health effects, then exposures need to be considered in the context of the entire oxidant environment in which individuals find themselves and the relative oxidant capacity of the various components of that mixture. Li et al. (1)

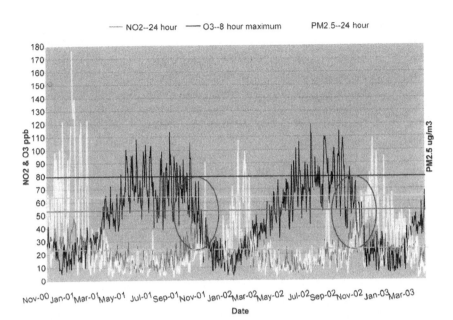

Figure 10 Time series of ambient pollutant data from Fresno, CA, November 1, 2000 through March 31, 2002. Solid black line, O_3 8-hr maximum standard; solid orange line, existing federal $PM_{2.5}$ 24-hr maximum; dashed orange line, California $PM_{2.5}$ 24-hr maximum standard; solid red line, federal NO_2 annual mean (California 1-hr maximum $= 250$ ppb). Circles define areas with relatively increased and fluctuating daily levels of O_3, NO_2, and $PM_{2.5}$. (From California Air Resources Board to author as part of ongoing study.)

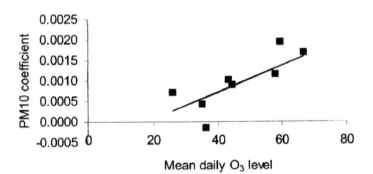

Figure 11 Regression coefficients for effects of daily changes in PM_{10} concentrations on respiratory hospital admissions in persons age 65+ from APHEA-2 cities vs. mean daily O_3 concentrations. (From Ref. 110.)

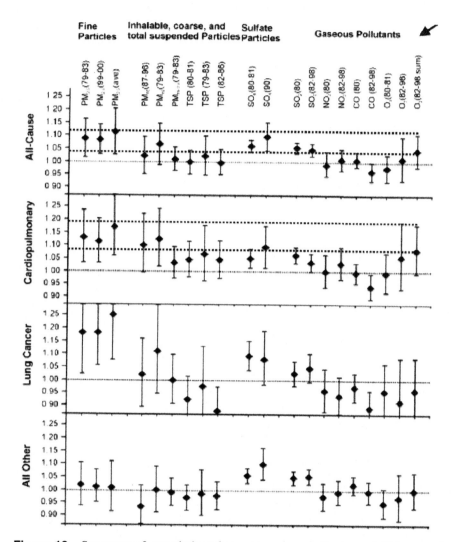

Figure 12 Summary of associations between various indicators of PM aerosol and gaseous pollutants for ACS study over different averaging periods. Mean annual O_3 concentration from 1982–1998 (column to left of arrow) 59.7($\pm$ 12.8)ppb. Column marked with arrow represents 3rd quarter ("summertime") O_3 concentrations. Dashed arrows project (current author's addition) the point estimates and the upper bound of the 95% confidence interval estimates for the effect of summertime O_3 on mortality. (From Ref. 50.)

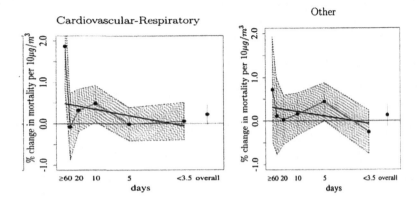

Figure 13 Pooled estimates of log relative rates of mortality at different time scales for cardiovascular-respiratory (left panel) and other causes of mortality (right panel) for four US cities (Pittsburgh, PA; Minneapolis, MN; Seattle, WA; Chicago, IL), 1987–1994. Shaded regions are ±2 standard errors of the estimates. Percentage increases in mortality were greater at longer than shorter exposure intervals before death (NB: greatest lags are near the origin of the x-axis. (From Ref. 59.)

evaluated the oxidant capacity of ambient air[c] from the Los Angeles basin that was used in an in vitro study of ultrafine PM and oxidant cell damage and demonstrated a close relationship between quinone reduction and triggering of host antioxidant defenses. Their analysis focused only on the contribution of quinone (a PAH) to the oxidative capacity of the ambient air. Other quinines also contribute to the oxidative burden. Ozone and NO_x also participate in a wide variety of reactions that also generate highly reactive radials that are capable of producing oxidative damage in vivo as noted above (6,8,9). The importance of this perspective for epidemiological studies is demonstrated by data from Fresno, CA in Fig. 10. During the transition from the summertime ozone season to the wintertime $PM_{2.5}$ season (wood burning, and time of frequent inversions that trap polluted air near the surface), there are numbers of days with relatively high $PM_{2.5}$, NO_2, and O_3 and differing time trends in the pollutant series. Clearly an appropriate summary of toxicological potential for this mixture to result in acute health effects (and chronic with repeated exposures over years) is not to be found by the measurement of the mass of each component or some particular component of $PM_{2.5}$. This point is reinforced by data from the APHEA-2 (Air Pollution on Health, a European Approach) studies on the effects of ambient pollution on respiratory hospital admissions (Fig. 11)

---

[c] Dithiothreitol assay based on the formation of reactive oxygen species by catalysis of quinone (2).

(110). The association between daily changes in respiratory hospital admissions and daily PM_{10} concentrations for persons aged 65+ were highly dependent on the concomitant O_3 concentrations. Similar inferences can be made for pollutant mixtures in the eastern United States, despite claims that gaseous pollutants appear to be acting as surrogates for PM-associated health effects (111).

V. Evidence for Health Effects Associated with Chronic Exposure to Oxidant Air Pollutants

While there is an extensive body of cross-sectional data that shows associations between ambient concentrations of oxidant air pollutants and health effects, cross-section studies are plagued with numerous problems with regard to inferences related to chronic exposure effects: (1) difficulties in the establishment of temporal sequence; (2) lack of data on duration of residence in the areas being studied; (3) survivor effects due to out-migration or early death from specific diseases of persons with heightened susceptibility to air pollution-related health effects; (4) assessment of exposure over short (mostly single) periods of time with the assumption that these exposures are representative past exposure; and (5) mixing of age, period, and cohort effects that can confound air pollution–disease associations. Therefore, the focus of this section is on the few cohort studies that have provided data on which to base inferences related to oxidant-induced health effects and data from time series studies that have evaluated mortality displacement and provide evidence for lingering effects that persist beyond the immediate exposure period.

A. Evidence for Associations with Mortality

In the 1990s, Dockery et al. (112) and Pope et al. (113) published landmark prospective, cohort studies that associated mortality with long-term exposure to ambient pollutant PM concentrations. In both studies, PM_{10} mass and sulfate were most closely associated with mortality. These studies have been discussed extensively and will not be reviewed further, since recent updates are available.

Pope et al. (50) published an update to the original American Cancer Society (ACS) cohort study (113). This update doubled the follow-up time to the year 1998, expanded the exposure data to include $PM_{2.5}$ and added new covariate data. In particular, data were available for NO_2 and O_3 as well as PM measures. Summertime O_3 concentrations were associated with all-cause and cardiopulmonary mortality, and the effects clearly overlap those for $PM_{2.5}$ (Fig. 12). For cardiopulmonary mortality, there is substantial overlap between the estimated effect for annual O_3 concentrations and those for

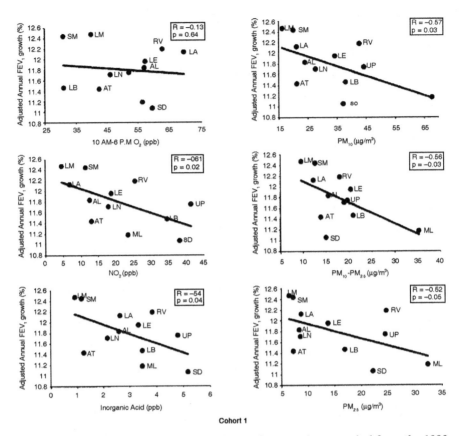

Figure 14 Relationship between FEVi growth over a 4-year period from the 1993 (cohort 1) and the 1996 (cohort 2) Children's Health Study cohorts. Acid vapors refer to (HCl + HNO₃). (From Refs. 52,53.)

$PM_{2.5}$. For subjects who lived well east of the Mississippi River, it would be difficult to separate the $PM_{2.5}$ effects from those of O_3 in the summer months that are characterized by photochemical smog and PM from local generation and transport from power plants in the mid-west. Synergistic effects likely occur, which cannot be measured by current analytic techniques. It is difficult to evaluate O_3 effects in the original Six Cities data, since the range of concentrations from O_3 is very narrow (21–28 ppb) compared to a nearly three-fold range (11–30 μg/m³) for $PM_{2.5}$ (112). However, even over this narrow range, there is a suggestion of O_3 effects at $PM_{2.5}$ levels 15 μg/m³ (Fig. 3 of Ref. 112), which again suggests that it is the total pollutant, oxidant environment rather a single component that is the "cause" of the associations.

The Adventist Study of Smog (AHSMOG) evaluated mortality from a cohort of Seventh Day Adventists in California observed from 1979–1992

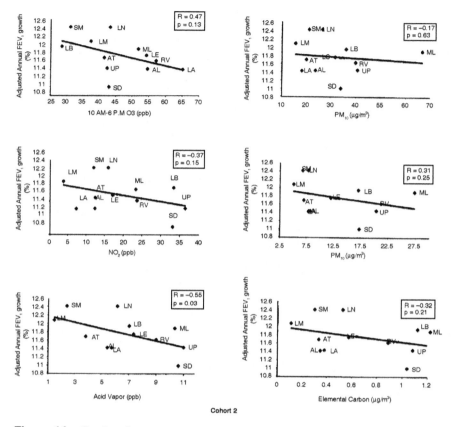

Figure 14 *Continued*

(114). Individual estimates of exposure were developed based on residence, commuting patterns, and several other factors (115,116), which differ from the purely ecological estimates used in the Six Cities and ACS studies. For all-cause mortality in males, the text notes only an association with PM_{10}. However, inspection of their Table 3 indicates that there is an association with O_3 whose point estimates and 95% confidence intervals are nearly identical to the "significant" PM_{10} association. The same interpretation occurs with deaths in males due to any nonmahgnant respiratory disease (Table 3). In the case of lung cancer mortality, the largest effect estimate in males is for number of days of O_3 per year $> 100\,ppb$ (Table 3), despite statistically significant effects for PM_{10} metrics. In females, only mean SO_2 and NO_2 levels are associated with lung cancer mortality (Table 3). These data are more properly interpreted as demonstrating health effects that most likely are associated with the complex $PM–O_3–NO_2$ environment that characterizes the areas in California in which the subjects resided rather than to any single pollutant.

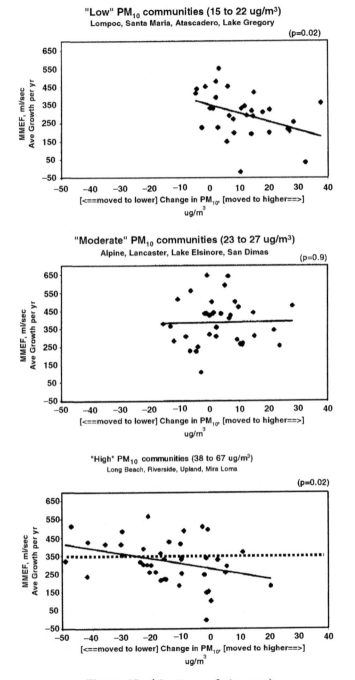

Figure 15 (*Caption on facing page*)

Table 3 Selected Results[a] from Table 3 of the AHSMOG of Mortality, 1977–1992: Adjusted Relative Risks and 95% Confidence Intervals

	Pollutant average 1973 to censoring date			
	PM_{10} days $> 100\,\mu g/m^3$	PM_{10} mean concentration	O_3 hr/yr $> 100\,ppb$	O_3 mean concentration
IQR[b]	43 days/year	24.1 $\mu g/m^3$	551 hr/year	12 ppb
All cause				
Males	1.12 (1.01, 1.24)	1.11	1.14 (0.98, 1.32)	1.09 (0.95, 1.25)
Respiratory				
Males[c]	1.28 (1.03, 1.57)	1.23 (0.94,1.61)	1.20 (0.88, 1.64)	1.12, (0.85, 1.47)
Lung cancer				
Males	2.38 (1.42, 3.97)	3.36 (1.57, 7.19)	4.19 (1.81, 9.69)	2.10 (0.99, 4.44)
Females[d]				

[a]Results presented for association report as statistically significant for at least one measure of PM_{10}.
[b]IQR—interquartile (25th–75th percentile) range for each pollutant.
[c]Defined as "any mention of nonmalignant respiratory disease" on the death certificate.
[d]For females, statistically significant effects were observed for mean SO_2 concentration (IQR = 3.7 ppb) 3.01 (1.88, 4.84) and mean NO_2 concentration (IQR = 19.8 ppb) 2.81 (1.15, 6.89). *Source*: From Ref. 115.

Investigators from the Netherlands reported associations between mortality and indicators of traffic-related air pollution in a cohort study from 1986 to 1994 (117). Pollutant exposures were partitioned into "regional background," "urban background," and "traffic-related" concentrations. The latter were based on residential location within 100 m of a major freeway or 50 m of an major urban road (117). Data for NO_2, and black smoke (BS), were provided but no data for O_3. There were consistent associations between exposure both to background and traffic-related BS and NO_2 and cardiopulmonary mortality, with the magnitude of the associations being similar for BS and NO_2 [RR/10 $\mu g/m^3$ increase for residence near major road: BS = 1.95 (95% confidence interval: 1.09, 3.51); NO_2 = 1.94 (95% CI: 1.08, 3.48). RR/10 $\mu g/m^3$ increase in background: BS = 1.34 (95% CI: 0.68, 2.64); NO_2 = 1.54 (95% CI: 0.81, 2.92)]. Since

Figure 15 (*Facing Page*) Effects on maximum mid-expiratory flow (MMEF) of moving from a Children's Health Study community to a community with differing levels of ambient pollutants stratified by level of PM10 in the CHS community. Dashed line is the author's approximate projection of the average growth rates for CHS children from "moderate" CHS communities (middle panel). (From Ref. 88.) (Note there is a conflict between the text and the lower panel with regard to the *p* value for the regression. The text indicates a *p*- value of 0.09, which differs from that in the lower panel.)

BS and NO_2, in this study, are equivalent markers for traffic-related pollutants, it is not surprising that the results for each component are nearly identical. Again, these results are most consistent with the interpretation that it is the complex environment, rather than any single component of that environment, that most likely is related to the observed associations.

If we take it as a given that some part of PM-related health effects are related directly to oxidant properties of PM as well as to the oxidant properties of the products of atmospheric chemical processes that involve oxides of nitrogen and ozone, then we can draw further support for the likelihood of effects related to chronic oxidant exposure from explorations of the issue of "harvesting" in studies of health effects related to daily changes in ambient PM concentrations. In the end, overall health impact of the associations between daily changes in PM aerosol and daily mortality depends upon the extent to which life expectancy is shortened by exposure (118). If the people who are dying were those whose deaths are advanced by only a few days, then a phenomenon that has been termed "harvesting" or mortality displacement would be the sole explanation for the increase in deaths and would not support the occurrence of a meaningful impact on overall mortality as measured by loss of life expectancy (55). There is general agreement (see Ref. 118 for alternative view) that the daily increases in mortality with increases in daily PM are not due simply to harvesting (55–59). Schwartz (56) carried out analyses based on smoothing windows of 15, 30, 45, and 60 days and observed that the percentage increases in mortality (years 1979–1986) per $10 \, \mu g/m^3$ increase in $PM_{2.5}$ in Boston peaked at 15, 60, and 60 days for COPD, pneumonia, and ischemic heart disease (IHD) deaths, respectively Chronic obstructive lung disease, showed evidence of harvesting at the 60-day averaging window, and pneumonia showed evidence of short-term harvesting, followed by increased percentage in mortality. These data imply that COPD deaths are being brought forward by about 2 months, while deaths from pneumonia and IHD are not due to harvesting and may reflect "enrichment" of the at-risk pool as a consequent of persistent exposure to increased average levels of PM (56). An analysis of the APHEA project, based on distributed lag models applied to 10 cities, failed to find strong evidence for mortality displacement for total daily mortality (58). Moreover, the effect estimate for mortality for exposures 11–60 days before death was more than two-thirds as large as that for the 10 days just prior to death (0.688 ± 0.261 vs. 0.922 ± 0.184, respectively—both estimates are $\times 10^3$). A further analysis of the APHEA-2 data that evaluated cause-specific deaths, stratified by age, again failed to find evidence of mortality displacement and did find evidence for more prolonged effects of PM on mortality (Table 4) (119). The magnitude of the estimated population affected increased with the number of lags considered up to 40 days, with estimates based on 40 days considerably greater than the effect estimate

Table 4 Effect of Lag Structure on Estimated Percentage Increase in Cause-Specific Mortality of PM on Mortality from the APHEA-2 Project

	Estimated percentage decrease (95% CI)	
	Cardiovascular diseases	Respiratory diseases
Unrestricted distributed lag		
20 lags	1.34 (0.89, 1.79)	1.71 (−0.65, 4.12)
30 lags	1.72 (1.20, 2.25)	2.62 (0.19, 5.11)
40 lags	1.97 (1.38, 2.55)	4.20 (1.08, 7.42)
Ages 65–74 years (40 days of lags)		
4th degree polynomial lag	2.06 (1.05, 3.09)	NA
Unrestricted lag	1.62 (0.54, 2.70)	
Ages ≥75 years (40 days of lags)		
4th degree polynomial lag	2.35 (1.42, 3.29)	4.57 (1.25, 7.99)
Unrestricted lag	2.52 (1.57, 3.48)	4.52 (0.89, 8.28)

Source: From Ref. 119.

of 0.78% increase for lags 0.1 (95% CI: −0.17, 1.66%) (119). Similar results were observed by Dominici et al. (59) in a study of daily mortality in four U.S. cities between 1987 and 1994 (Fig. 13). Results were similar for frequency-domain and time-scale estimates. The observations that effect estimates for any given day's exposure are greatest at times up to 2 months removed when taken together with the observation of autocorrelation between daily measures of air pollutants (see Fig. 10 for example), strongly suggests the occurrence of cumulating effects over time that are likely to increase the risk of manifest disease and induction and/or aggravation of the pathophysiological processes that underlie the development of disease etiology and exacerbation.

B. Evidence for Associations with Asthma

Many studies have documented the adverse effects of daily increases in ambient pollutants on symptoms and lung function in children with asthma who live in environments characterized by periods of high PM and O_3 (most recently, see Refs. 120–123). In contrast, there is very little evidence from prospective studies that ambient air pollution plays a role in the primary etiology of asthma.

The AHSMOG (Adventist Health and Smog Study) was one of the first prospective studies to observe an association between long-term exposure to ambient pollutant concentrations on the occurrence of incident asthma (124). Once again cumulative individual exposure estimates were made based on interpolation of monthly statistics from fixed site monitoring stations to residential and work location zip code centroids and cumulated over the period of follow-up. Mean sulfate concentrations were associated with the occurrence of new cases of self-reported doctor diagnosed asthma plus wheezing over the years 1977–1987 in subjects ages 27–95 in 1977 (average age = 56 years) (see Table 2 from Ref. 124). New onset was not related to sex. However, there also was an association between the report of chronic bronchitis or asthma before age 16 and "new" asthma in the study interval. No data were provided to distinguish associations with truly incident asthma vs. asthma that recurred after having been in remission for some years. A later study by these same investigators that covered the years 1977–1992 reported that new onset asthma (same definition as in previous study) was associated in males only with 20-year mean 8-hr O_3 concentrations [RR/27 ppb increase = 2.1 (1.03, 4.2) (125)]. A significant interaction was observed between mean 8-year ozone concentration and a doctor's diagnosis of asthma in 1997 for both males and females, which led the authors to conclude that their data were consistent with effects related to truly incident as well as recrudescent cases but the relative strengths of the associations could not be separated. It should be noted that, over the period of follow-up, there was a substantial correlation between mean PM_{10} mass and mean O_3 concentrations ($r = 0.77$) but less so for mean sulfate and O_3 ($r = 0.33$) (114). The use of monthly means to create the 20-year means should have mitigated bias toward more precisely estimated O_3 associations (O_3 concentrations were available on a daily basis) compared to the every sixth day PM measurements. Nonetheless, if the data from the two studies are taken together, the most reasonable conclusion is that the total pollutant mixture is most likely responsible for the associations rather than any single component.

Additional evidence that the ambient pollutant mixture could contribute to the incidence of asthma comes from a 4-year follow-up of the CHS (51). This study observed and the highest crude incidence of new onset asthma over a 4-year period in "high" O_3 communities among children who participated in three or more outdoor sports (Table 5). A smaller increase in risk was seen for high PM communities (same as high NO_2 communities). Division of communities into high O_3–low other pollutants and high O_3–high other pollutants did not provide evidence for interaction with other pollutants [RR for ≥3 sports: high–low = 4.2 (1.6, 10.7) and 3.3 (1.6, 6.9), respectively] (Table 5). Moreover, there was little effect in low ozone communities, irrespective of the levels of other pollutants (51). These data do point to the photochemical processes that involve O_3 formation and a variety of highly oxidant species as being paramount in the observed associations. Since these reactions are driven by hydrocarbons found as part of PM, the data point to the aggregate oxidant environment as a major contributor to the observed associations. A study of incident bronchitis over a 4-year period in children with asthma for same population

Table 5 Adjusted Relative Risks (95% CI) of New Onset Asthma Based on 4-Year Follow-up of the Children's Health Study

Number of sports played	PM effects		Ozone effects	
	Low PM communities		Low O_3 communities	High O_3 communities
0	1.0 (0.023)[a]	1.0 (0.021)	1.0 (0.027)	1.0 (0.018)
1	1.5 (1.0, 2.2)	1.1 (0.7, 1.7)	1.3 (0.9, 1.3)	1.3 (0.8,2.0)
2	1.2 (0.7, 1.9)	0.9 (0.5, 1.7)	0.8 (0.5, 1.4)	1.3 (0.7, 2.3)
≥3	1.7 (0.9, 3.2)	2.0 (1.1, 3.6),	0.8 (0.4, 1.6)	3.3 (1.9, 5.8),
	(0.033)[a]	(0.033)	(0.019)	(0.050)

Based on 4-year mean concentrations in each of 12 communities in southern California: high-pollution communities—8-hr $O_3 = 40(\pm 8)$ ppb, $PM_{10} = 22$ (± 4) $\mu g/m^3$, $PM_{2.5} = 8$ (± 1) $\mu g/m^3$, $NO_2 = 11(\pm 5)$ ppb, acid (inorganic hydrochloric acid and nitric acid vapor) $= 2(\pm 1)$ ppb; low-pollution communities—8-hr $O_3 = 60(\pm 5)$ ppb, $PM_{10} = 43$ (± 12) $\mu g/m^3$, $PM_{2.5} = 21(\pm 6)$ $\mu g/m^3$, $NO_2 = 29(\pm 9)$ ppb, acid (inorganic hydrochloric acid and nitric acid vapor) $= 4(\pm 1)$ ppb; high- and low-PM and ozone communities were not the same; high- and low-PM and NO_2 communities were the same.
[a]Incidence based on person years of follow-up
Source: From Ref. 51.

observed increased within community odds ratios for occurrence of incident bronchitis for NO_2, O_3, $PM_{2.5}$, and organic carbon (OC) (per unit deviation of annual mean from 4-year mean for each pollutant $= 1.07$, 1.06, 1.09, 1.41, respectively; lower bound of all confidence intervals ≥1.00) with trends toward increased odds for PM_{10}, $PM_{10-2.5}$, inorganic and organic acids, and elemental carbon (1.04, 1.02, 1.20, 1.19, and 2.63, respectively; lower bounds of CIs < 1.00). Examination of the correlation coefficient between all of the other pollutants and O_3 (exclusive of $PM_{10-2.5}$, range 0.64 for PM_{10}–0.81 for OC) reinforces the view that the effect reported most likely is due to the aggregate pollutant environment, with its oxidant components likely playing an important role. Bronchitis symptoms (increased cough and phlegm production) in the children with asthma often reflect exacerbations of asthma, which would suggest that the ambient pollutant environment contributes to disease severity as defined by the National Asthma Education and Prevention Program (126) and likely adds additional oxidative stress due to acute inflammation. In summary, the findings from the CHS are consistent with the interpretation that the observed health effects most likely are due the complex oxidant environments and its enhancement of inflammatory reactions and the augmentation of immune responses that are central to the pathogenesis and pathophysiology of asthma (Fig. 2).

Ozone, NO_2, and diesel exhaust particles (particularly the PAH components) have been shown to enhance responses to inhaled allergens (127–129). Jenkins et al. (128) demonstrated that the $PD_{20}FEV_1$ to mite allergen was not altered by controlled exposure to an O_3 concentration of 100 ppb or an NO_2 concentration of 200 ppb when each was administered separately but was reduced when concentrations of both gases were administered together. In an infant rhesus monkey model, Schlegele et al. (130) demonstrated that cyclic inhalation of O_3 and house dust mite allergen (HDMA) produced a marked increase in IgE and airway eosinophilia not seen with HDMA sensitization alone and greater degrees of airway hyperresponsiveness and structural remodeling than observed in animals exposed and sensitized only to HDMA. A series of studies have shown that components of diesel exhaust (PAHs, in particular) are capable of driving the immune response to inhaled antigens toward an IgE response (131,132). Of particular interest for the pathogenesis of new onset allergic respiratory disease is the observation that diesel PM can induce sensitization to a neoantigen in persons already sensitized to an allergen that triggers IgE-induced allergic response (133). Coupled with ability of both O_3 and NO_2 to enhance physiological responses to inhaled allergen, these findings add to the likelihood that the observed associations in CHS may represent one causal mechanism that contributes to the risk of asthma. Moreover, the study by Schelegle et al. (130) when coupled with the results of Kunzli et al. (109), cited previously, add credibility to the likelihood that long-term exposure to oxidant pollutants can produce persistence structural damage to the lung.

One additional prospective epidemiological study provides support for a connection between oxidant pollutants and asthma etiology. Brauer et al. (134) evaluated the relationship between "traffic-related pollutants" (soot by filter absorbance, $PM_{2.5}$, NO_2—all three pollutants highly correlated, $r > 0.90$) on the occurrence an asthma diagnosis over the first 24 months of life[d] in a birth cohort study of 4146 children in the Netherlands. Home-based individual exposure assignments were based on previously validated model based on geographical information system (GIS) data and a pollutant measurement and modeling exercise (135). Over the first 24 months of life, the adjusted odds ratio for new asthma for an interquartile increase ($3.2 \, \mu g/m^3$) in $PM_{2.5}$ exposure was $\sim$1.2 with the lower bound of the 95% CI just below 1 (data estimated from Fig. 2 of Ref. 135, exact OR and CI not given).

---

[d] The diagnosis of asthma may be difficult in the first few years of life. However, it can be assumed that these children at least had recurrent and severe episodes of wheezing.

C. Associations with Alterations in Growth of Lung Function in Children

Studies from two separate cohorts in the southern California CHS illustrate the potential fallacy of inference about air pollution health effects based on consideration of single pollutants. Data for FEV_1 from the first 1993 cohort (left panel of Fig. 14) were interpreted as showing significant deficits in lung growth relative to 4-year average community levels of NO_2 and inorganic acid vapor $(HCl + HNO_3)$ with little effect associated with community levels of O_3 (52). The NO_2 and inorganic acid vapor $(HCl + HNO_3)$ associations were greatest for measures of small airway function (FEF_{75}) (data not shown), with the regression coefficients being nearly identical for each (52). Results from the second cohort were considered to provide corroborative evidence for the results from cohort 1 (right panel of Fig. 14) (53), although the relationships clearly differ for O_3, and PM_{10}, and $PM_{2.5}$. For both cohorts, the most consistent effect is for inorganic acids (see Table 7 from Ref. 53). The HNO_3 component results from photochemistry that involves O_3, NO_x (specifically the reaction of NO_2 with the OH radical), and the organic component of $PM_{2.5}$. Formation of HCl also depends, in part, on reaction of chloride ions (from sea salt) with OH radical (136) that are derived from photochemical reactions the involve O_3 $[O_3 + h\nu \rightarrow O_2 + O(^1D); O(^1D) + H_2O \rightarrow 2 \text{ OH}$, where $O(^1D)$ is excited oxygen (9). After consideration of other sources of oxidant pollutants (gas stoves, second-hand smoke exposure, pets as a source of allergen and endotoxin), annual growth of FEV_1 between the communities with the highest and lowest community levels of PM_{10} was associated with NO_2 concentrations only for children with asthma.

While the above data are consistent with long-term effects of chronic exposure to ambient pollutants, they do not imply necessarily irreversible effects. Avol et al. (88) were able to study 110 of 149 children who moved from the CHS communities. Subjects were assigned pollution scores based on their former and new communities of residence (Fig. 15). On average, children who came from "high" PM_{10} CHS communities and moved to lower PM_{10} communities experienced increases in their growth of maximum mid-expiratory flow (MMEF, FEF_{25-75}) rates (annual increase in MMEF = 19 mL/sec per 10 μg/m^3 increase in PM_{10}—lower panel of Fig. 15). However, many children moved to communities where they would be expected, on average to have continued deficits of lung function growth (compare low and middle panels of Fig. 15). Subjects who moved from a low-PM community to a high communities (top panel of Fig. 15) experienced a 54.9 mL/sec decreased in rate of growth of MMEF for each 10 μg/m^3 increase in PM_{10}. Duration away from the CHS community was associated with a trend toward increasing PM_{10} effect. Although PM_{10} was the only pollutant whose effect was statistically significant, the direction of effects for O_3 and NO_2 were in the same direction as those for PM_{10}. In aggregate, these results indicate that some effects of exposure to oxidant environments on lung function are reversible and that growth rates are not likely, on average to make up all of past deficits when children move to communities with lower levels of ambient oxidant pollutants (compare middle and lower panels of Fig. 15).

D. Associations with Cancer and Cardiovascular Disease

Despite the data reviewed in Sec. I.A. related to the role of oxidative stress in the production of DNA damage and the role of oxidative mechanisms in the pathogenesis of atherosclerotic cardiovascular disease, there are no data from prospective epidemiological, cohort studies to document the role of long-term exposure to oxidant ambient pollutants and the incidence of cancers and cardiovascular disease. However, the data related to mortality displacement do provide some support for a role of ambient oxidant pollution in the ongoing pathogenesis of cardiovascular disease. This is especially the case when considered in conjunction with epidemiological data that show associations between daily changes in ambient pollutant levels and heart rate variability (137), changes in blood viscosity (138), sequestration of red blood cells in the circulation (139) and data on alterations of endothelial function (140,141).

VI. Summary and Conclusions

This chapter has summarized the limited data related to the occurrence of health effects that are most likely attributable to chronic exposure to oxidant ambient pollutant mixtures. Despite its limited scope, the data on birth outcomes, the mortality data derived from the ACS cohort and the data on asthma occurrence from the CHS make a strong argument in support such relationship. The emerging body of experimental data on the role of oxidant stress and cellular damage and disease pathogenesis provide a strong base of support for the epidemiological data and should serve as a stimulus to fill the current gaps in current knowledge and to highlight the need to consider the potential effects of today's concentrations of ambient pollutants on the future health of populations.

With regard to exposure, direct measurements of the oxidant burden of a given ambient mixture such as those applied by Li et al. (2) need wider application in epidemiological studies and expansion to include additional chemical components and/or to reflect products of specific atmospheric chemistry of ambient mixtures in various meteorological settings. Epidemiological studies that contrast areas with large differences in the sources or atmospheric chemistry that contribute to the total oxidant burden of the air would be most useful in terms of the development of data for specific quantitative risk assessment and to determine whether or not sources and specific atmospheric environments are even relevant, with respect to the oxidant burdens that they impose, to such risk assessment. Additional studies that focus on the mass concentrations of pollutants or groups of pollutants are not likely to provide any insights with regard to the relationship between chronic exposure to oxidant pollutants and human health.

With regard to the epidemiological data, issues of feasibility, time and cost quickly temper any suggestions for additional cohort studies to expand the database related to effects of long-term exposures on cancer and cardiovascular diseases in particular but also asthma, chronic obstructive lung disease and birth outcomes. Existing cohort studies in children and adolescents that are collecting data on intermediates on the pathway to these diseases represent potential targets to provide support for chronic exposure and cardiovascular disease outcomes as do studies of individuals with specific genetic constellations that put them at high risk for adverse health outcomes as illustrated by the data for GSTM1 cited previously.

References

1. Marnett LJ. Health effects of aldehydes and alcohols in mobile source emissions. In: Watson AY, Bates RR, Kennedy D, eds. Air Pollution, The Automobile and Public Health. Washington, D.C.: National Academy Press, 1988: 579–603.
2. Li N, Sioutas C, Cho A, Schmitz D, Misra C, Sempf J, Wang M, Oberley T, Froines J, Nel A. Ultrafine particulate pollutants induce oxidative stress and mitochondnal damage. Environ Health Perspect 2003; 111:455–460.
3. Leikauf GD, Zhao Q, Zhou S, Santrock J. Ozonolysis products of membrane fatty acids activate eicosanoid metabolism in human airway epithelial cells. Am J Respir Cell Mol Biol 1993; 9:594–602.
4. Pryor WA, Squadrito GL, Friedman M. The cascade mechanism to explain ozone toxicity: the role of lipid ozonation products. Free Rad Biol Med 1995; 19:935–941.
5. Kafoury RM, Pryor WA, Squadrito GL, Salgo MG, Zou X, Friedman M. Induction of inflammatory mediators in human airway epithelial cells by lipid ozonation products. Am J Respir Crit Care Med 1999; 160:1934–1942.
6. Mudway IS, Kelly FJ. Ozone and the lung: a sensitive issue. Mol Aspects Med 2000; 21:1–48.
7. Winters RS, Burnette-Vick BA, Johnson DA. Ozone, but not nitrogen dioxide, fragments elastin and increases its susceptibility to proteolysis. Am J Respir Crit Care Med 1994; 150:1026–1031.
8. Postlethwait EM, Langford SD, Jacobson LM, Bidani A. NO_2 reactive absorption substrates in rat pulmonary surface lining fluids. Free Rad Biol Med 1995; 19:553–563.

9. U.S. Environmental Protection Agency. Air Quality Criteria For Oxides of Nitrogen Vol I of III, EPA/600/8-9l/049aF. Research Triangle Park, NC: Environmental Criteria and Assessment Office, 1993:5–1, 5–61.

10. Avissar NE, Reed CK, Cox C, Frampton MW, Finkelstein JN. Ozone, but not nitrogen dioxide, exposure decreases glutathione peroxidases in epithelial lining fluid of human lung. Am J Respir Crit Care Med 2000; 162:1342–1347.

11. Azadniv M, Utell MJ, Morrow PE, Gibb FR, Nichols J, Roberts NJ Jr, Speers DM, Torres A, Ts Y, Abraham MK, Voter KZ, Frampton MW. Effects of nitrogen dioxide exposure on human host defenses. Inhal Toxicol 1998; 10:585–601.

12. Gaston B, Drazen JM, Loscalzo J, Stamler JS. The biology of nitrogen oxides in the airways. Am J Respir Crit Care Med 1994; 149:538–551.

13. Ghio AJ, Stonehuerner J, Pritchard RJ, Piantodosi CA, Dreher KL, Costa DL. Humic-like substances in air pollution particulates correlate with concentrations of transition metals and oxidant generation. Inhal Toxicol 1996; 8:479–494.

14. Pritchard RJ, Ghio AJ, Lehmann JR, Winsett DW, Tepper JS, Park P, Gilmour MI, Dreher KL, Costa DL. Oxidant generation and lung injury after particulate air pollutant exposure increase with concentration of associated metals. Inhal Toxicol 1996; 8:457–477.

15. Dreher KL, Jaskot RH, Lehmann JR, Richards JH, McGee JK, Ghio AJ, Costa DL. Soluble transition metals mediate residual oil fly ash induced acute lung injury. J Toxicol Environ Health 1997; 50:285–305.

16. Ghio AJ, Meng HH, Hatch GE, Costa DL. Luminol-enhanced chemiluminescence after in vitro exposures of rat alveolar macrophages to oil fly ash is metal dependent. Inhal Toxicol 1997; 9:255–271.

17. Dye JA, Lehmann JR, McGee JK, Winsett DW, Ledbetter AD, Everitt JI, Ghio AJ, Costa DL. Acute pulmonary toxicity of particulate matter filter extracts in rats: coherence with epidemiologic studies in Utah Valley residents. Environ Health Perspect 2001; 109(suppl 3):395–403.

18. Aust AE, Ball JC, Hu AA, Lighty JS, Smith KR, Straccia AM, Veranth JM, Young WC. Particle characteristics responsible for effects on human lung epithelial cells. Res Rep Health Eff Inst 2002:1–65; discussion 67–76.

19. Tyler W, Tyler N, Last J, Gillespie M, Barstow T. Comparison of daily and seasonal exposures of young monkeys to ozone. Toxicology 1988; 50:131–144.

20. Harkema JR, Plopper CG, Hyde DM, St, George JA, Wilson DW, Dungworth DL. Response of macaque bronchiolar epithelium to ambient concentrations of ozone. Am J Pathol 1993; 143:857–866.

21. Niewoehner DE, Leinerman J, Rice DB. Pathologic changes in the peripheral airways of 12 young cigarette smokers. New Engl J Med 1974; 291: 755–758.

22. Cheng T-J, Kao H-P, Chan C-C, Chang WP. Effects of ozone on DNA single-strand breaks and 8-oxoguanine formation in A549 cells. Environ Res 2003; In press, www.sciencedirect.com.

23. Bermudez E, Ferng S-F, Castro CE, Mustafa MG. DNA strand breaks caused by exposure to ozone and nitrogen dioxide. Environ Res 1999; 81:72–80.

24. Kumagai Y, Arimoto T, Shinyashiki M, Shimojo N, Nakai Y, Yoshikawa T, Sagai M. Generation of reactive oxygen species during interaction of diesel exhaust particle components with NADPH-cytochrome P450 reductase and involvement of the bioactivation in the DNA damage. Free Rad Biol Med 1997; 22:479–487.

25. Seagrave J, McDonald JD, Gigliotti AP, Nikula KJ, Seilkop SK, Gurevich M, Mauderly JL. Mutagenicity and in vivo toxicity of combined particulate and semivolatile organic fractions of gasoline and diesel engine emissions. Toxicol Sci 2002; 70:212–226.

26. Moller P, Daneshvar B, Loft S, Wallin H, Poulsen HE, Autrup H, Ravn-Haren G, Dragsted LO. Oxidative DNA damage in vitamin C-supplemented guinea pigs after intratracheal instillation of diesel exhaust particles. Toxicol Appl Pharmacol 2003; 189:39–44.

27. Ma JY, Ma JK. The dual effect of the particulate and organic components of diesel exhaust particles on the alteration of pulmonary immune/inflammatory responses and metabolic enzymes. J Enviorn Sci Health Part C Environ Carcinog Ecotoxicol Rev 2002; 20:117–147.

28. Calderon-Garciduenas L, Osnaya-Brizuela N, Ramirex-Martinez L, Villarreal-Calderon A. DNA strand breaks in human nasal respiratory epithelium are induced upon exposure to urban pollution. Environ Health Perspect 1996; 104:160–168.

29. Calderon-Garciduenas L, Osnaya N, Rodriguez-Alcaraz A, vilarreal-Calderon A. DNA damage in nasal respiratory epithelium from children exposed to urban air pollution. Env Molec Mutagenesis 1997; 30:11–20.

30. Calderon-Garciduenas L, Wen-Wang L, Zhang YJ, Rodriguez-Alcaraz A, Osnaya N, Villarreal-Calderon A, Santella RM. 8-Hydroxy-2'-deoxyguanosine, a major mutagenic oxidative DNA lesion, and DNA strand breaks in nasal respiratory epithelium of children exposed to urban pollution. Environ Health Perspect 1999; 107:469–474.

31. Steinberg D. Low density lipoprotein oxidation and its significance. J Biol Chem 1997; 272:20963–20966.

32. Nemmar A, Hoet PH, Vanquickenborne B, Dinsdale D, Thomeer M, Hoylaerts MF, Vanbilloen H, Mortelmans L, Nemery B. Passage of inhaled particles into the blood circulation in humans. Circulation 2002; 105: 411–414.

33. Ross R. Atherosclerosis—An inflammatory disease. New Engl J Med 1999; 340:115–126.

34. Mukae H, Hogg JC, English D, Vincent R, van Eeden SF. Phagocytosis of particulate air pollutants by human alveolar macrophages stimulates the bone marrow. Am J Physiol Lung Cell Molec Physiol 2000; 279:L924–L931.

35. Mukae H, Vincent R, Quinlan K, English D, Hards J, Hogg JC, van Eeden SF. The effect of repeated exposure to particulate air pollution (PM10) on the bone marrow. Am J Respir Crit Care Med 2001; 163:201–209.

36. Tan WC, Qiu D, Liam BL, Ng TP, Lee SH, van Eeden SF, D'Yachkova Y, Hogg JC. The human bone marrow response to acute air pollution caused by forest fires. Am J Respir Crit Care Med 2000; 161:1213–1217.

37. van Eeden SF, Tan WC, Suwa T, Mukae H, Terashima T, Fujii T, Qui D, Vincent R, Hogg JC. Cytokines involved in the systemic inflammatory response induced by exposure to particulate matter air pollutants (PM 10). Am J Respir Crit Care Med 2001; 164:826–830.

38. Ridker PM, Hennekens CH, Buring JE, Fifai N. C-reactive protein and other makers of inflammation in the prediction of cardiovascular disease in women. New Engl J Med 2000; 342:836–843.

39. Repine JE, Bast A, Lankhorst I. and the Oxidative Stress Study Group. Oxidative stress in chronic obstructive pulmonary disease. Am J Respir Crit Care Med 1997; 156:341–357.

40. Kim CS, Kang TC. Comparative measurement of lung deposition of inhaled fine particles in normal subjects and patients with obstructive airway disease. Am J Respir Grit Care Med 1997; 155:899–905.

41. Foster WM, Silver JA, Groth ML. Exposure to ozone alters regional function and particle dosimetry in the human lung. J Appl Physiol 1993; 75: 1938–1945.

42. Romieu I, Meneses F, Ramirez M, Ruiz S, Perez Padilla R, Sienra JJ, Gerber M, Grievink L, Dekker R, Walda I, Brunekreef B. Antioxidant supplementation and respiratory functions among workers exposed to high levels of ozone. Am J Respir Crit Care Med 1998; 158:226–232.

43. Romieu I, Sienra-Monge JJ, Ramirez-Aguilar M, Tellez-Rojo MM, Moreno-Macias H, Reyes-Ruiz NI, del Rio-Navarro BE, Ruiz-Navarro MX, Hatch G, Slade R, Hernandez-Avila M. Antioxidant supplementation and lung functions among children with asthma exposed to high levels of air pollutants. Am J Respir Crit Care Med 2002; 166:703–709.

44. Grievink L, Jansen SM, van't Veer P, Brunekreef B. Acute effects of ozone on pulmonary function of cyclists receiving antioxidant supplements. Occup Environ Med 1998; 55:13–17.

45. Grievink L, Zijlstra AG, Ke X, Brunekreef B. Double-blind intervention trial on modulation of ozone effects on pulmonary function. Am J Epidemiol 1999; 149:306–314.

46. Trenga CL, Koenig JQ, Williams PV. Dietary antioxidants and ozone-induced bronchial 20 hyperresponsiveness in adults with asthma. Arch Environ Health 2001; 56:242–249.

47. Samet JM, Hatch GE, Horstman D, Steck-Scott S, Arab L, Bromberg PA, Levine M, McDonnell WF, Devlin RB. Effect of antioxidant supplementation on ozone-induced lung injury in human subjects. Am J Respir Crit Care Med 2001; 164:819–825.

48. U.S. Enviromental Protection Agency. Review of the National Ambient Air Quality Standards for Particulate Matter: Policy Assessment of Scientific and Technical Information. Research Triangle Park: Office of Air Quality Planning and Standards, April, 1996: Chapter VI.

49. U.S. Environmental Protection Agency. Fourth External Review Draft of Air Quality Criteria for Particulate Matter (June 1, 2003)—Volume II. Research Triangle Park, NC: US EPA, 2003.

50. Pope CA III, Burnett RT, Thun MJ, Calle EE, Krewski D, Ito K, Thurston GD. Lung cancer cardiopulmonary mortality, and long-term exposure to fine particulate air pollution. JAMA 2002; 287:1132–1141.
51. McConnell R, Berhane K, Gilliland F, London SJ, Islam T, Gauderman WJ, Avol E, Margolis HG, Peters JM. Asthma in exercising children exposed to ozone: a cohort study. Lancet 2002; 359:386–391.
52. Gauderman WJ, McConnell R, Gilliland F, London S, Thomas D, Avol E, Vora H, Berhane K, Rappaport EB, Lurmann F, Margolis HC, Peters J. Association between air pollution and lung function growth in Southern California children. Am J Respir Crit Care Med 2000; 162:1383–1390.
53. Gauderman WJ, Gilliland GF, Vora H, Avol E, Stram D, McConnell R, Thomas D, Lurmann F, Margolis H, Rappaport EB, Peters JM. Association between air pollution and lung function growth in southern California Children—Results form a second cohort. Am J Respir Crit Care Med 2003; 166:76–84.
54. McConnell R, Berhane K, Gilliland F, Molitor J, Thomas D, Lurmann F, Avol E, Gauderman WJ, Peters JM. Prospective study of air pollution and bronchitic symptoms in children with asthma. Am J Respir Crit Care Med 2003; 168:790–797.
55. Zeger SL, Dominici F, Samet JM. Harvesting-resistent estimates of air pollution effects on mortality. Ann Epidemiol 1999; 10:171–175.
56. Schwartz J. Harvesting and long term exposure effects in the relation between air pollution and mortality. Am J Epidemiol 2000; 151:440–448.
57. Schwartz J. Is there harvesting in the association of airborne particles with daily deaths and hospital admissions. Epidemiology 2001; 12:55–61.
58. Zanobetti A, Schwartz J, Samoli E, Gryparis A, Touloumi G, Atkinson R, Le Tertre A, Bobros J, Celko M, Goren A, Forsberg B, Michelozzi P, Rabczenko D, Aranguez Ruiz E, Katsouyanni K. The temporal pattern of mortality responses to air pollution: a multicity assessment of mortality displacement. Epidemiol 2002; 13:87–93.
59. Dominici F, McDermott A, Zeger SL, Samet JM. Airborne particulate matter and mortality: timescale effects in four US cities. Am J Epidemiol 2003; 157:1055–1065.
60. Churg A, Brauer M, Avila-Casado MDC, Fortoul TI, Wright JL. Chronic exposure to high levels of particulate air pollution and small airway remodeling. Environ Health Perspect 2003; 111:714–718.
61. Frank R, Tankersley C. Air pollution and daily mortality: a hypothesis concerning the role of impaired homeostasis. Environ Health Perspect 2002; 110:61–65.
62. U.S. Environmental Protection Agency. Air Quality Criteria for Ozone and Related Photochemical Oxidants, EPA/600/P-93/004cF. Vol. I of III. Research Triangle Park, NC, 1996.
63. Levin H. Indoor air quality by design. In: Spengler JD, Samet JM, McCarthy JF, eds. Indoor Air Quality Handbook. New York: McGraw-Hill, 2001: 60.5.
64. U.S. Environmental Protection Agency. Latest Findings on National Air Quality-2002, Status and Trends. Research Triangle Park, NC: Office of

Air Quality Planning and Standards, Emissions Monitoring and Analysis Division, EPA 454/K-03–001, August, 2003.

65. Baldasano JM, Valera E, Jimenez P. Air quality data from large cities. Sci Total Environ 2003; 307:141–165.

66. Wark K, Warner CF. Air Pollution Its Origin and Control. New York: Harper Collings, 1981:143–151.

67. Neas LM, Dockery DW, Ware JH, Spengler JD, Speizer FE, Ferris BG Jr. Association of indoor nitrogen dioxide with respiratory symptoms and pulmonary function in children. Am J Epidemiol 1991; 134:204–219.

68. Lee K, Xue J, Geyh AS, Ozkaynak H, Leaderer BP, Weschler CJ, Spengler JD. Nitrous acid, nitrogen dioxide, and ozone concentrations in residential environments. Environ Health Perspect 2002; 110:145–150.

69. Levy JI, Lee K, Yanagisawa Y, Hutchinson P, Spengler JD. Determinants of nitrogen dioxide concentrations in indoor ice skating rinks. Am J Publ Health 1998; 88:1781–1786.

70. Pereira LAA, Loomis D, Conceicoa GMS, Braga ALF, Areas RM, Kishi JS, Singer JM, Bohm GM, Saldiva PHN. Association between air pollution and intrauterine mortality in Sao Paulo, Brazil. Environ Health Perspect 1998; 106:325–329.

71. Wang X, Ding J, Ryan L, Xu X. Association between air pollution and low birth weight: a community-based study. Environ Health Perspect 1997; 105:514–520.

72. Bobak M, Leon DA. Pregnancy outcomes and outdoor air pollution: an ecological study in districts of the Czech Republic 1986–8. Occup Environ Med 1999; 56:539–543.

73. Rogers JF, Thompson SJ, Addy CL, McKeown RE, Cowen DJ, Decoufle P. Association of very low birth weight with exposures to environmental sulfur dioxide and total suspended particulates. Am J Epidemiol 2000; 151:602–613.

74. Wilhelm M, Ritz B. Residential proximity to traffic and adverse birth outcomes in Los Angeles county, California, 1994–1996. Environ Health Perspect 2003; 111:207–216.

75. Perera FP, Rauh V, Tsai WY, Kinney P, Camann D, Barr D, Bernert T, Garfinkel R, Tu YH, Diaz D, Dietrich J, Whyatt RM. Effects of transplacental exposure to environmental pollutants on birth outcomes in a multiethnic population. Environ Health Perspect 2003; 111:201–205.

76. Liu S, Krewski D, Shi Y, Chen Y, Burnett RT. Association between gaseous ambient air pollutants and adverse pregnancy outcomes in Vancouver, Canada. Environ Health Perspect 2003; 111:1773–1778.

77. Xu X, Ding H, Wang X. Acute effects of total suspended particles and sulfur dioxides on preterm delivery: a community-based cohort study. Arch Environ Health 1995; 50:407–415.

78. Ritz B, Yu F, Chapa G, Fruin S. Effect of air pollution on preterm birth among children born in southern California between 1989 and 1993. Epidemiology 2000; 11:502–511.

79. Dejmek J, Solansky I, Benes I, Lenicek J, Sram RJ. The impact of polycyclic aromatic hydrocarbons and fine particles on pregnancy outcome. Environ Health Perspect 2000; 108:1159–1164.

80. Loomis D, Castillejos M, Gold DR, McDonnell W, Borja-Aburto VH. Air pollution and infant mortality in Mexico City. Epidemiology 1999; 10: 118–123.
81. Bobak M, Leon DA. Air pollution and infant mortality in the Czech Republic, 1986–88. Lancet 1992; 340:1010–1014.
82. Woodruff T, Grillo J, Schoendorf K. The relationship between selected causes of postneonatal infant mortality and particulate air pollution in the United States. Environ Health Perspect 1997; 105:608–612.
83. Bobak M, Leon DA. The effect of air pollution on infant mortality appears specific for respiratory causes. Epidemiology 1999; 10:666–670.
84. Dolk H, Pattenden S, Vrijheid M, Thakrar B, Armstrong B. Perinatal and infant mortality and low birth weight among residents near cokeworks in Great Britain. Arch Environ Health 2000; 55:26–30.
85. Annesi-Maesano I, Moreau D, Strachan D. In utero and perinatal complications preceding asthma. Allergy 2001; 56:491–497.
86. Steffensen FH, Sorensen HT, Gillman MW, Rothman KJ, Sabroe S, Fischer P, Olsen J. Low birth weight and preterm delivery as risk factors for asthma and atopic dermatitis in young adult males. Epidemiology 2000; 11: 185–188.
87. Mortimer KM, Tager IB, Dockery DW, Neas LM, Redline S. The effect of ozone on inner-city children with asthma: identification of susceptible subgroups. Am J Respir Crit Care Med 2000; 162:1838–1845.
88. Avol EL, Gauderman WJ, Tan SM, London SJ, Peters JM. Respiratory effects of relocating to areas of differing air pollution levels. Am J Respir Crit Care Med 2001; 164:2067–2072.
89. Barker DJ, Godfrey KM, Fall C, Osmond C, Winter PD, Shaheen SO. Relation of birth weight and childhood respiratory infection to adult lung function and death from chronic obstructive airways disease. Brit Med J 1991; 303:671–675.
90. Mann SL, Wadsworth MEJ, Colley JRT. Accumulation of factors influencing respiratory illness in members of a national birth cohort and their offspring. J Epidemiol Commun Health 1992; 46:286–292.
91. Ward PA, Warren JS, Johnson KJ. Oxygen radicals, inflammation, and tissue injury. Free Rad Biol Med 1988; 5:403–408.
92. Chow CW, Herrera Abreu MT, Suzuki T, Downey GP. Oxidative stress and acute lung injury. Am J Respir Cell Mol Biol 2003; 29:427–431.
93. Djukanovic R, Roche WR, Wilson JW, Beasley CR, Twentyman OP, Howarth RH, Holgate ST. Mucosal inflammation in asthma. Am Rev Respir Dis 1990; 142:434–457.
94. Wanner A, Boushey H, Lee TH, eds. Inflammation in Chronic Obstructive Lung Disease. Am J Respiratory Critical Care Med 1999; 160(2):S1–S79.
95. Sohal RS, Weindruch R. Oxidative stress, caloric restriction, and aging. Science 1996; 273:59–63.
96. Eaton DL, Bammler TK. Concise review of the glutathione S-transferases and their significance to toxicology. Toxicol Sci 1999; 49:156–154.
97. Hayes JD, Strange RC. Glutathione S-transferase polymorphisms and their biological consequences. Pharmacology 2000; 61:154–166.

98. Romieu I, Sienra-Monge JJ, Ramirez M, Moreno-Macias H, Reyes-Ruiz NI, del Rio-Navarro BE, Hernandez-Avila M, London S J. Genetic polymorphism of GSTMI and antioxidant supplementation influence lung function in relation to ozone exposure among asthmatic children in Mexico City. Thorax—In press 2003.

99. Nebert DW, Petersen DD, Fornace AJ Jr. Cellular responses to oxidative stress: The [*Ah*] gene battery as a paradigm. Environ Health Perspect 1990; 18:13–25.

100. Schulz WA, Eickelmann P, Sies H. Free radicals in toxicology: redox cycling and NAD(P)H:quinone oxidoreductase. Arch Toxicol Suppl 1996; 18:217–222.

101. Bergamaschi E, De Palma G, Mozzoni P, Vanni S, Vettori MV, Broeckaert F, Bernard A, Mutti A. Polymorphism of quinone-metabolizing enzymes and susceptibility to ozone-induced acute effects. Am J Respir Crit Care Med 2001; 163:1426–1431.

102. Corradi M, Alinovi R, Goldoni M, Vettori M, Folesani G, Mozzoni P, Cavazzini S, Bergamaschi E, Rossi L, Mutti A. Biomarkers of oxidative stress after controlled human exposure to ozone. Toxicol Lett 2002; 134:219–225.

103. Gilliland FD, Gauderman WJ, Vora H, Rappaport E, Dubeau L. Effects of glutathione-*S*-transferase Ml, Tl, and PI on childhood lung function growth. Am J Respir Crit Care Med 2002; 166:710–716.

104. Blankenberg S, Rupprecht HJ, Bickel C, Torzewski M, Hafner G, Tiret L, Smieja M, Cambien F, JMeyer J, Lackner KJ. for the AtheroGene Investigators. Glutathione peroxidase 1 activity and cardiovascular events in patients with coronary artery disease. New Engl J Med 2002; 349:1605–1613.

105. Künzli N, Lurmann F, Segal M, Ngo L, Balmes J, Tager IB. Reliability of lifetime residential history and activity measures as elements of cumulative ambient ozone exposure assessment. J Exp Anal Environ Epidemiol 1996; (In press).

106. Gonzales M, Ngo L, Hammond KS, Tager IB. Validation of a questionnaire and microenvironmental model for estimating past exposures to ozone. Int J Environ Health Res 2003; 13:249–260.

107. U.S. Environmental Protection Agency. Air Quality Criteria for Ozone and Related Photochemical Oxidants, EPA/600/P-93/004cF. Vol. III of III. Research Triangle Park, NC, 1996.

108. U.S. Environmental Protection Agency. Air Quality Criteria for Particulate Matter Volume II. Air Quality Criteria for Particulate Matter Volumes I–III. Washington, DC: National Center for Environmental Assessment Office of Research and Development, U.S. EPA, 1996 EPA/600/P-95–001bF.

109. Kunzli N, Lurmann F, Segal M, Ngo L, Balmes J, Tager IB. Association between lifetime ambient ozone exposure and pulmonary function in college freshman—Results of a pilot study. Environ Res 1997; 72:8–23.

110. Atkinson RW, Anderson HR, Sunyer J, Ayres J, Baccini M, Vonk JM, Boumghar A, Forastiere F, Forsberg B, Touloumi G, Schwartz J, Katsouyanni K. Acute effects of particulate air pollution on respiratory admissions: results from APHEA 2 project. Air pollution and health: a European approach. Am J Respir Crit Care Med 2001; 164:1860–1866.

111. Sarnat JA, Schwartz J, Catalano PJ, Suh HH. Gaseous pollutants in particulate matter epidemiology: confounders or surrogates? Environ Health Perspect 2001; 109:1053–1061.

112. Dockery DW, Pope Ad, Xu X, Spengler JD, Ware JH, Fay ME, Ferris BJ, Speizer FE. An association between air pollution and mortality in six U.S. cities [see comments]. New Engl J Med 1993; 329:1753–1759.

113. Pope CA, Thun MJ, Namboodiri MM, Dockery DW, Evans JS, Speizer FE, Heath CW. Particle air pollution as a predictor of mortality in a prospective study of U.S. adults. Am J Respir Crit Care Med 1995; 151:669–674.

114. Abbey DE, Nishino N, McDonnell WF, Burchette RJ, Knutsen SF, Lawrence Beeson W, Yang JX. Long-term inhalable particles and other air pollutants related to mortality in nonsmokers. Am J Respir Crit Care Med 1999; 159:373–382.

115. Abbey D, Mills P, Petersen F, Beeson W. Long-term ambient concentrations of total suspended particulates and oxidants as related to incidence of chronic disease in California Seventh-Day Adventists. Environ Health Perspect 1991; 94:43–50.

116. Abbey D, Petersen F, Mills P, Beeson W. Long-term ambient concentrations of total suspended particulates, ozone, and sulfur dioxide and respiratory symptoms in a nonsmoking population. Arch Environ Health 1993; 48:33–46.

117. Hoek G, Brunekreef B, Goldbohm S, Fischer P, van den Brandt PA. Association between mortality and indicators of traffic-related air pollution in the Netherlands: a cohort study. Lancet 2002; 360:1203–1209.

118. Murray CJ, Nelson RN. State-space modeling of the relationship between air quality and mortality. J Air Waste Manag Assoc 2000; 50:1075–1080.

119. Zanobetti A, Schwartz J, Samoli E, Gryparis A, Touloumi G, Peacock J, Anderson RH, Le Tertre A, Bobros J, Celko M, Goren A, Forsberg B, Michelozzi P, Rabczenko D, Hoyos SP, Wichmann HE, Katsouyanni K. The temporal pattern of respiratory and heart disease mortality in response to air pollution. Environ Health Perspect 2003; 111:1188–1193.

120. Gold DR, Damokosh AI, Pope CA III, Dockery DW, McDonnell WF, Serrano P, Retama A, Castillejos M. Particulate and ozone pollutant effects on the respiratory function of children in southwest Mexico City [see comments] [published erratum appears in Epidemiology 1999 Jul;10(4):470]. Epidemiology 1999; 10:8–16.

121. Romieu I, Meneses R, Ruiz S, Sienra JJ, Huerta J, WHite MC, Etzel RA. Effects of air pollution on the respiratory health of asthmatic children living in Mexico City. Am J Respir Crit Care Med 1996; 154(pt l):300–307.

122. Mortimer KM, Neas LM, Dockery DW, Redline S, Tager IB. The effect of summer ozone on inner city children with asthma. Eur Respir J 2002; 19:699–705.

123. Gent JF, Triche EW, Holford TR, Belanger K, Bracken MB, Beckett WS, Leaderer BP. Association of low-level ozone and fine particles with respiratory symptoms in children with asthma. JAMA 2003; 290:1859–1867.

124. Abbey DE, Petersen FF, Mills PK, Kittle L. Chronic respiratory disease associated with long term ambient concentrations of sulfates and other air pollutants. J Exp Anal Environ Epidemiol 1993; 3:99–115.

125. McDonnell WF, Abbey DE, Nishino N, Lebowitz MD. Long-term ambient ozone concentration and the incidence of asthma in non-smoking adults: the Ahsmog Study. Environ Res 1999; 80:110–121.

126. National Heart Lung and Blood Institute. National Asthma Education and Prevention Program, Expert Panel Report 2: Guidelines for the Diagnosis and Management of Asthma. Bethesda, MD: National Institutes of Health, 1997.

127. Tunnicliffe WS, Burge PS, Ayres JG. Effect of domestic concentrations of nitrogen dioxide on airway responses to inhaled allergen in asthmatic patients. Lancet 1994; 344:1733–1736.

128. Jenkins HS, Devalia JL, Mister RL, Bevan AM, Rusznak C, Davies RJ. The effect of exposure to ozone and nitrogen dioxide on the airway response of atopic asthmatics to inhaled allergen: dose- and time-dependent effects. Am J Respir Crit Care Med 1999; 160:33–39.

129. Torres R, Nowak D, Magnussen H. The effect of ozone exposure on allergen responsiveness in subjects with asthma or rhinitis. Am J Respir Crit Care Med 1996; 153:56–64.

130. Schelegle ES, Miller LA, Gershwin LJ, Fanucchi MV, Van Winkle LS, Gerriets JE, Walby WF, Mitchell V, Tarkington BK, Wong VJ, Baker GL, Pantle LM, Joad JP, Pinkerton KE, Wu R, Evans MJ, Hyde DM, Plopper CG. Repeated episodes of ozone inhalation amplifies the effects of allergen sensitization and inhalation on airway immune and structural development in Rhesus monkeys. Toxicol Appl Pharmacol 2003; 191:74–85.

131. Tsien A, Diaz-Sanchez D, Ma J, Saxon A. The organic component of diesel exhaust particles and phenanthrene, a major polyaromatic hydrocarbon constituent, enhances IgE production by IgE-secreting EBV-transformed human B cells in vitro. Toxicol Appl Pharmacol 1997; 142:256–263.

132. Nel AE, Diaz-Sanchez D, Ng D, Hiura T, Saxon A. Enhancement of allergic inflammation by the interaction between diesel exhaust particles and the immune system. J Allergy Clin Immunol 1998; 102:539–554.

133. Diaz-Sanchez D, Garcia MP, Wang M, Jyrala M, Saxon A. Nasal challenge with diesel exhaust particles can induce sensitization to a neoallergen in the human mucosa. J Allergy Clin Immunol 1999; 104:1183–1188.

134. Brauer M, Hoek G, Van Vliet P, Meliefste K, Fischer PH, Wijga A, Koopman LP, Neijens HJ, Gerritsen J, Kerkhof M, Heinrich J, Bellander T, Brunekreef B. Air pollution from traffic and the development of respiratory infections and asthmatic and allergic symptoms in children. Am J Respir Grit Care Med 2002; 166:1092–1098.

135. Brauer M, Hoek G, van Vliet P, Meliefste K, Fischer P, Gehring U, Heinrich J, Cyrys J, Bellander T, Lewne M, Brunekreef B. Estimating long-term average particulate air pollution concentrations: application of traffic indicators and geographic information systems. Epidemiology 2003; 14:228–239.

136. Finlayson-Pitts BJ, Pitts JN. Atmospheric Chemistry: Fundamentals and Experimental Techniques. New York: John Wiley & Sons, 1986:678–679.

137. Gold DR, Litonjua A, Schwartz J, Lovett E, Larson A, Nearing B, Allen G, Verrier M, Cherry R, Verrier R. Ambient pollution and heart rate variability. Circulation 2000; 101:1267–1273.

138. Peters A, Doring A, Wichmann H-E, Koenig W. Increased plasma viscosity during an air pollution episode: a link to mortality. Lancet 1997; 349: 1582–1587.

139. Seaton A, Soutar A, Crawford V, Elton R, McNerlan S, Cherrie J, Watt M, Agius R, Stout R. Particulate air pollution and the blood. Thorax 1999; 54:1027–1032.

140. Bouthillier L, Vincent R, Goegan P, Adamson IY, Bjarnason S, Stewart M, Guenette J, Potvin M, Kumarathasan P. Acute effects of inhaled urban particles and ozone: lung morphology, macrophage activity, and plasma endothelin-1. Amer J Pathol 1998; 153:1873–1884.

141. Brook RD, Brook JR, Urch B, Vincent R, Rajagopalan S, Silverman F. Inhalation of fine particulate air pollution and ozone causes acute arterial vaso constriction in healthy adults. Circulation 2002; 105:1534–1536.

142. Li N, Kim S, Wang M, Froines J, Sioutas C, Nel A. Use of a stratified oxidative stress model to study the biological effects of ambient concentrated and diesel exhaust particulate matter. Inhal Toxicol 2002; 14:459–486.

143. Tager IB. Health effects of aerosols: mechanisms and epidemiology. In: Ruzer L, ed. Aerosols Handbook: Measurement, Dosimetry, and Health Effects. Boca Raton: CRC Press, In press.

144. Hiura TS, Kaszubowski MP, Li N, Nel AE. Chemicals in diesel exhaust particles generate reactive oxygen radicals and induce apoptosis in macrophages. J Immunol 1999; 163:5582–5591.

145. Hiura TS, Li N, Kaplan R, Horwitz M, Seagrave JC, Nel AE. The role of a mitochondrial pathway in the induction of apoptosis by chemicals extracted from diesel exhaust particles. J Immunol 2000; 165:2703–2711.

146. Li N, Venkatesan MI, Miguel A, Kaplan R, Gujuluva C, Alam J, Nel A. Induction of heme oxygenase-1 expression in macrophages by diesel exhaust particle chemicals and quinones via the antioxidant-responsive element. J Immunol 2000; 165:3393–3401.

147. Li N, Wang M, Oberley TD, Sempf JM, Nel AE. Comparison of the pro-oxidative and proinflammatory effects of organic diesel particle chemical in bronchial epithelial cells and macrophages. J Immunol 2002; 169:4531–4541.

9

Pulmonary Toxicity of Occupational and Environmental Exposures to Fibers and Nano-Sized Particulate

DAVID B. WARHEIT

DuPont Haskell Laboratory, Newark, Delaware, U.S.A.

I. Introduction

Occupational and environmental exposures to inhaled fibers and particulates can result in the development of lung disease. In this regard, recent epidemiological studies have demonstrated an association between elevated levels of particulate urban air pollution and adverse health effects in humans; particularly in susceptible individuals with pre-existing respiratory and cardiovascular disease (1–3). The components of particulate matter in urban air pollution have been characterized into three modes—namely, ultrafine particulates (i.e., <0.1 μm diameter), fine particles (ranging from −0.1 μm to 2.5 μm), and coarse particles (>2.5 μm). Ultrafine particles contribute very little to the overall mass, but are disproportionate in particle number. Epidemiological studies suggest that ultrafine and fine-mode particles are better correlated with adverse health effects when compared to coarse particles (4). Oberdorster (5) has postulated that urban source ultrafine particles, consisting of a carbonaceous core with surface attached inorganic and organic materials, are the major cause of adverse health effects in compromised individuals during high air pollution days.

In addition to the ambient environment, exposures to ultrafine particles are known to occur in occupational settings and often are manifested as fumes generated from smelting processes of metals. Adverse acute health effects in exposed workers include metal-fume fever, flu-like symptoms, nausea, and headaches (5–9). Exposure concentrations to these particles at the workplace are significantly higher when compared to urban atmospheres. The higher concentrations may predispose the ultrafine particles at the workplace to agglomerate into larger sized particles. When comparing the potential adverse health effects of ultrafine particles in occupational settings vs. ambient environmental concentrations, it is important to emphasize that the exposed populations in the workplace generally are represented by healthy individuals, while in the general environment, the impact of air pollutants is most significant in affecting compromised individuals in the urban setting.

This brief chapter is designed to focus on several of the pertinent issues and raise questions regarding the mechanisms of pulmonary toxicity following exposures to fibrous and nonfibrous particulates, both in the ambient environmental and occupational settings. In this regard, numerous epidemiological studies have clearly demonstrated a correlation between air pollution events and enhanced morbidity/mortality in the affected populations. Yet, the toxicological mechanisms associated with the PM-induced adverse health effects remain to be clearly defined. In contrast, occupational exposures to cytotoxic particulates such as silica particles and asbestos fibers have produced serious lung injury and the pathogenetic mechanisms are generally well understood. Moreover, in pulmonary toxicity studies, silica and asbestos exposures to experimental animals such as rats produce lesions similar to those observed in exposed humans. Thus, from a mechanistic perspective, it would appear that the pathogenetic mechanisms and corresponding adverse health effects related to occupational exposures to toxic dusts are better understood when compared to the adverse health impacts resulting from exposures to ambient air pollution. What is the reason for this apparent discrepancy? Several factors may be operative herein and these include the following: (1) as discussed above, the pathogenetic mechanisms of lung disease associated with occupational exposures to silica and asbestos fibers are well recognized; (2) furthermore, similar lesions can be produced in experimental animals; (3) exposures to the PM components of air pollution clearly must be a mixture and are not well defined; (4) exposures to "carbonaceous-type" (combustion-related) particulates, and acidic-type (sulfate) particles are not particularly toxic to experimental animals and can produce adverse pulmonary effects in rats (the most sensitive species) only at high exposure concentrations; (5) it seems likely that the PM components in air pollution may produce adverse impacts only in sensitive or compromised individuals with pre-existing cardiopulmonary disease and this sensitivity is difficult to model in experimental animals; (6) some ultrafine particulates may not be as toxic as the conventional wisdom would suggest; and finally (7) PM effects may act synergistically with other components of air pollution (e.g., oxidants such as ozone and nitrogen dioxide, carbon monoxide, aldehydes, and VOCs) to produce adverse health impacts.

In the following sections, current and established concepts related to the development of occupational lung diseases are discussed. Subsequently, current understandings of the health impacts of low solubility particles and nano or ultrafine particles are reviewed. As noted below, it is obvious that the toxicological database on occupational diseases caused by asbestos and silica is far more robust than the currently available hazard information on particles which may represent particulate matter components of ambient air pollution.

II. Occupational Lung Diseases

Pulmonary responses to inhaled particulates such as crystalline silica or asbestos have long been considered to be major occupational hazards causing disability and death among workers in a variety of industries. In this respect, the various forms of asbestos fibers have been associated with the development of pulmonary fibrosis (i.e., asbestosis), lung cancer, and mesothelioma. In addition, the causal relationship between inhalation of dusts containing crystalline silica and pulmonary inflammation and the consequent development of silica-induced pulmonary fibrosis (i.e., silicosis) are well known (10–12).

A. Asbestos and other Fibrous Particulates—Concepts of Fiber Toxicology

Fibrous particulates are a health concern because inhalation exposures to some pathogenic dusts, such as asbestos fibers, are associated with fibrotic lung disease and cancer. Moreover, hazard assessments of fibers generally are more complex than those of nonfibrous particulates, because fiber toxicity is strongly influenced by both chemical composition and physical characteristics, i.e., aspect ratio (length/diameter). The World Health Organization (WHO) has defined a respirable fiber (one that can be inhaled and deposit into the alveolar regions of the lung) as a particulate with an aspect ratio (length:diameter ratio) of at ≥3:1; along with fiber lengths >5 μm and diameters <3 μm. Fiber dimensions are known to impact the dose to the respiratory tract and greatly influence both lung biopersistence (length of time fibers persist in the lung) as well as biological reactivity. The characteristic long and thin geometry of straight or curly aerosolized fibers can pose problems for lung clearance by alveolar macrophages, as the long fibers (>20 μm in length) of very durable compositions can remain in the lung indefinitely (Fig. 1). Longer fibers may also be more biologically reactive

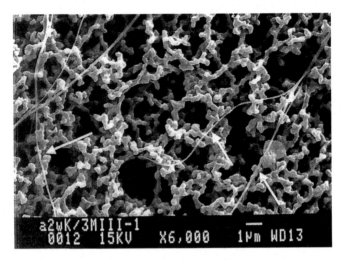

Figure 1   Scanning electron micrograph demonstrating chrysotile asbestos fibers (arrows) recovered from the lungs of a rat 3 months after a 2-week inhalation exposure. Note that the fibers are predominantly long as the bulk of the shorter asbestos fibers have been cleared by the 3-month postexposure period.

than short fibers (13). In support of this concept, rats were exposed for one year by inhalation to aerosols of amosite asbestos that had been processed to be either "short" (<5 μm in length) or long (>20 μm). No significant histopathological pulmonary effects were observed in rats exposed to the short fibers, but one-third of the rats exposed to similar mass concentrations of long fibers developed lung tumors and pulmonary fibrosis (14). In other studies, similar fiber-length-related effects were observed in rats exposed by inhalation for one year to long or short chrysotile asbestos fibers (15).

Deposition of inhaled fibers in the distal lung (at the level of the bronchoalveolar junctions) is the initial event that can lead to the development of fiber-related lung disease. Size, shape, and density are also important factors in influencing deposition characteristics. The primary fiber deposition mechanisms in the lung are impaction, sedimentation, and interception. Impaction is enhanced under conditions of high flow velocity and occurs primarily in the larger airways. Sedimentation occurs primarily under conditions of low-flow velocity, long residence time, and small airway size. The likelihood of interception is enhanced with increasing fiber length. The early pulmonary effects associated with fiber-induced lung diseases are probably related to the initial patterns of fiber deposition in the lung. In humans, the development of asbestosis is known to be initiated at the level of the respiratory bronchiole, the likely preferential site of asbestos fiber deposition in the distal lung. Studies using rodents have demonstrated that inhaled particulates and fibers small enough to pass through the rodent airways deposit primarily on the epithelial surfaces of alveolar duct bifurcations and at the junctions of terminal bronchioles and alveolar ducts, perhaps as a consequence of air flow characteristics (Fig. 2a–d).

Fiber biopersistence can be defined in its broadest sense as the ability of inhaled fibers to resist changes in number, dimension, surface chemistry, chemical composition, surface area, and other characteristics. Any or all of

(a)
Rat Lung Microdissecction

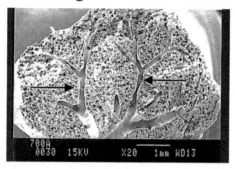

(b)
Rat Lung – Junction of Terminal Bronchiole and Alveolar Dust

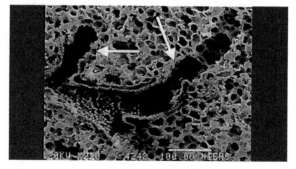

Figure 2 (a) Scanning electron micrograph of a left lung of a rat demonstrating a microdissection of the major airways (arrows) moving in a distal direction to the bronchoalveolar junctions—preferential sites of inhaled particle and fiber deposition in the distal lung. (b) Scanning electron micrograph of section of dissected distal lung tissue of a rat demonstrating the bronchoalveolar junctions (arrows), i.e., the end of the terminal bronchiole and beginning of the alveolar ducts. These are the preferential sites of inhaled particle and fiber deposition in the distal lung. (c) Scanning electron micrograph demonstrating deposition of inhaled carbonyl iron particles (arrows) at the alveolar duct bifurcations in the distal lung of a rat. (d) Scanning electron micrograph demonstrating deposition of inhaled chrysotile asbestos fibers (arrows) in the distal lung of a rat. *(Continued next page)*

^(c)   Particle Deposition at Junction of
Terminal Bronchiole and Alveolar Dust

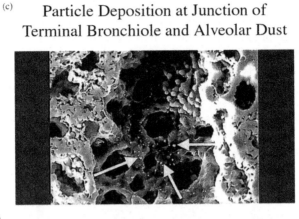

^(d) **Chrysotile Asbestos Fiber Deposition
on Alveolar Duct Bifurcation**

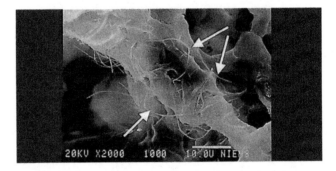

Figure 2 (*Continued*)

these parameters can be altered during a fiber's residence in the lung, and
such alterations affect the lung's long-term response to the fiber.

III. Crystalline Silica

The pulmonary response to inhaled silica has long been considered to be a
major occupational hazard, causing disability and deaths among workers in
a variety of industries. Some of the processes and work environments which
are frequently associated with silica exposure include mining, sandblasting
of abrasive materials, quarrying and tunneling, stonecutting, glass and pot-
tery manufacturing, metal casting, boiler scaling, and vitreous enameling
(16). Ambient silica particles are emitted into the environment as a

fractional component of particulate emissions. Silica particle emissions in the environment can arise from natural, industrial, and farming activities. There are only limited data on ambient air concentrations of either crystalline or amorphous silica particles, due, in part, to the limits in accurately quantifying crystalline silica and to the inability, under existing measurement methods, of separating the identity of crystalline silica from other particulate matter. In addition, concern about nonoccupational or ambient silica exposure, specifically crystalline silica, has emerged only recently, principally from populations in the western United States, and particularly from the state of California.

Silica is one of the most common substances to which workers have been exposed. There are at least four polymorphs or forms of crystalline silica dust. These include quartz, cristobalite, tridymite, and tripoli. The causal relationship between inhalation of dust containing crystalline silica and pulmonary inflammation and the consequent development of silica-induced pulmonary fibrosis (i.e., silicosis) is well established (10–12). During the acute phase of exposure, a pulmonary inflammatory response develops and may progress to alveolar proteinosis and a granulomatous-type pattern of disease in rats and other rodent species. A pattern of nodular fibrosis occurs in chronically exposed animals and humans (10–12,16). In 1997, the International Agency for Research on Cancer (IARC) classified crystalline silica (quartz and cristobalite) as Group I carcinogens— and concluded that there was sufficient evidence of carcinogenicity in experimental animals and in humans to warrant this classification (17).

A. Concepts in the Pathogenic Development of Silica-Related Lung Disease

Exposures to crystalline silica are associated with the development of chronic inflammation and pulmonary fibrosis (i.e., silicosis) in humans (10,16) and in experimental animals (11,16,18–22). The pathogenetic mechanisms of silica-induced lung injury have not been fully elucidated; however, it is well known that silica exposures result in cell injury, cytokine release, and corresponding inflammation. Similar to asbestos fibers, inhaled silica particles deposit at the level of the bronchoalveolar junctions and interact with macrophages and epithelial cells stimulating cell injury and inflammatory responses (Fig. 3a–b). This leads to a cascade of events which include oxidative stress which may cause mutations in epithelial cells and upregulation of proinflammatory genes (17,23). Cellular injury and the generation of inflammatory cell-derived growth factors lead to enhanced epithelial cell proliferation and hyperplasia which may contribute to the development of tumors. Because clearance of inhaled quartz particles is impaired, this cytotoxic dust accumulates in the lung and the aforementioned cycle continues (24).

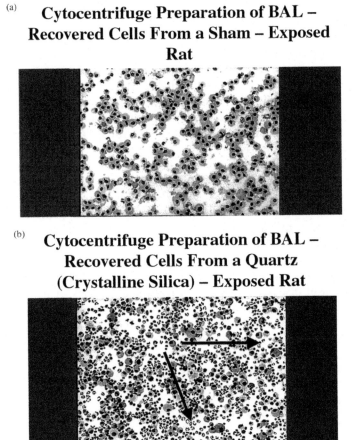

(a) Cytocentrifuge Preparation of BAL – Recovered Cells From a Sham – Exposed Rat

(b) Cytocentrifuge Preparation of BAL – Recovered Cells From a Quartz (Crystalline Silica) – Exposed Rat

Figure 3 (a) Cytocentrifuge preparation of bronchoalveolar lavaged cells recovered from the lung of a rat exposed to room air. The cell population is comprised of alveolar macrophages. (b) Cytocentrifuge preparation of bronchoalveolar lavaged cells recovered from the lung of a rat exposed to an aerosol of quartz—crystalline silica particles. Note the significant number of inflammatory cells—primarily neutrophils (arrows), but also lymphocytes, in addition to the resident population of alveolar macrophages.

B. Crystalline Silica vs. Amorphous Silica Pulmonary Toxicity

It is interesting to note that comparative studies have shown that crystalline silica particles are more inflammogenic and cytotoxic than amorphous types of silica particles of similar chemical composition. In one study, pulmonary responses in crystalline and amorphous-exposed rats were compared after short-term inhalation exposure to polymorphs of silica dust. Groups of rats were exposed 6 hr/day for 3 days at 10 or 100 mg/m^3 to crystalline silica in the forms of quartz or cristobalite particles or to amorphous silica in the form of precipitated silica particles. Another group was exposed to ultrafine Ludox colloidal silica (particle size = 22 nm) at 10, 50 or 150 mg/m^3 6 hr/day, 5 day week for two or four weeks. Pulmonary inflammation and cytotoxicity were assessed using bronchoalveolar lavage methodologies and histopathology of lung tissues. Both forms of crystalline silica produced persistent pulmonary inflammatory responses characterized by neutrophil recruitment and consistently elevated biomarkers of cytotoxicity in bronchoalveolar lavage fluids; in addition, progressive histopathological lesions were observed within one month of the exposure. Exposures to both amorphous silica particulate-types (precipitated and ultrafine colloidal) produced transient pulmonary inflammation. The results demonstrated that inhaled crystalline silica dust produced significantly greater pulmonary toxicity when compared to the amorphous types, including ultrafine colloidal silica particles (25,26).

IV. Poorly Soluble Particulate Matter

While the toxic effects of silica and asbestos are well established, with few exceptions (e.g., coal dust) the epidemiological and toxicological data base in humans for other dusts is rather sparse. As a consequence, rodent inhalation bioassays have become the preferred method for evaluating potential health hazards, and thus estimating human health risks from exposures to airborne particulates. Increasing numbers of inhalation studies in rats have demonstrated that chronic exposures to high concentrations of insoluble particulates result in the development of pulmonary inflammation, fibrosis, and lung tumors (27,28). The application of the concept of inhalation bioassays for estimating these health risks for humans is complicated by interspecies differences in dosimetry and pulmonary responses. One issue that is troublesome stems from the fact that carcinogenic effects have been produced in rats by test materials ranging from the biologically active (e.g., silica) to those generally considered to be biologically inert such as titanium dioxide particles. Indeed, with few exceptions, most materials of low solubility and low toxicity have produced lung tumors in rats following long-term exposures at high concentrations. Due to the sensitivity in response, the rat inhalation bioassay has been challenged for its appropriateness as a model to extrapolate to humans (27).

   As discussed in Sec. I, epidemiological reports demonstrate a correlation between enhanced ambient air particulate matter (PM) and increased morbidity and mortality. In attempting to ascertain the possible mechanisms for PM-induced adverse health effects, several investigators have evaluated the pulmonary impacts of residual oil fly ash (ROFA), which is derived from the combustion of oil and residual fuel oil and may significantly contribute to the ambient air particle burden for certain locations (reviewed in Ref. 29). Pulmonary exposures to ROFA in experimental animals are effective in producing acute lung injury. ROFA samples often contain significant amounts of toxic transition metals such as vanadium and nickel. Whether ROFA is truly representative of ambient air particulate matter is controversial; ROFA may represent a significant PM component in the areas bordering power plants.

Some recent studies have combined the exposure effects of ROFA with exposures in compromised animal models in an attempt to simulate the sensitive human populations who are thought to be at greatest risk to be adversely impacted by exposures to PM-related air pollution. Some of the "compromised" models include spontaneously hypersensitive rats, cardiovascular compromised rats, rat models of bronchitis, rat models of monocrotaline-induced hypertension, and endotoxin/lipopolysaccharide exposed, young and old rats and mice (30–36). The synergistic effects of a toxic PM exposure such as ROFA combined with a compromised animal model appear to enhance the acute, adverse cardiopulmonary health effects, and these parameters can be measured. The connection between these possible experimental responses and the adverse health effects in PM-exposed humans remains controversial.

A. Species Differences in Lung Responses to Inhaled Low-Toxicity Dusts

The relevance for human health effects of the rat lung tumor response to overload particle concentrations (i.e., exceeding the ability to maintain pulmonary clearance of particles) in inhalation bioassays is a controversial issue (28). The results of numerous bioassays have demonstrated that chronic inhalation exposures of rats, hamsters, or mice to dusts at high concentrations lead to impairment of particle clearance or so-called lung particle overload effects. In rats, but not to any degree in mice or hamsters, chronic exposures to low solubility particulates lead to dust overload-related lung pathology, resulting in epithelial hyperplasia, metaplasia, and subsequently the development of lung tumors. It has been postulated by many investigators that particle-induced, persistent pulmonary inflammation and cellular proliferation are important factors in the development of lung tumors. In addition, based upon the existing coal dust epidemiology data, it has been considered that the human response to dust overload concentrations may be very different from the pulmonary responses observed in dust-exposed rats. Indeed, this view was supported by the EPA's Clean

Air Science Advisory Committee (CASAC) (37), a group of independent scientists who suggested to the EPA Administrator that the mechanisms associated with the rat pulmonary tumor response to diesel exhaust may be unique to that species and that these studies are not relevant for risk assessments in humans. This idea is also supported by experimentalists who have concluded that the dust-induced lung tumors may well be rat specific and thus problematic for human risk evaluation (38).

Snipes (39) reviewed the available literature comparing the pulmonary clearance and distribution effects of high concentrations of inhaled dusts in rodent and nonrodent mammalian species. He concluded that the clearance of inhaled dusts in rats is relatively rapid. In contrast, larger mammals, including humans, exhibit slower lung clearance patterns following exposures to inhaled dusts. Moreover, in rats, a large proportion of the inhaled dust burden is contained within alveolar macrophages, while the larger, nonrodent species retained dust particulates predominantly in the pulmonary interstitium. As a consequence, high dose and long-term inhalation of dusts by the larger mammalian species is likely to result in dust accumulation patterns which are different from those observed in rats, and this clearly would have a significant impact on the manifestation of overload-related effects. In this regard, it is possible in the larger species for normal particle clearance patterns to be operative despite the accumulation of large dust burdens. The results of long-term inhalation studies with uranium dioxide particles in the rat, monkey, and dog demonstrated that pulmonary clearance patterns were not altered in the monkey or dog under long-term exposure conditions which produced pulmonary clearance impairment in the rat. Snipes suggested that the responses of species to inhaled overload dust exposures may be influenced to a greater degree by the pattern of dust accumulation in the lung rather than the amount (i.e., mass, particle number or surface area) of the accumulated dust. It was concluded that the limited data obtained from dust-exposed monkeys, dogs, and humans, which demonstrated significant species differences in responses to high dust burdens when compared to rodents, indicated that lung overload effects in rats may not be relevant for larger mammals, including humans.

Nikula et al. (40) compared the anatomical patterns of particle retention and the lung tissue responses of F344 rats and cynomolgus monkeys exposed for 2 years to high concentrations of diesel exhaust (2 mg soot/m^3; MMAD 0.2–0.4 µm), coal dust (2 mg/m^3; MMAD = 40% <7 µm) and a combination of the two pollutants (1 mg soot and 1 mg respirable coal dust/m^3). For normalization purposes, the relative volume density of particulate material in the lung and the distribution of dust among selected pulmonary compartments were determined using morphometric techniques. The results demonstrated that for coal dust and coal dust-diesel-exposed groups, significantly greater dust burdens were retained in the lungs of monkeys when compared with rats (the results for exposure to diesel dust alone were equivalent in the two species). Nikula et al. also reported the patterns of dust accumulation differed between the two species, a similar conclusion to that of Snipes (39). However, within each species, the sites of particle retention and pulmonary reactions were consistent for the three dust materials that were tested (coal dust, diesel soot, and combined coal dust and diesel soot). The anatomic pattern of particle retention in the lungs of rats was observed to be within the lumens of alveolar ducts and alveoli, whereas in the monkey lung, the dust was preferentially sequestered in the interstitial compartment. The authors reported that the pulmonary response of rats, but not monkeys, was associated with alveolar inflammation, epithelial hyperplasia, and septal fibrosis. In the monkey, particle-associated inflammation was significantly less common than in the rat. It was concluded that the responses of the rat to high concentrations of low-solubility dusts are not likely to be predictive of retention patterns and pulmonary histopathologic responses in similarly exposed primates.

More recently, Nikula et al. (41) studied the influence of exposure concentration or dose on the distribution of particulate material in rat and human lungs. They used morphometric techniques to examine the influence of exposure concentration on particle retention by analyzing histological lung sections from rats and humans. The rats had been exposed for 24 months to diesel exhaust at 0.35, 3.5, or 7.0 mg soot/m^3. The human subjects were: (1) nonsmokers who did not work as miners, (2) nonsmoking coal miners who worked under the current standard of 2 mg/m^3 for 10–20 mean years (mean = 14 years), and (3) nonsmoking coal miners who worked under the former standard of <10 mg dust/m^3 for 33–50 years (mean = 40 years). The distribution of retained particles within the lung compartments was markedly different between species. In all three groups of rats, 82–85% of the retained particulate material was located in the alveolar and alveolar duct lumens, primarily in alveolar macrophages. In humans, 57%, 68%, and 91% of the retained particulate material were located in the interstitium of the lung in the nonminers, coal miners under the current standard, and coal miners under the former standard, respectively. The authors suggested that the results show that chronically inhaled diesel soot is retained predominately in the airspaces of rats over a wide range of exposures, whereas in humans chronically inhaled particulate material is retained primarily in the interstitial compartment. In humans, the percentage of particles in the interstitium is enhanced with increasing dose (exposure concentration, years of exposure, and/or lung burden). This difference in distribution may bring different lung cells into contact with the retained particles or particle-containing macrophages in rats and humans, and may account for differences in species response to inhaled particles. A summary of comparisons of species differences in response to inhaled particles is presented in Table 1 (42).

Table 1 Comparison of Attributes of Lung Overload in the Rat, Monkey, Dog, and Humans

Classical attributes and sequelae of lung overload	Rats	Dog, monkey, and man
Chronic lung inflammation	Yes	Uncertain
Hyperplasia of macrophages and epithelial cells	Yes	Uncertain
Altered lung clearance (overwhelmed macrophage-mediated clearance)	Yes	Probably not
Enhanced pulmonary burdens of particles	Yes	Probably not
Enhanced interstitialization of deposited particles	Yes	Yes
Enhanced translocation of particles from lung to thoracic lymph nodes	Probably	Probably
Interstitial lung disease (fibrosis)	Yes	Yes but less severe
Development of lung tumors	Yes	No

B. Ultrafine and/or Nanoparticles

Studies in rats demonstrate that ultrafine particles (generally synonymous with "nanoparticles" and defined as particles in the size range <100 nm) administered to the lung cause a greater inflammatory response when compared to larger particles at equivalent mass concentrations (1,5). Surface properties (surface chemistry–surface area) appear to play an important role in ultrafine particle toxicity. Contributing to the effects of ultrafine particles is their very high size-specific deposition when inhaled as singlet ultrafine particles rather than as aggregated particles. Some evidence suggests that inhaled ultrafine particles, after deposition in the lung, largely escape alveolar macrophage surveillance and gain access to the pulmonary interstitium (1,5).

A number of studies have been reported which used inhalation of ultrafine particles by laboratory animals at very high particle concentrations. These hazard-based toxicity studies were designed to investigate pulmonary effects caused by lung particle overload, i.e., induction of lung tumors in rats at high retained particulate lung burdens. Specifically, chronic inhalation studies with ultrafine and fine TiO_2 particles (average primary particle sizes $\sim$20 and $\sim$250 nm) have shown that less than one-tenth the inhaled mass concentrations of the aggregated ultrafine particles, compared with the fine particles, are sufficient to produce an equivalent amount of tumor-induction in rats in these long-term studies (approximately 20–30%) (43,44). In addition, pulmonary toxicity studies have been performed with aggregates of ultrafine and fine carbon black, nickel, as well as TiO_2 particles in rats

(45–48), and results demonstrated the significantly enhanced lung inflammatory potency of the ultrafine particles when compared to fine-sized particulates of similar composition. When the instilled doses were expressed in terms of particle surface area, the responses of the ultrafine and fine TiO_2 particles fell on the same dose–response curve. This is because a given mass of ultrafine particles has a much greater surface area than the same mass of fine, yet respirable particles and therefore is more likely to cause particle overload in the lung. Thus, from a toxicological and regulatory viewpoint, it is important to separate the pulmonary effects of ultrafine particles at overload vs. nonoverload conditions.

Furthermore, the fate of ultrafine particles following deposition in the alveolar regions of the rat lung may be very different from that of larger particles. It appears that deposited ultrafine particles are not as readily phagocytized by alveolar macrophages as are larger particles, and as a consequence, penetrate much more rapidly to interstitial sites, possibly including the endothelium.

Obviously, there are a number of open questions which still need to be investigated with respect to the toxicity of ultrafine particles. One is related to the translocation of deposited ultrafine particles to interstitial and extra-pulmonary tissues, which has still not been shown convincingly at this point. Another is an elucidation of the mechanisms of effects of ultrafine particles at a cellular and molecular level.

Mechanistic hypotheses need to be investigated to consider the local effects elicited in the lung as well as systemic effects, for example, the cardiovascular system, since people with pre-existing cardiopulmonary diseases have been found to be most susceptible to ambient particulate pollution.

C. Species Differences in Lung Responses to Inhaled Ultrafine TiO_2 Particles

The results of two recently completed inhalation toxicity studies (49,50) have provided important insights into the following:

1. (rodent) species differences in lung responses to inhaled fine-sized and ultrafine titanium dioxide particles;
2. comparisions of rat lung responses and potency comparisons between pigment-grade (fine-sized-particle size = ~300 nm) and ultrafine (particle-size = 15–40 nm) TiO_2 particles.

With the exception of exposure concentrations, the experimental designs of the two studies were nearly identical. In the ultrafine TiO_2 study, female rats, mice, and hamsters were exposed by inhalation to 0.5, 2.0, or 10 mg/m^3 ultrafine (uf) TiO_2 particles (10–40 nm in diameter for 13 weeks, 6 hr/day, 5 days/week). Following the exposure period, the lungs of animals were evaluated immediately after, as well as 4, 13, 26 or 52 weeks (49 weeks for the uf-TiO_2-exposed hamsters) and at each time point uf-TiO_2 burdens in the lung and lymph nodes; and biomarkers of lung injury, including inflammation, cytotoxicity, lung cell proliferation and histopathologic alterations were assessed. Mice and rats had similar retained particle lung burdens at the end of the exposures, whereas hamsters had retained lung burdens that were significantly lower. Lung burdens in all three species decreased with time following completion of exposure, and 1 year later, the percentages of the lung particle burden remaining in the high dose exposure group ($10 \, mg/m^3$) group were 57%, 45%, and 3% for rat, mouse, and hamster, respectively. The retardation of particle clearance from the lungs in mice and rats of the $10 \, mg/m^3$ groups is evidence of pulmonary particle overload. Significant pulmonary inflammation was evident, particularly in rats, as well as in mice exposed to $10 \, mg/m^3$ (Fig. 4a–c) concomitant with increased concentrations of soluble biomarkers of cell injury in bronchoalveolar lavage fluids (BALF). The initial neutrophil response in rats was far greater than in mice and the response of hamsters was minimal. At the highest exposure concentration, $10 \, mg/m^3$, consistent increases in bronchoalveolar lavage fluid biomarkers of lung injury (e.g., LDH and protein) were highest in rats>mice>hamsters and diminished with time postexposure. It was noteworthy that progressive epithelial and fibroproliferative alterations were observed in the lungs of rats but not in mice or hamsters. These lesions were characterized by foci of alveolar epithelial proliferation of metaplastic epithelial cells or alveolar bronchiolization surrounding areas of heavily particle-laden macrophages. Other observations included interstitial particle accumulation and alveolar septal fibrosis. These lesions became more pronounced with increasing time postexposure. The authors concluded that there were significant species differences in the pulmonary responses to inhaled ultrafine TiO_2 particles. Under conditions of equivalent particle lung burdens, rats developed a more severe inflammatory response than mice and subsequently developed progressive epithelial and fibroproliferative changes. These findings were consistent with the results of a companion study using inhaled pigment-grade (fine mode) TiO_2 (49). These species differences can be explained both by pulmonary response and by particle dosimetry differences between these rodent species (50).

To summarize the points raised in this section, on a per mass basis, ultrafine particles produce greater inflammogenic, fibrogenic, and tumorigenic pulmonary responses in the lungs of rats when compared to fine-sized particles (>100 nm in diameter) of similar composition. In addition, it seems clear that the pulmonary inflammatory and tumorigenic responses of the rat to long-term inhalation of high concentrations of low-toxicity dusts is significantly enhanced in comparison with similarly exposed mice and hamsters. It has been postulated that the "inappropriate" response of enhanced pulmonary inflammation, cell proliferation, and inflammatory-derived mutagenesis in the rat could account for the development of

(a) **Pulmonary Inflammation in BAL Fluids of Female Rats Exposed to Ultrafine TiO2 Particles**

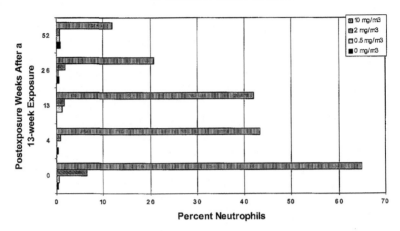

Figure 4 (a) Pulmonary inflammation in BAL fluids of female rats exposed to 0, 0.5, 2, and 10 mg/m^3 aerosolized ultrafine TiO$_2$ particles for a 13-week exposure period. Lung inflammation in particle and control rats is represented by % neutrophils (PMN) in BAL fluids immediately after exposure, as well as 4 weeks, 13, 26 and 52 weeks postinhalation exposure (pe). Values presented are mean values of percent neutrophils in BAL fluids. High dose overload exposures (10 mg/m^3) to ultrafine TiO$_2$ particles produced a potent pulmonary inflammatory response (>60% PMNs at the end of exposure), which, at comparable dust loads, was significantly greater than the effects measured in mice or hamsters. (b) Pulmonary inflammation in BAL fluids of female mice exposed to 0, 0.5,2, and 10 mg/m^3 aerosolized ultrafine TiO$_2$ particles for a 13-week exposure period. Lung inflammation in particle and control rats is represented by % neutrophils (PMN) in BAL fluids immediately after exposure, as well as 4 weeks, 13, 26 and 52-week postinhalation exposure (pe). Values presented are mean values of percent neutrophils in BAL fluids. High dose overload exposures (10 mg/m^3) to ultrafine TiO$_2$ particles produced a less potent pulmonary inflammatory response (<16% PMNs at the end of exposure), which, at comparable dust loads, was significantly less than the effects measured in rats. (c) Pulmonary inflammation in BAL fluids of female hamsters exposed to 0, 0.5, 2, and 10 mg/m^3 aerosolized ultrafine TiO$_2$ particles for a 13-week exposure period. Lung inflammation in particle and control rats is represented by % neutrophils (PMN) in BAL fluids immediately after exposure, as well as 4 weeks, 13, 26 and 45 weeks post inhalation exposure (pe). Values presented are mean values of percent neutrophils in BAL fluids. High dose overload exposures (10 mg/m^3) to ultrafine TiO$_2$ particles produced a less potent pulmonary inflammatory response ($\sim$10% PMNs at the end of exposure), which, at comparable dust loads, was significantly less than the effects measured in rats.

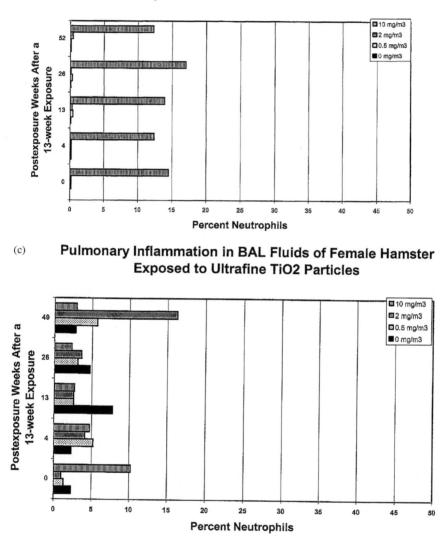

Figure 4 *Continued*

pulmonary tumors following exposures to a variety of particulate-types. Evidence from numerous studies suggests that the mouse and hamster do not develop pulmonary tumors following exposures to low-toxicity dusts. The available data in coal miners suggest that exposure to coal mine dust does not result in particle overload-related tumors in humans.

It is interesting to note that the threshold limit values (TLVs) set for particulates not otherwise classified (PNOC) are based, in large part, upon particle overload dynamics in the rat lung. It is important to note, however, that evidence is accumulating which indicates that the pulmonary responses of dogs, primates, and humans are very different from those observed in dust-exposed rodent species, and, in particular, the rat model. In this regard, the rat model demonstrates a faster particle clearance pattern concomitant with a greater proportion of the retained dust burden being contained within alveolar macrophages. In contrast, morphologic observations of the lungs of dust-exposed monkeys and humans indicate that the larger mammalian species demonstrated a slower particle clearance pattern and a greater tendency to interstitialize the retained lung burden. It would seem reasonable to assume that: (1) a slower clearance pattern corresponding to a greater retained dust burden in the lung, concomitant with (2) enhanced interstitilization (considered to be a vulnerable compartment for the development of interstitial inflammation and fibrosis) should provide stimuli for an enhanced likelihood of developing dust-induced pathogenic pulmonary effects in particle-exposed primates and humans. However, the limited evidence available in autopsy lung samples of coal miners and in exposed primates suggests that the lungs of larger mammals are less responsive to the dust burden insult than the rat model. If these conclusions are confirmed, they are likely to have a significant influence on risk assessment determinations for low-toxicity dusts.

D. Other Variables/Issues Related to Nanoparticle Pulmonary Toxicology

As discussed earlier, there is a common perception that exposures to ultrafine or nanoparticles produce significantly greater pulmonary toxicity when compared to equivalent concentrations of fine-sized particles of identical composition. It must be noted that the toxicological database upon which this common perception rests is based primarily on the results of studies with three particle-types: namely titanium dioxide, carbon black, and diesel particulates. In addition to the issue of species differences, two additional variables may play an important role in the toxicity of ultrafine particles: These are the following: (1) Whether the nanoparticles, which commonly aggregate in the ambient aerosol disaggregate following deposition in the distal lung. If the ultrafine particles disaggregate upon interaction with alveolar lung fluids, then they could behave as discrete individual particles; (2) Surface coatings on particles are likely to play an important role in pulmonary effects. In this respect, using a pulmonary bioassay toxicity methodology, we recently assessed the pulmonary toxicity of a number of commercial formulations of fine-sized titanium dioxide (TiO_2) particles— each with different surface coatings/treatments. The results demonstrated that one of the surface coatings on the TiO_2 particle produced enhanced pulmonary inflammation and cytotoxicity when compared to the other formulations containing different surface treatments (51).

The presence, absence, or composition of surface coatings may serve to complicate our perceptions regarding the toxicity of nanoparticles. As noted previously, most comparative lung toxicity studies have reported that ultrafine or titanium dioxide particles produced greater pulmonary inflammation when compared with fine-sized TiO_2 particles. However, recent preliminary studies have indicated that pulmonary exposures to uncoated TiO_2 nanorods and nanodots (particle size $\sim$50 nm) did not produce enhanced lung inflammation in rats when compared to fine-sized TiO_2 particles (particle size $\sim$300 nm) (Fig. 5a and b). Similar preliminary findings have been reported when comparing uncoated nanoquartz particles (50 nm) vs. fine-sized quartz particles (particle size $\sim$1.6 μm). In pulmonary instillation studies, at equivalent mass doses, the nanoquartz particles produced a less intensive pulmonary inflammatory and cytotoxic response vs. the Min-U-Sil quartz particles (52). This result is intriguing since quartz crystalline silica is classified as a Category 1 human carcinogen by the International Agency for Research on Cancer (IARC) (17). The preliminary finding suggests that particle size is only one factor in determining pulmonary toxicity.

An additional factor which may influence the hazard evaluation and corresponding risk to engineered nanoparticulates is the electrostatic attraction/aggregation or agglomeration potential of some nanoscale materials, and in particular, single wall carbon nanotubes (SWCNT). Two pulmonary bioassay studies, in mice (53) and in rats (54) with SWCNT, were recently reported. Individual SWCNT have dimensions of 1 nm (diameter) by >1 μm (length). However, SWCNT rarely, if ever, exist as discrete individual particles, and due to their strong electrostatic attraction, form agglomerates of "nanoropes" or "nanomats," consisting of 10–200 individual SWCNT (54). In a recent study, rats were intratracheally instilled with multiple doses of either SWCNT, quartz particles (positive control), or carbonyl iron particles (negative control). Exposures to high dose (5 mg/kg) SWCNT produced mortality in $\sim$15% of the instilled rats within 24 hr postinstillation exposure. This mortality resulted from mechanical blockage of the large airways by the instilled aggregate. The bronchoalveolar lavage and cell proliferation results demonstrated that lung exposures to quartz particles produced significant increases vs. controls in pulmonary inflammation, cytotoxicity, and lung parenchymal cell proliferation indices; while exposures to SWCNT produced transient lung inflammation. Histopathological analyses revealed quartz particles produced inflammation, foamy alveolar macrophage accumulation, and tissue thickening. In contrast, pulmonary exposures to SWCNT produced a non-dose-dependent series of multifocal granulomas, which was evidence of a foreign tissue body

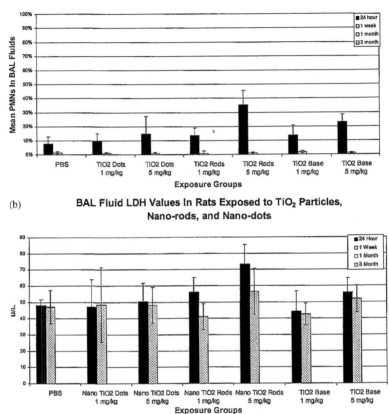

(a) Percent Neutrophils In BAL Fluids of Rats Exposed to TiO₂ Particles, Nano-rods, and Nano-dots

(b) BAL Fluid LDH Values In Rats Exposed to TiO₂ Particles, Nano-rods, and Nano-dots

Figure 5 (a) Pulmonary inflammation in BAL fluids of male rats exposed to 1 or 5 mg/kg base TiO₂ particles (300 nm), uncoated NanoTiO₂ dots (50 nm), or uncoated NanoTiO₂ rods. Lung inflammation in particle and control rats is represented by % neutrophils (PMN) in BAL fluids 24 hr as well as 1-week postintratracheal instillation exposure (pe). Values presented are mean values of percent neutrophils in BAL fluids. Pulmonary exposures to base or NanoTiO₂ dots and rods produced a transient lung inflammatory response at 24 hr postexposure. However, little or no inflammation was measured by 1 week postexposure. These preliminary results indicate that exposures to NanoTiO₂ dots and rods did not produce more inflammation than the fine-sized TiO₂ particles. (b) BAL fluid LDH values for male rats exposed to 1 or 5 mg/kg base TiO₂ particles (300 nm), uncoated NanoTiO₂ dots (50 nm), or uncoated NanoTiO₂ rods at 24 hr and 1 week postintratracheal instillation exposures (pe). BAL fluid LDH is a biomarker for lung cytotoxicity values. No significant increases in BALF LDH vs. controls were measured in the NanoTiO₂ dots or rods-exposed rats when compared to the fine-sized TiO₂ particles. These preliminary results indicate that exposures to NanoTiO₂ dots and rods did not produce more lung cytotoxicity when compared to the fine-sized TiO₂ particles.

reaction. In the center of each of the granulomas were agglomerated carbon nanotubes surrounded by mononuclear cell-types (54). Similar findings were reported by Lam et al. (53) in SWCNT-exposed mice. It is noteworthy that, unlike the results with quartz particles, the finding of unusual pulmonary lesions (i.e., multifocal granulomas) in rats was not consistent with the following: enhanced cell proliferation indices, sustained lung inflammation, a dose–response relationship; and a uniform and progressive distribution of lesions (54). In addition, the results of two recent exposure assessment studies indicate very low respirable (55) aerosol SWCNT concentration exposures at the workplace. Thus, the physiological relevance of these findings remains to be determined by conducting an inhalation toxicity study in rats with aerosols of SWCNT. It is also important to note herein that single wall carbon nanotubes, due to their unique electrostatic characteristics, do not appear to be representative of other nanoscale particulates.

V. Conclusions

- Epidemiological studies demonstrate that a correlation exists between air pollution events and enhanced morbidity/mortality.

  - The toxicological mechanisms associated with the PM-induced adverse health effects remain to be clearly defined.

- In contrast, occupational exposures to silica particles and asbestos fibers have produced serious lung injury, and the pathogenetic mechanisms are generally well understood.

  - In pulmonary toxicity studies, silica and asbestos exposures to experimental animals such as rats produce lung lesions similar to those observed in exposed humans.
  - However, in pulmonary toxicity studies with low solubility particles (likely constituents of ambient air PM), only high, overload doses produce pulmonary lesions in rats, the most sensitive species, and these may have limited relevance for humans, due to species differences.
  - It seems likely that the PM components may produce adverse health impacts only in sensitive or compromised individuals with pre-existing cardiopulmonary disease and this sensitivity is difficult to model in experimental animals.
  - PM-derived ultrafine particles are generally considered to be more toxic than fine-sized particulates due to surface area and oxidant stress considerations; however, other factors such as aggregation/disaggregation potential and surface coatings may be important variables in influencing toxicity.

- Perhaps the most significant reason why the mechanisms of PM-induced adverse effects are so difficult to define is because PM effects likely act synergistically with other components of air pollution (e.g., oxidants such as ozone and nitrogen dioxide, carbon monoxide, aldehydes, VOCs, ambient temperatures, etc.) to produce adverse health effects in compromised individuals. Thus, both components of the equation, i.e., air pollution constituent mixtures, concomitant with sensitive individuals having pre-existing cardiopulmonary disease, are very difficult to model in experimental studies.

  - On a mass basis, nano or ultrafine particles (i.e., $<100 \, nm$) are considered to produce greater pulmonary toxicity when compared to fine-sized particles (i.e., size range $-100 \, nm$ $>3 \, \mu m$) of identical composition. This conclusion has been derived based only on comparisons of two or three particle-types.
  - It seems likely that in addition to particle size; other factors such as surface coatings, aggregation/disaggregation potential, and origin of composition (gas phase (fumed) vs. liquid phase (colloidal/precipitated)) will have a significant impact on the potential toxicity of inhaled engineered nanoparticles.

References

1. Donaldson K, Stone V, Clouter A, Renwick L, MacNee W. Ultrafine particles Occup Environ Med 2001; 58:211–216.
2. Donaldson K, Brown D, Clouter A, Duffin R, MacNee W, Renwick L, Tran L, Stone V. The pulmonary toxicology of ultrafine particles. J Aerosol Med 2002; 15:213–220.
3. Oberdorster G. Pulmonary effects of inhaled ultrafine particles. Int Arch Occup Environ Health 2001; 74:1–8.
4. US EPA 1996. Air quality criteria for particulate matter. Vol III EPA/600/ P-95/001cF.
5. Oberdorster G. Toxicology of ultrafine particles: in vivo studies. Phil Trans R Soc London A 2000; 358:2719–2740.
6. Drinker P, Thomson RM, Finn JL. Metal fume fever. II. Resistance acquired by inhalation of zinc oxide on two successive days. J Ind Hygiene Toxicol 1927; 9:98–105.
7. Gordon T, Chen LC, Fine JM, Schlesinger RB, Su WY, Kimmel TA, Amdur MO. Pulmonary effects of inhaled zinc oxide in human subjects, guinea pigs, rats and rabbits. Am Ind Hygiene Assoc J 1992; 53:503–509.
8. Goldstein M, Weiss H, Wade K, et al. An outbreak of fume fever in an electronics instrument testing laboratory. J Occup Med 1987; 29:746–749.

9. Rosenstock L, Cullen MR. Clinical Occupational Medicine. Philadelphia, PA: Saunders, 1986:28–32.
10. Spencer H. The Pathology of the Lung. Oxford: Pergamon, 1977.
11. Morgan A, Moores SR, Homes A, Evans JC, Evans NH, Black A. The effect of quartz, administered by intratracheal instillation on the rat lung 1. The cellular response. Environ Res 1980; 22:1–2.
12. Bowden DH. Macrophages, dust and pulmonary disease. Exp Lung Res 1987; 12:89–107.
13. Warheit DB, Hart GA, Hesterberg TW. Fibers. In: Marquardt H, Schafer SG, McClellan RO, Welsch F, eds. Toxicology. San Diego, CA: Academic Press, 1999:833–850 [chapter 34].
14. Davis JMG, Addison J, Bolton RE, Donaldson K, et al. The pathogenicity of long vs. short fiber samples of amosite asbestos administered to rats by inhalation or intraperitoneal injection. Br J Exp Pathol 1986; 67:415–430.
15. Davis JMG, Jones AD. Comparison of the pathogenicity of long and short fibers of chrysotile asbestos in rats. Br J Exp Pathol 1988; 69:717–737.
16. Ziskind M, Jones RN, Weill H. Silicosis. Am Rev Respir Dis 1976; 113: 643–665.
17. IARC Monograph. IARC Monograph on the Evaluation of the Carcinogenic Risk of Chemicals to Humans. Vol. 68. Silica, Some Silicates, Coal Dust and Para-Aramid Fibrils. Lyon, France: IARC Press, 1997.
18. Allison AC, Harrington JS, Birbeck M. An examination of the cytotoxic effects of silica on macrophages. J Exp Med 1966; 124:141.
19. Burns CA, Zarkower A, Ferguson FG. Murine immunological and histological changes in response to chronic silica exposure. Environ Res 1980; 21:298–307.
20. Lugano EM, Dauber JH, Daniele RP. Acute experimental silicosis: lung morphology, histology, and macrophage chemotaxin secretion. Am J Pathol 1982; 109:27–36.
21. Warheit DB, Gavett SH. Current concepts in the pathogenesis of particulate-induced lung injury. In: Warheit DB, ed. Fiber Toxicology. San Diego: Academic Press, 1993:305–322.
22. Donaldson K, Bolton RE, Jones A, Brown GM, Robertson MD, Slight J, Cowie H, Davis JMG. Kinetics of the bronchoalveolar leucocyte response in rats during exposure to equal airborne mass concentrations of chrysotile asbestos or titanium dioxide. Thorax 1988; 43:525–533.
23. Borm PJA, Driscoll KD. Particles, inflammation and respiratory tract carcinogenesis. Toxicol Lett 1996; 88:109–113.
24. Donaldson K, Borm PJA. The quartz hazard: a variable entity. Ann Occup Hyg 1998; 42:287–294.
25. Warheit DB, Carakostas MC, Kelly DP, Hartsky MA. Four-week inhalation toxicity study with Ludox colloidal silica in rats: pulmonary cellular responses. Fundam Appl Toxicol 1991; 16:590–601.
26. Warheit DB, McHugh TA, Hartsky MA. Differential pulmonary responses in rats inhaling various forms of silica dust (i.e., crystalline, colloidal and amorphous). Scand J Work Environ Health 1995; 21(suppl 2):19–21.
27. Hext PM. Current perspectives on particuiate induced pulmonary tumours. Hum Exp Toxicol 1994; 13:700–715.

28. ILSI. The relevance of the rat lung response to particle overload for human risk assessment: a workshop consensus report. Inhal Toxicol 2000; 12:1–17.

29. Ghio AJ, Silbajoris R, Carson JL, Samet JM. Biological effects of oil fly ash. Environ Health Perspect 2002; 110(suppl 1):89–94.

30. Kodavanti UP, Jackson MC, Ledbetter AD, Richards JR, Gardner SY, Watkinson WP, Campen MJ, Costa DL. Lung injury from intratracheal and inhalation exposures to residual oil fly ash in a rat model of monocrotaline-induced pulmonary hypertension. J Toxicol Environ Health A 1999; 57:543–563.

31. Kodavanti UP, Mebane R, Ledbetter A, Krantz T, McGee J, Jackson MC, Walsh L, Hilliard H, Chen BY, Richards J, Costa DL. Variable pulmonary responses from exposures to concentrated ambient air particles in a rat model of bronchitis. Toxicol Sci 2000; 54:441–451.

32. Kodavanti UP, Schladweiler MC, Richards JR, Costa DL. Acute lung injury from intratracheal exposure to fugitive residual oil fly ash and its constituents metals in normo- and spontaneously hypertensive rats. Inhal Toxicol 2001; 13:37–54.

33. Campen MJ, Nolan JP, Shladweiler MC, Kodavanti UP, Costa DL, Watkinson WP. Cardiac and thermoregulatory effects of instilled particulate matter-associated transition metals in healthy and cardiopulmonary-compromised rats. J Toxicol Environ Health A 2002; 65:1615–1631.

34. Elder ACP, Johnston C, Finkelstein J, Oberdorster G. Induction of adaptation to inhaled lipopolysacchardie in young and old rats and mice. Inhal Toxicol 2000; 12:225–243.

35. Elder ACP, Gelein R, Finkelstein J, Cox C, Oberdorster G. Endotoxin priming affects the lung response to inhaled ultrafine particles and ozone in young and old rats. Inhal Toxicol 2000; 12(suppl1):85–98.

36. Elder ACP, Gelein R, Finkelstein J, Cox C, Oberdorster G. The pulmonary inflammatory response to inhaled ultrafine particles is modified by age, respiratory tract sensitization, and disease. Inhal Toxicol 2000; 12(suppl 4):227–246.

37. Clean Air Science Advisory Committee (CASAC). May 4–5 Meeting ,1995.

38. Levy LS. Squamous lung lesions associated with chronic exposure by inhalation of rats to p-aramid fibrils (fine fiber dusts) and to titanium dioxide: findings of a pathology workshop. In: Mohr U et al, eds. Toxic and Carcinogenic Effects of Solid Particles in the Respiratory Tract. Washington, DC: ILSI Press, 1994:473–478.

39. Snipes MB. Current information on lung overload in nonrodent mammals: contrast with rats. Inhal Toxicol 1996; 8(suppl):91–109.

40. Nikula KJ, Avila KJ, Griffith WC, Mauderly JL. Lung tissue responses and sites of particle retention differ between rats and cynomolgus monkeys exposed chronically to diesel exhaust and coal dust. Fundam Appl Toxicol 1997; 37:37–53.

41. Nikula KJ, Vallyathan V, Green FH, Hahn F. Influence of exposure concentration or dose on the distribution of particulate material in rat and human lungs. Environ Health Perspect 2001; 109:311–318.

42. Warheit DB. Mechanistic considerations for toxicity assessments: in vivo. In: Report to the Medical Research Council at the IEH (Institute for Environment and Health, UK). IEH Report on Approaches to Predicting Toxicity from

Occupational Exposure to Dusts. Report R11. Norwich, United Kingdom: Page Bros, 1999:68–77.

43. Lee KP, Trochimomicz HJ, Reinhardt CF. Pulmonary response of rats exposed to titanium dioxide (TiO_2) by inhalation for two years. Toxicol Appl Pharmacol 1985; 79:179–192.

44. Heinrich U, Fuhst R, Rittinghausen S, Creutzenberg O, Bellmann B, Koch W, Levsen K. Chronic inhalation exposure of Wistar rats and two different strains of mice to diesel engine exhaust, carbon black, and titanium dioxide. Inhalation Toxicol 1995; 7:533–556.

45. Ferin J, Oberdorster G, Penney DP. Pulmonary retention of ultrafine and fine particles in rats. Am J Respir Cell Mol Biol 1992; 6:535–542.

46. Oberdorster G, Ferin J, Lehnert BE. Correlation between particle size, in vivo particle persistence, and lung injury. Environ Health Perspect 1994; 102(suppl 5):173–179.

47. Li XY, Gilmour PS, Donaldson K, MacNee W. Free radical activity and proinflammatory effects of particulate air pollution (PM10) in vivo and in vitro. Thorax 1996; 51:1216–1222.

48. Zhang Q, Kusaka Y, Zhu X, Sato K, Mo Y, Kluz T, Donaldson K. Comparative toxicity of standard nickel and ultrafine nickel in lung after intratracheal instillation. J Occup Health 2003; 45:23–30.

49. Bermudez E, Mangum JB, Asgharian B, Wong BA, Reverdy EE, Janszen DB, Hext PM, Warheit DB, Everitt JI. Long-term pulmonary responses of three laboratory rodent species to subchronic inhalation of pigmentary titanium dioxide particles. Toxicol Sci 2002; 70:86–97.

50. Bermudez E, Mangum JB, Wong BA, Asgharian B, Hext PM, Warheit DB, Everitt Jl. Pulmonary responses of mice, rats, and hamsters to subchronic inhalation of ultrafine titanium dioxide particles. Toxicol Sci 2004; 77:347–357.

51. Warheit DB, Webb TR, Reed KL. Pulmonary toxicity studies with TiO_2 particles containing various commercial coatings. Toxicologist 2003; 72(No.1):298A.

52. Warheit DB, Webb TR, Reed KL, Colvin V, Sayes CM. Assessing the pulmonary hazards and health risks of nano (ultrafine) particles and carbon nanotubes: Lung toxicity studies in rats and relevance of these findings for humans. Abstract of papers, 227th ACS National Meeting, Anaheim, CA, United States, March 28-April 1, 2004.

53. Lam CW, James JT, McCluskey R, Hunter RL. Pulmonary toxicity of single-wall carbon nanotubes in mice 7 and 90 days after intratracheal instillation. Toxicol Sci 2004; 77:126–134.

54. Warheit DB, Laurence BR, Reed KL, Roach DH, Reynolds GA, Webb TR. Comparative pulmonary toxicity assessment of single-wall carbon nanotubes in rats. Toxicol Sci 2004; 77:117–125.

55. Maynard AD, Baron PA, Foley M, Shvedova AA, Kisin ER, Castranova V. Exposure to carbon nanotube material: aerosol release during the handling of unrefined single-walled carbon nanotube material. J Toxicol Environ Health A 2004; 67:87–107.

10

Biological Airborne Pollutants

HARRIET A. BURGE

Harvard School of Public Health, Harvard University,
Boston, Massachusetts, U.S.A.

I. Introduction

Bioaerosols include viruses, bacteria and their relatives, fungal spores, pollen and other plant particles, and many fragments released from living organisms. Bioaerosols have long been considered to be "natural" and therefore not pollutants. For the most part, this is true. The organisms that are part of or produce the aerosol are a natural part of the earth's environment, and most are probably essential to the functioning of the earth's ecosystem. Humans have evolved in the presence of bioaerosols, and also have evolved to withstand their onslaught. It is probably true that some bioaerosol exposure is essential to the proper functioning of the human immune system and fungal exposure may have other protective effects (1).

These natural components of the earth's environment do become pollutants when, by human action, exposure patterns are modified so that excess disease results. Human disturbance that has led to detrimental changes in exposure include changing plant ecosystems resulting in monocultures of aerosol-producing organisms, and the development of built environments that foster the development of communities of aerosol-producing organisms leading to unusual human exposure. In addition, human travel has allowed broad distribution of organisms that can have devastating effects in new environments.

This chapter is an overview of the latest information on bioaerosols as it relates to human respiratory disease. In cases where there are many citations that could be used to document an observation, the choice has been to reference the most recent rather than the landmark initial observations.

II. Bioaerosol Disease Burdens

Because virtually, everyone develops one or more airborne viral infections over their lifetime, all of the other bioaerosols (and for that matter any other aerosol) become less important with respect to disease burdens. However, fortunately, most of the airborne viral diseases are relatively mild, depending on the susceptibility of the host. However, many viruses do cause significant morbidity, and in some populations, exceptionally virulent influenza strains have led to major epidemics with high mortality. Worldwide, at least 30–40 million people died in the 1918 Spanish influenza epidemic. Given a tripling of the world's population, such an epidemic could kill 100 million people today (2). Influenza continues to be an important cause of excess mortality, especially in the winter months, with death rates of approximately 12,000 people per year (3–5).

Hypersensitivity diseases rank high with respect to morbidity. As many as 40% of some populations have allergies, and about 6% of the population of the United States have asthma. Asthma has become such a common disease in children that many hospitals have set up asthma triage programs. Nearly 4500 deaths from asthma were reported in the United States for the year 2000 (6).

If other bioaerosols were ranked with respect to airborne disease burden, bacterial infections (causing *Mycoplasma pneumonia* and tuberculosis), or infectious fungi (causing histoplasmosis, *Pneumocystis carinii* pneumonia, and others). Far down on the list are bioaerosol-related inhalation toxicoses.

III. Definitions
A. Bioaerosols

By definition, bioaerosols are airborne particles derived from living organisms. Each particle in a bioaerosol may be the organisms itself, a reproductive unit of the organism (e.g., a spore), or a fragment of the organism.

B. Agents, Sources, and Reservoirs

A bioagent is the actual particle or biochemical that ultimately leads to disease once an appropriate dose has been accumulated. Thus, *Alt a* 1 is

Table 1 Agents, Sources, and Reservoirs for Some Important Bioaerosols

Agent	Source	Primary reservoir	Secondary reservoir
Alt a 1	*Alternaria alternata*	Dead plant material	Dust or soil
Der p 1	*Dermatophagoides pteronyssinus*	Dust	Dust
Fel d 1	*Felis domesticus*	*Felis domesticus*	Dust
Bacillus anthracis	*Bacillus anthracis*	Infected animal	Soil, dust
Influenza vims	Influenza virus	Infected person	???
Aflatoxin	*Aspergillus flavus*	Moldy corn	Corn dust

the protein that leads to the allergic response commonly attributed to the spore of the fungus *Alternaria alternata*. The source of the bioagent is the living organism that originally produced the agent. In the case of *Alt a* 1, the source is the fungus *A. alternata*. For bacteria and viruses, the agent and the source are the same, since in each case the organism is the agent. The primary reservoir is the place where the source organism is living. Again using *Alt a* 1, the primary reservoir could be dead plant material represented by the paper on gypsum board. The secondary reservoir is the place where particles containing the agent have accumulated. For *Alt a* 1, the secondary reservoir could be dust (indoors) or soil (outdoors). It should be noted that these are arbitrary divisions, and the delimitations between them are often blurred. Table 1 outlines agents, sources, and reservoirs for some important bioaerosols.

C. Exposure and Dose

For the purposes of this paper, exposure is represented by measurements up to the point of entry into the respiratory tract. Dose is the actual amount of the agent that reaches the site within the respiratory tract where it can cause its effect. Thus, exposure is a measure of concentrations in air over the time a person actually spends in an aerosol. Dose is the number of particles that enter the respiratory tract and reach an appropriate site times the amount of agent/particle. Obviously, in order to determine dose, one needs to know the time exposed to the aerosol, the number of particles in the aerosol, the size of individual aerosol particles, the amount of agent/particle, and the location in the respiratory tract where the particle must impact in order to be effective. Thus, for *Amb a* 1 (ragweed allergen) dose would be the sum of all the allergen that was released anywhere in the respiratory tract, while for *Mycobacterium tuberculosis,* only those living organisms that reach the alveoli are counted.

IV. Overview of Diseases Related to Bioaerosol Exposure
A. Airborne Infectious Disease
1. Infectious Agents

All airborne infectious disease, by definition, is related to bioaerosol exposure. In order to transmit such disease, the organism has to become
airborne, and be able to remain infective in the airborne state.
Organisms that fall into this category include bacteria, viruses, and fungi.
Many factors influence whether or not an organism can cause disease via
the airborne route. They include:

  a. A mechanism for aerosolization of the organism,
  b. The ability to survive in the airborne state, and
  c. The ability to cause disease via respiratory tract exposure.

Aerosolization mechanisms can be coughs that occur as symptoms of
some infectious diseases, or mechanical disturbance of environmental
reservoirs, and depend on the specific type of disease. The ability to survive
in the airborne state depends on the viability of the micro-organism, the
material in which it becomes aerosolized, and the nature of the air environment. Many environmental factors affect aerosol survival, including humidity, ultraviolet light, and the "open air factor." A number of studies have
demonstrated that the ability to survive as an aerosol is unique to each
organism and condition, and there are no generalities that allow extrapolation from one organism to another (7,8).

Infectious agents may be either virulent or opportunistic. The virulent
agents infect all exposed people who do not have specific immunity. Opportu-
nists infect only people with some degree of damage to their innate immunity

A truly airborne infection is considered to spread more than 3 ft from
the host. Large respiratory droplets from coughing and sneezing should settle within this distance, while only dry droplet nuclei should be able to travel
further. However, this is an arbitrary measure. Some common airborne diseases from each type of infectious organism are presented in Table 2.
Opportunistic organisms are marked with an asterisk.

2. Person-to-Person Transmission

Humans are not sources (as far as we know) of any agent affecting human
health. However, they are very important primary reservoirs for bacterial
and viral agents of disease. Any human infection that involves the
respiratory tract and leads to coughing and sneezing could be spread via droplets and droplet nuclei as a bioaerosol. The droplets consist of respiratory
secretions entraining the viral or bacterial particles. These secretions tend to
protect the organism from environmental damage (9–11). Most respiratory
droplets dry very quickly to small ($\sim 2\,\mu m$) droplet nuclei. Common diseases
transmitted via these droplet nuclei include measles, whooping cough,

Table 2 Common Airborne Infections

Bacteria	Viruses	Fungi
Bordetella pertussis (whooping cough)	Influenza	*Pneumocystis carinii*[a] (pneumonia)
Mycobacterium tuberculosis (tuberculosis)	Adeno viruses (common colds)	*Histoplasma capsulatum* (histoplasmosis)
Francisella tularensis (tularemia)	Rhinovirus (common colds)	*Coccidiodes immitis* (coccidioidomycosis)
Coxiella burnetii (Q fever)	Variola (smallpox)	*Blastomyces dermatididis* (blastomycosis)
Bacillus anthracis (anthrax)	Varicella (chickenpox)	*Cryptococcus neoformans*[a] (Cryptococcosis)
Legionella pneumophila[a] (legionnaires' disease)	Rubella (German measles), Rubeola (measles)	*Aspergillus fumigatus*[a] (invasive aspergillosis)
Yersinia pestis (pneumonic plague)		

[a]Opportunistic organisms.

tuberculosis, influenza, some common colds, etc. (5,12–15). Requirements for airborne spread of such diseases include the ability of the organism to survive airborne transport, and its ability to cause infection by inhalation. Another probable requirement is either that the infection can result from a relatively low dose (small number of organisms) or that the disease process results in aerosols with large numbers of infectious units. Thus, tuberculosis is spread on small droplet nuclei that penetrate deep into the lung. Evidence suggests that a single organism of *M. tuberculosis* could cause infection (16).

Some infectious agents are hardy enough to survive transport through ventilation systems. Epidemics of measles and tuberculosis resulting from ventilation system transport have been reported (12,17).

Infectious aerosols can also be produced occasionally by diseases that normally do not lead to respiratory symptoms. The vomiting that is stimulated by some gastrointestinal viruses can lead to droplet formation and inhalational exposure and disease (18).

In addition to respiratory droplets, human occupants of indoor spaces release skin scales with adherent bacteria. Skin scales that carry bacteria are a significant problem in hospitals where exposure during surgeries may lead to dangerous infections (19,20).

3. Animal-to-Person Transmission

Animals may also act as primary reservoirs for infectious agents that infect humans. Thus, the primary natural reservoir from which exposure to *Bacillus anthracis* (anthrax) occurs is animals. Most of the "natural" cases of human anthrax have resulted from inhalation of aerosols resulting from handling of animal skins (21,22). Tularemia and Q fever are other human infections that result from exposure to infected rabbits and sheep, respectively (23–25).

4. Environment-to-Person Transmission

Most human infectious agents do not reproduce outside the host, and most of those that do require highly specialized environments. A majority of environmental-source infections result from some human-driven changes that have occurred. The so-called "emerging infectious diseases" are considered to result from disruption of natural habitats and broad travel (26).

Many naturally occurring environmental agents are opportunistic, requiring that the host have some sort of immune deficiency for infection to occur. In this category are *Cryptococcus*, *Legionella*, and *Aspergillus*.

Legionella pneumophila is a common bacterium that inhabits warm water, for example, in shallow parts of streams. Human intervention has provided habitats from which aerosolization and human exposure can occur, resulting in infection. It is important as a cause of nosocomial infections along with several other agents (27,28). *Aspergillus fumigatus* is another agent that is responsible for nosocomial infections resulting from environmental disturbance. Construction activities in hospitals are especially problematic (29).

Dental machinery and laser devices are suspected to produce infectious viral aerosols (30). Finally, laboratory accidents can produce aerosols containing infectious agents that would otherwise be very unlikely to become airborne (31–33).

5. Biowarfare Infectious Agents

Unfortunately, the current state of the world mandates a brief discussion of infectious agents as weapons. The anthrax outbreaks related to mailed spores has put the world on alert about the potential for the use of micro-organisms as mechanisms of terror (34).

Anthrax could be considered the "ideal" microbiological weapon. Very few people are immune. The illness is severe, often fatal, and once symptoms occur little can be done for the victim. The dose (the number of infectious units necessary to initiate infection) is not large (about 8000 cells, perhaps less). Finally, the organism is easy to produce and makes endospores, which are extremely resistant to environmental stresses, and can survive for many years in the dry state. Given all of this, it is actually surprising that more people exposed to the postoffice aerosols were not infected. Since it is difficult to reclose Pandora's box, there are likely to occur additional outbreaks of this disease in the future. Vigilance and eventual immunization are our current defense.

Other infectious agents are also on the "list" of potential weapons. These include plague, smallpox, tularemia, the hemorrhagic fevers, and others (35–38). None of these have all of the advantages of anthrax, none live in aerosols as well, and all are more difficult to produce in mass.

B. Hypersensitivity Diseases

Allergens are generally proteins that are able to elicit a specific immune response that results in a predisposition to hypersensitivity disease. The illnesses differ from infections in which specific genetic predisposition factors are probably necessary for the disease to occur, and exposure without this predisposition generally will not cause illness regardless of its intensity.

Potentially, allergenic proteins are probably produced by all living organisms. Whether or not a particular allergen actually causes sensitization probably depends both on the potency of the allergen and nature of the exposure. The biological-source allergens are generally proteins, and are often enzymes that facilitate the organisms' interaction with the environment. As proteins, the agents are not, in themselves, alive. In some cases, however, the source organism may need to be alive in order to release the allergen (e.g., some fungal spores) (39).

1. IgE-Mediated Allergic Disease

Because of the increasing prevalence of asthma, many studies have been initiated that seek to discover risk factors. Many of these studies focus on environmental exposures to bioaerosols. While it appears clear that bioaerosols are intrinsically involved with both the development and the expression of asthma, results tend to be inconsistent with respect to the specific bioaerosols that are involved. Results vary with populations, geographic locations, and economic status, to name a few factors.

Probably all nonhuman animals produce material that can induce hypersensitivity responses in some people. There are reports of allergy to such divergent creatures as reindeer (40) and sewer flies (41). Fortunately, most people come into continuous contact with only a few animals that shed copious allergens.

a. Mammals

Dogs and cats are common sources for potent allergens. Dog allergens (e.g., *Can f* 1 and *Can f* 2) are lipocalin proteins produced orally in dogs and spread through saliva (42). Several cat allergens have been characterized. *Fel d* 1 is produced in the skin of the cat and is also abundant in lacrimal fluid and saliva (43,44). Its biological activity, aside from its allergenicity, is unclear. *Fel d* 3 is also formed in and released from cat skin, and is a cysteine protease inhibitor (45). Approximately half of airborne cat allergen is carried on particles larger than 9 μm which settle

quickly. However, a reasonable amount is also associated with small particles that remain airborne for long periods following removal of the cat
(46,47).

Skin reactivity to cat and dog allergens is clearly a risk factor for pulmonary effects related to exposure (48–50). On the other hand, a number of
studies have now reported that early exposure to pet allergens protects children from asthma (51–54). It appears that sensitization occurs most often in
children living without these pets, and exposure to the allergen occurs
primarily outside the home (55).

Rat and mouse urinary proteins (*Rat n* 1 and *Mus m* 1, respectively)
are other important mammalian allergens that are involved in occupational
allergy among laboratory animal handlers, as well as possibly playing a role
in inner city asthma (56–58).

b. Arthropods

Dust mites are barely visible acarids that produce allergen-rich fecal material. Dust mites are found wherever temperature and moisture conditions
support their life style. Dust mites do not drink water, but rather absorb
it through their exoskeleton (59). They are quite fond of human beds, especially in humid climates. They also may be abundant in carpet and furniture
dust. The allergens are primarily found in fecal particles.

The feces are formed into membrane-bound balls that are about
20 μm in diameter (60). Most of the allergens are contained in these balls,
and because they settle rapidly, dust mite allergen is rarely recovered from
the air. Dust mites produce a variety of species-specific allergens (*Der f* 1, 2,
etc.; *Der p* 2; *Blo t* 1, *Blo t* 3, and *Eur m* 1). *Der p* 1 is proteolytic, a characteristic that enhances its allergenicity (61). Dust mite allergens are clearly
important in both children and adults (62–64) and many others.

Cockroaches are true bugs (Hemiptera) that are among the best-
adapted creatures on earth (65). They are present wherever food, water,
and shelter are consistently available and where they are not rigorously
eliminated.

Cockroaches produce a number of cross-reactive and species-specific
allergens. *Blatella germanica*, the German cockroach, is the most common
household insect pest in the United States, and measures of either *Bla g* 1 or
2 are made in most studies seeking to discover relationships between
environmental exposures and asthma. Other important cockroaches include
Periplaneta americana (American cockroach), which produces *Per a* 1, and
the oriental cockroach (*Blatta orientalis*) (66). Particle size for cockroach
allergen exposure is not well established.

The primary reservoir for cockroach allergen is secretions, feces, and
body parts of the cockroaches. Secondary reservoir is dust. Cockroaches
have long been considered to carry infectious diseases. While allergen exposure is probably the most important risk associated with cockroach

infestation, evidence does exist that cockroaches can be secondary reservoirs for some infectious agents (67–70).

Cockroach allergens are also important sensitizers, especially in low income inner city populations and many others (62,71–73).

c. Plants

Plants are important sources for outdoor allergen aerosols. Pollen is the main particle type carrying these allergens, but some plant allergens are also borne on small pieces of pollen, bare cytoplasm particles, and adhered to other small particles (74,75).

Outdoor pollen concentrations, and hence allergen concentrations, have a very strong seasonal component and individual allergens are virtually absent from the air outside of the period during which pollen is being produced. The population of pollen types in the air is controlled primarily by local vegetation types, and secondarily by long distance transport (76).

Pollen readily penetrates naturally ventilated interiors, and outdoor air is the secondary reservoir for indoor pollen allergens. Production of pollen by indoor plants is relatively rare except in greenhouse environments (77).

Pollen has historically been considered responsible for hay fever symptoms but not asthma (78). However, recent studies have implicated pollen exposure in acute asthma exacerbation (79,80).

Natural rubber latex derived from the plant *Hevia brasiliensis* contains numerous allergens (81–83). Exposure to latex was common in hospital settings, both among health care workers and patients. For health care workers, powered latex gloves appear to be the primary culprit (84,85).

d. Fungi

In addition to causing infections, fungi also produce allergens. The allergens are probably digestive enzymes secreted by the spore in preparation for germination. There are 200,000 species of fungi that have been identified, and probably more than a million overall. Of these, only a very few have been studied for allergenicity, and these are not necessarily those to which people are most commonly exposed. The best known of the allergen producing fungi is *Alternaria alternata,* which produces *Alt a* 1 (among other allergens). *Alt a* 1 is produced by a number of different related fungi (e.g., *Stemphylium*). Other fungi that have been studied for allergen content include *Penicillium chrysogenum* (*Pen c* 1), *Aspergillus fumigatus* (*Asp f* 1), *Cladosporium herbarum* (*Cla h* 1), *Psilocybe cubensis* (*Psi c* 1), and *Coprinus comatus* (*Cop c* 1). The latter two are members of the basidiomycetes, species of which produce massive spore aerosols during wet weather (86). Another group of abundant spores are produced by ascomycetes. None of these have been evaluated for allergen content. Enolase allergens that cross-react broadly have been recovered from several fungal species (87).

Most fungal allergens are proteins involved in the search for and digestion of food. Many are expressed only when the fungus has sufficient water for spore germination, and when the appropriate food source is present. Thus, these allergens are released only as the spore germinates (88). With respect to exposure, the living spore probably lands on the respiratory mucosa, begins to germinate (after minutes or hours), then releases allergens.

Fungal spores and their allergens are abundant in outdoor air. Their prevalence is controlled primarily by meteorological factors, although some are seasonal as well. They also can be abundant indoors when damp conditions remain for more than a week or two.

For fungal allergens, the source is the spore, the primary reservoir the fungal colony from which the spore was released, and secondary reservoirs are dust, soil, and other materials that trap fungal spores.

2. Hypersensitivity Pneumonitis

Hypersensitivity pneumonitis (HP) is a cell-mediated response to highly reactive chemicals and small particle antigens. The antigens are generally derived from bacteria, especially thermophilic actinomycetes, and fungi. Hypersensitivity pneumonitis is primarily an occupational illness, and individual outbreaks are generally named by the type of work being done. Thus, farmer's lung disease is HP caused by exposure to hay contaminated with a thermophilic actinomycete. Cheese worker's lung involves exposure to molds; machining fluid lung is probably related to exposure to *Mycobacterium* aerosols. Table 3 presents some of the cases of HP and their causes that have been published.

More important than the specific organism, however, appears to be the conditions under which exposure occurs. Apparently relatively intense exposure to a small particle antigen is necessary, and wherever this occurs, the disease may present itself. It also may be that some coexposure is important. Endotoxin, for example, is always present in machining coolants, and probably also in bird droppings and mushroom compost.

3. Toxicoses

Bioaerosol toxicoses also do not depend on the presence of living organisms, but only on the toxins they generate. Exposure generally results in illness in a dose-dependent fashion as for nonbiological toxins.

a. Endotoxin

The best known bacterial toxin that is considered important as an aerosol is bacterial endotoxin. Endotoxin is a lipopolysaccharide (LPS) that forms part of the cell wall of gram-negative bacteria. All gram-negative bacteria have LPS, but only some is toxic and can be called endotoxin (89).

(1) **Direct effects**: Endotoxin challenges in normal subjects induce transient pulmonary function changes (90,91). In sensitive laboratory

Table 3 Hypersensitivity Pneumonitis Antigens

Name of disease	Agent	Reservoir for agent	References
Machinists lung	*Mycobacterium immunogenum*	Machining fluid	89
Suberosis	*Penicillium frequentans, Aspergillus fumigatus,* cork dust	Cork	90
Feather duvet lung	Goose feathers	Duvet	91
Bird fanciers' lung	Pigeon antigen	Pigeons	92
Summer type HP	*Trichosporon asahii*	Home contamination	93
Mushroom workers' lung	Thermoactinomyces spp.	Mushroom compost	94
	Tricholoma conglobatum	Mushrooms	95
Hot tub lung	*Mycobacterium avium* complex	Hot tub contamination	96

animals, low levels of endotoxin induce airway remodeling (92). Exposure to endotoxin may also be responsible for relatively low lung cancer mortality in farmers (93).

Endotoxin is especially abundant in farming environments or other situations where organic material is handled, and evidence is strong that these exposures lead to inflammatory lung disease (94,95). Byssinosis, a respiratory disease of cotton workers, is the illness that was first identified as related to endotoxin aerosol exposure. Although the exposure is complex in these environments, symptoms correlate independently with the level of endotoxin exposure (96). Endotoxin-associated inflammatory lung disease has also been documented in those working with corn (97), soybeans (98), cotton (99), jute (100), swine (101), poultry (102), and in many other situations.

(2) **Synergistic effects:** Endotoxin exposure appears to enhance the response to allergens, possibly by making the respiratory mucosa more receptive to the allergens through inflammation (103), and endotoxin concentrations in indoor living environments are among the correlates of asthma symptoms (104,105). Endotoxin also exacerbates the effects of *A. fumigatus* exposure in horses (106), and probably plays a role in pulmonary effects induced by exposure to microbially contaminated machining fluids (107).

b. Mycotoxins

Mycotoxins are secondary metabolites produced by many fungi during digestion of specific substrates. Probably all fungal species produce some mycotoxins. However, even the most important toxin producers do not consistently produce the toxin. For example, about 40% of the strains of *Stachybotrys chartarum* that have been examined can produce mycotoxins. Mycotoxins are well known as food toxicants, causing a broad range of acute and chronic illness following ingestion (108). Notable are cancers related to aflatoxin and ochratoxin ingestion, alimentary toxic aleukia from trichothecene ingestion, abortions, gangrene, convulsions, and hallucinations from ergot poisoning (109–111). Only a very few studies have documented inhalation exposure sufficient to cause illness. These have occurred exclusively in agricultural environments such as workers handling moldy grain (110,112–114).

Mycotoxin exposure in residential, office, and school environments continues to be a public concern, in spite of very little evidence of toxin exposure, even when toxigenic fungi are abundant. The history of this concern dates from an outbreak of hemosiderosis in babies in a Cleveland inner city neighborhood. A CDC study mentioned the possibility that fungal toxins could be involved, and a subsequent report by some of the investigators identified *Stachybotrys atra* (*chartarum*) specifically (115–117). Subsequently, the CDC reanalyzed the data from the initial investigation, and concluded that a connection between mycotoxin exposure and the illness had not been documented (118). Subsequent studies have documented that, in fact, some strains of *S. chartarum* do produce very toxic metabolites under some circumstances, and that these metabolites could cause pulmonary bleeding if sufficient dose were to be achieved (119–121). However, no study has yet documented that sufficient exposure has occurred to cause these experimental effects. In addition, limited evidence is available that very high spore concentrations would be necessary to result in acute illness, and that volatile components of the growth of toxic fungi do not have a direct effect (122).

The primary source for mycotoxins is the spore or mycelial fragment that includes the toxin. Primary reservoirs are the fungal colonies and the substrates on which they are growing (e.g., food). Mycotoxins may also accumulate in dust which then becomes a secondary reservoir. Aerosolization of mycotoxins occurs with spore release, and when substrate material is disturbed.

c. Plant Toxins

Plant toxins have not seriously been considered as bioaerosols except as biological warfare agents. Ricin, a toxin derived from castor bean (*Ricinus communis*) was discovered in an envelope in a South Carolina postal facility in 2003 (123). Its dust has also been recovered from the Senate Office building in February 2004. It is a protein synthesis inhibitor, and enters cells by binding to cell surface carbohydrates. The most hazardous routes of administration for ricin are injection and inhalation, with a lethal dose being approximately 5–10 µg/kg. The inhalation lethal dose is probably in the upper part of this range (124).

V. Important Environmental Reservoirs
A. Dead Organic Materials

Dead organic materials are primary reservoirs for many fungi and bacteria. The fungi, in particular, use dead plant material for food. Many common activities disturb dead organic materials and produce bioaerosols. Outdoors, lawn mowing, gardening, spreading of mulch, and raking leaves are all important aerosol generating activities (39,125).

Bioaerosols are especially important in farming environments and compost sites, both with large concentrations of nonliving organic material (126–128). Field crops are allowed to die in the fields before harvest. During harvesting operations, dense clouds of spores are released into the air (98). These aerosols have probably changed the nature of the ambient fungal aerosol because of changing agricultural practice.

Stored grain is another major primary and secondary reservoir for fungi. Exposure to such dust can lead to organic dust toxic syndrome that is believed to be caused, in part, by fungal toxins (129,130). Toxin concentrations have been measured in airborne dust during harvesting and grain unloading (0.04–$92 \, ng/m^3$) and during animal feeding (5–$421 \, ng/m^3$).

A. fumigatus and the thermophilic actinomycetes are particularly abundant in compost because they are able to grow at the high temperatures that develop within the piles. Disturbance of the piles releases clouds of spores, causing concern for adjacent residents (131,132).

Most of the materials used in building houses and in interior finishes of larger buildings are essentially dead organic material. When these materials become wet, they support fungal growth and become primary reservoirs for spores and their allergens. Construction activities produce fungal aerosols even in the absence of measurable growth. Epidemics of aspergillosis have occurred related to construction activities in hospitals (29).

B. Water

Water is a primary reservoir for bacteria such as *Legionella*. The bacteria grow within amoebae in biofilms on surfaces in contact with the water. The organisms are washed from the biofilms, and released in water droplets. Cooling towers are an important reservoir for legionellae (133). Another important reservoir from which legionellae are aerosolized is from shower heads (134,135).

Humidifiers that do not boil water become primary reservoirs for bacteria and yeasts (136). These organisms, along with eluted antigens, are sprayed into the air by the action of the humidifier causing intense small particle aerosols. Exposure to these aerosols has been reported to cause HP (137,138).

c. House Dust

House dust is composed of fibers, starch granules, skin scales, insect fragments, all of the "indoor" allergens (cat, dog, dust mite, cockroach, and fungal). Endotoxin can also be abundant in dust. Some fungi may grow even in the low water conditions available in house dust. Yeasts, for example, are especially abundant in dust.

House dust is considered to be representative of long-term exposures in the indoor environment, and dust samples are often used as exposure surrogates in epidemiological studies. This may be acceptable for agents for which dust is the primary reservoir for exposure (e.g., dust mite allergens). However, for fungi (for example), there are multiple exposure reservoirs. In addition, house dust may develop its own ecosystem from which little exposure occurs (139,140).

VI. Measurements

Measuring exposure to bioaerosols, as for other kinds of aerosols, can be accomplished at several levels each with differing levels of representativeness, sensitivity, and specificity. Which approach one uses depends on the hypothesis under consideration. Developing measurement strategies without prior hypothesis generation has led to innumerable problems in the bioaerosols world.

Measurement approaches include visual observation, collection of bulk and/or surface samples, air samples, and human samples for biomarker determination. How, when, where, and how many samples are collected determines the representativeness of the data for the given environment. The type of analysis chosen determines the sensitivity and specificity of the data.

Analytical methods range from microscopic observation of intact bulk material, to measurement of specific DNA. Table 4 summarizes some of the most important analytical approaches used for bioaerosols.

Some of these analytical approaches reveal information about the actual agents of disease (e.g., culture or gene probes for specific infectious agents, immunoassays for allergens, and chemical assays for specific toxins) (141–143). Some look for the presence of any agents that cause specific effects. The rest are indicators for exposure to the disease agents. Thus, counting or culturing *Alternaria* and *Stachybotrys* spores is used as a surrogate for exposure to *Alternaria* allergens and *Stachybotrys* toxins, respectively.

Measurements of markers of human exposure in serum, urine, or saliva are used for many types of environmental exposures. Measurement of specific IgE in human serum is indicative of sensitizing exposures to allergens, although such measurements are not good measures of where or when

Table 4 Data Derived from Different Bioaerosol Analytical Approaches

Approach	Data retrieved	Good usage example
Microscopy	Counts of particle types	Fungal spore and pollen exposure indoors and out on air samples and some source samples
Culture	Counts of culturable particles	Concentrations of specific culturable organisms such as *Aspergillus fumigatus* or *Staphylococcus aureus* in hospitals
Immunoassays	Concentrations of specific molecules (e.g., allergens)	Concentrations of specific allergens in air or source samples
Other bioassays	Units of effector agents (e.g., Limulus assay for endotoxin)	Concentrations of endotoxin in air or bulk samples
Chemical analysis	Amounts of specific chemicals	Concentration of specific toxin (e.g., endotoxin, specific mycotoxin) in air or bulk sample
Genetic probes	Presence of specific DNA sequences	Presence of specific strain of *Aspergillus fumigatus* implicated in outbreak of infection

the exposure might have occurred. Results of recent efforts to use IgG as an exposure measure have produced conflicting results (144,145). Assays have also begun to be developed to attempt to measure specific mycotoxins in human serum (146).

Recent concerns about biowarfare have prompted research into new methods for detection of biological aerosol clouds. Many of these involve laser detection of fluorescing materials in biological particles. These methods provide indications of the presence and concentrations of total bioaerosols, and identification of specific types relies on other methods (primarily DNA probes) (147).

VII. Control

Control of bioaerosol-induced disease is specific for the type of disease, and can range from immunization to source control.

A. Contagious Disease

Airborne contagious disease is controlled by immunization. A prime example of this approach is the eradication of smallpox that was accomplished with widespread immunization (148). Personal protection is also common practice, especially in health care settings. The use of air disinfection has been tested for efficacy in controlling tuberculosis outbreaks (149).

B. Source Control

For environmental source infectious and the other bioaerosol-induced diseases, source control is the primary approach for control. Disinfection of cooling towers and water systems are used to control *Legionella* (150,151).

Fungal contamination is removed by removing substrates supporting mold growth and by washing hard surfaces (152,153). Still controversial is the use of sealants to cover fungal growth that cannot be easily removed (154).

Allergen control also focuses on source removal, although evidence for the efficacy of control is weak. Encasing mattresses and pillows appears to prevent exposure to dust mite allergen (155). However, cockroach allergen control appears to be more problematic (156). Cat allergen level reductions do appear to reduce symptoms in sensitized patients (157). However, vacuuming apparently increases cat allergen exposure during cleaning (158).

C. Exposure Control

Exposure control involves cleaning the air either at a personal or ambient level. As mentioned above, tuberculosis control has utilized ultraviolet air cleaning. Air cleaning for allergens has had mixed results. For cat, significant amounts of allergen are removed using HEPA filtration when the cat is in the room, but the filter unit had only marginal effects when the cat was elsewhere (159). Filtration does not have an effect on dust mite allergen, probably because the particles are large and do not remain airborne.

VIII. Conclusions

Although we spend our lives immersed in a sea of bioaerosols, for the most part they do us little harm, and perhaps some good. By far the majority of damage done by bioaerosols is via infectious disease. While such diseases have always been with us, generally it is changing patterns of human contact that currently lead to epidemics of old and newly emergent infections. Likewise, with allergens and potentially toxic bioaerosols, human intervention has provided the environments where exposures are sufficient to lead to significant disease. Studies of the human lifestyle are and will continue to be important in attempting to control these significant sources of morbidity and mortality.

Based on environmental science and mycology, a greater emphasis is being placed on the importance of the fungi as instigators and exacerbators of allergic disease. The major problem associated with both the diagnosis and control of fungal-related allergy is the lack of good allergen preparations for diagnosis and treatment. Although this is a difficult area, it is also historically an underfunded one. Still to be accomplished are the accumulation of data on the species of fungi to which people are commonly exposed; the dynamics of allergen production in these species; the nature of the allergens themselves; and the preparation of highly potent, stable allergen preparations. Until these goals have been accomplished, the diagnosis and treatment of fungal allergy will continue to frustrate physicians, researchers, and, most important, the patients suffering from these conditions.

References

1. Slamenova D, Labaj J, Krizkova L, Kogan G, Sandula J, Bresgen N, Eckl P. Protective effects of fungal $(1\rightarrow3)$-beta-D-glucan derivatives against oxidative DNA lesions in V79 hamster lung cells. Cancer Lett 2003; 198:153–160.
2. Barry JM. The site of origin of the 1918 influenza pandemic and its public health implications. J Transl Med 2004; 2:3.
3. Tillett HE, Nicholas S, Watson JM. Unusual pattern of influenza mortality in 1989/90. Lancet 1991; 338:1590–1591.
4. Fleming DM, van der Velden J, Paget WJ. The evolution of influenza surveillance in Europe and prospects for the next 10 years. Vaccine 2003; 21:1749–1753.
5. Bridges CB, Kuehnert MJ, Hall CB. Transmission of influenza: implications for control in health care settings. Clin Infect Dis 2003; 37:1094–1101.
6. Self-reported asthma prevalence and control among adults—United States, 2001. MMWR Morb Mortal Wkly Rep 2003; 52:381–384.
7. Ijaz MK, Brunner AH, Sattar SA, Nair RC, Johnson-Lussenburg CM. Survival characteristics of airborne human coronavirus 229E. J Gen Virol 1985; 66(Pt 12):2743–2748.
8. Akers TG, Bond S, Goldberg LJ. Effect of temperature and relative humidity on survival of airborne Columbia SK group viruses. Appl Microbiol 1966; 14:361–364.
9. Ko G, First MW, Burge HA. The characterization of upper-room ultraviolet germicidal irradiation in inactivating airborne microorganisms. Environ Health Perspect 2002; 110:95–101.
10. Ko G, Burge HA, Nardell EA, Thompson KM. Estimation of tuberculosis risk and incidence under upper room ultraviolet germicidal irradiation in a waiting room in a hypothetical scenario. Risk Anal 2001; 21:657–673.
11. Ko G, First MW, Burge HA. Influence of relative humidity on particle size and UV sensitivity of *Serratia marcescens* and *Mycobacterium bovis* BCG aerosols. Tuber Lung Dis 2000; 80:217–228.

12. Bloch AB, Orenstein WA, Ewing WM, Spain WH, Mallison GF, Herrmann KL, Hinman AR. Measles outbreak in a pediatric practice: airborne transmission in an office setting. Pediatrics 1985; 75:676–683.

13. Gehanno JF, Pestel-Caron M, Nouvellon M, Caillard JF. Nosocomial pertussis in healthcare workers from a pediatric emergency unit in France. Infect Control Hosp Epidemiol 1999; 20:549–552.

14. Nicas M. Respiratory protection and the risk of *Mycobacterium tuberculosis* infection. Am J IndMed 1995; 27:317–333.

15. Goldmann DA. Transmission of viral respiratory infections in the home. Pediatr Infect Dis J 2000; 19:S97–S102.

16. Riley RL. Aerial dissemination of pulmonary tuberculosis. Am Rev Tuberc 1957; 76:931–941.

17. Houk VN. Spread of tuberculosis via recirculated air in a naval vessel: the Byrd study. Ann N Y Acad Sci 1980; 353:10–24.

18. Chadwick PR, McCann R. Transmission of a small round structured virus by vomiting during a hospital outbreak of gastroenteritis. J Hosp Infect 1994; 26:251–259.

19. Weber S, Herwaldt LA, McNutt LA, Rhomberg P, Vaudaux P, Pfaller MA, Perl TM. An outbreak of *Staphylococcus aureus* in a pediatric cardiothoracic surgery unit. Infect Control Hosp Epidemiol 2002; 23:77–81.

20. Wang JT, Chang SC, Ko WJ, Chang YY, Chen ML, Pan HJ, Luh KT. A hospital- acquired outbreak of methicillin-resistant *Staphylococcus aureus* infection initiated by a surgeon carrier. J Hosp Infect 2001; 47:104–109.

21. Penn CC, Klotz SA. Anthrax pneumonia. Semin Respir Infect 1997; 12: 28–30.

22. Pfisterer RM. [An anthrax epidemic in Switzerland. Clinical, diagnostic and epidemiological aspects of a mostly forgotten disease]. Schweiz Med Wochenschr 1991; 121:813–825.

23. Elkins KL, Cowley SC, Bosio CM. Innate and adaptive immune responses to an intracellular bacterium, *Francisella tularensis* live vaccine strain. Microbes Infect 2003; 5:135–142.

24. Madariaga MG, Rezai K, Trenholme GM, Weinstein RA. Q fever: a biological weapon in your backyard. Lancet Infect Dis 2003; 3:709–721.

25. Asano K, Suzuki K, Nakamura Y, Asano R, Sakai T. Risk of acquiring zoonoses by the staff of companion-animal hospitals. Kansenshogaku Zasshi 2003; 77:944–947.

26. Greiser-Wilke I, Haas L. [Emergence of "new" viral zoonoses]. Dtsch Tierarztl Wochenschr 1999; 106:332–338.

27. Squier C, Yu VL, Stout JE. Waterborne nosocomial infections. Curr Infect Dis Rep 2000; 2:490–496.

28. Steinert M, Hentschel U, Hacker J. *Legionella pneumophila*: an aquatic microbe goes astray. FEMS Microbiol Rev 2002; 26:149–162.

29. Cooper EE, O'Reilly MA, Guest DI, Dharmage SC. Influence of building construction work on *Aspergillus* infection in a hospital setting. Infect Control Hosp Epidemiol 2003; 24:472–476.

30. Moreira LB, Sanchez D, Trousdale MD, Stevenson D, Yarber F, McDonnell PJ. Aerosolization of infectious virus by excimer laser. Am J Ophthalmol 1997; 123:297–302.
31. Sajo E, Zhu H, Courtney JC. Spatial distribution of indoor aerosol deposition under accidental release conditions. Health Phys 2002; 83:871–883.
32. Nikitin NI, Nesterenko AA. [Method of qualitative evaluation of the danger aerosol formation in a microbiological laboratory]. Gig Sanit 1994:50–52.
33. Pike RM. Past and present hazards of working with infectious agents. Arch Pathol Lab Med 1978; 102:333–336.
34. Higgins JA, Cooper M, Schroeder-Tucker L, Black S, Miller D, Karns JS, Manthey E, Breeze R, Perdue ML. A field investigation of *Bacillus anthracis* contamination of U.S. Department of Agriculture and other Washington, D.C., buildings during the anthrax attack of October 2001. Appl Environ Microbiol 2003; 69:593–599.
35. Deresinski S. *Coccidioides immitis* as a potential bioweapon. Semin Respir Infect 2003; 18:216–219.
36. Kagawa FT, Wehner JH, Mohindra V. Q fever as a biological weapon. Semin Respir Infect 2003; 18:183–195.
37. Bossi P, Bricaire F. [Tularemia, a potential bioterrorism weapon]. Presse Med 2003; 32:1126–1130.
38. Bossi P, Bricaire F. [The plague, possible bioterrorist act]. Presse Med 2003; 32:804–807.
39. Sporik RB, Arruda LK, Woodfolk J, Chapman MD, Platts-Mills TA. Environmental exposure to *Aspergillus fumigatus* allergen (*Asp f* I). Clin Exp Allergy 1993; 23:326–331.
40. Reijula K, Halmepuro L, Hannuksela M, Larmi E, Hassi J. Specific IgE to reindeer epithelium in Finnish reindeer herders. Allergy 1991; 46:577–581.
41. Gold BL, Mathews KP, Burge HA. Occupational asthma caused by sewer flies. Am Rev Respir Dis 1985; 131:949–952.
42. Konieczny A, Morgenstern JP, Bizinkauskas CB, Lilley CH, Brauer AW, Bond JF, Aalberse RC, Wallner BP, Kasaian MT. The major dog allergens, *Can f* 1 and *Can f* 2, are salivary lipocalin proteins: cloning and immunological characterization of the recombinant forms. Immunology 1997; 92: 577–586.
43. van Milligen FJ, van Swieten P, Aalberse RC. Structure of the major cat allergen *Fel d* I in different allergen sources: an immunoblotting analysis with monoclonal antibodies against denatured *Fel d* I and human IgE. Int Arch Allergy Immunol 1992; 99:63–73.
44. Mata P, Charpin D, Charpin C, Lucciani P, Vervloet D. *Fel d* I allergen: skin and or saliva? Ann Allergy 1992; 69:321–322.
45. Ichikawa K, Vailes LD, Pomes A, Chapman MD. Molecular cloning, expression and modelling of cat allergen, cystatin (*Fel d* 3), a cysteine protease inhibitor. Clin Exp Allergy 2001; 31:1279–1286.
46. Simpson A, Simpson B, Custovic A, Craven M, Woodcock A. Stringent environmental control in pregnancy and early life: the long-term effects on mite, cat and dog allergen. Clin Exp Allergy 2003; 33:1183–1189.

47. Custovic A, Simpson B, Simpson A, Hallam C, Craven M, Woodcock A. Relationship between mite, cat, and dog allergens in reservoir dust and ambient air. Allergy 1999; 54:612–616.

48. Nelson HS, Szefler SJ, Jacobs J, Huss K, Shapiro G, Sternberg AL. The relationships among environmental allergen sensitization, allergen exposure, pulmonary function, and bronchial hyperresponsiveness in the Childhood Asthma Management Program. J Allergy Clin Immunol 1999; 104:775–785.

49. Lieutier-Colas F, Purohit A, Meyer P, Fabries JF, Kopferschmitt MC, Dessanges JF, Pauli G, de Blay F. Bronchial challenge tests in patients with asthma sensitized to cats: the importance of large particles in the immediate response. Am J Respir Crit Care Med 2003; 167:1077–1082.

50. Jaen A, Sunyer J, Basagana X, Chinn S, Zock JP, Anto JM, Burney P. Specific sensitization to common allergens and pulmonary function in the European Community Respiratory Health Survey. Clin Exp Allergy 2002; 32: 1713–1719.

51. Hesselmar B, Aberg B, Eriksson B, Bjorksten B, Aberg N. High-dose exposure to cat is associated with clinical tolerance—a modified Th2 immune response?. Clin Exp Allergy 2003; 33:1681–1685.

52. Bacharier LB, Strunk RC. Pets and childhood asthma—how should the pediatrician respond to new information that pets may prevent asthma? Pediatrics 2003; 112:974–976.

53. Perzanowski MS, Ronmark E, Platts-Mills TA, Lundback B. Effect of cat and dog ownership on sensitization and development of asthma among preteenage children. Am J Respir Crit Care Med 2002; 166:696–702.

54. Holscher B, Frye C, Wichmann HE, Heinrich J. Exposure to pets and allergies in children. Pediatr Allergy Immunol 2002; 13:334–341.

55. Ritz BR, Hoelscher B, Frye C, Meyer I, Heinrich J. Allergic sensitization owing to 'second-hand' cat exposure in schools. Allergy 2002; 57:357–361.

56. Bayard C, Siddique AB, Berzins K, Troye-Blomberg M, Hellman U, Vesterberg O. Mapping of IgE binding regions in the major rat urinary protein, alpha 2u-globulin, using overlapping peptides. Immunol Invest 1999; 28:323–338.

57. Perry T, Matsui E, Merriman B, Duong T, Eggleston P. The prevalence of rat allergen in inner-city homes and its relationship to sensitization and asthma morbidity. J Allergy Clin Immunol 2003; 112:346–352.

58. Chew GL, Perzanowski MS, Miller RL, Correa JC, Hoepner LA, Jusino CM, Becker MG, Kinney PL. Distribution and determinants of mouse allergen exposure in low-income New York city apartments. Environ Health Perspect 2003; 111:1348–1351.

59. Arlian LG, Morgan MS. Biology, ecology, and prevalence of dust mites. Immunol Allergy Clin N Am 2003; 23:443–468.

60. Tovey ER, Chapman MD, Platts-Mills TA. Mite faeces are a major source of house dust allergens. Nature 1981; 289:592–593.

61. Gough L, Campbell E, Bayley D, Van Heeke G, Shakib F. Proteolytic activity of the house dust mite allergen *Der p* 1 enhances allergenicity in a mouse inhalation model. Clin Exp Allergy 2003; 33:1159–1163.

62. Celedon JC, Sredl D, Weiss ST, Pisarski M, Wakefield D, Cloutier M. Ethnicity and skin test reactivity to aeroallergens among asthmatic children in Connecticut. Chest 2004; 125:85–92.

63. Sears MR, Greene JM, Wiuan AR, Wiecek EM, Taylor DR, Flannery EM, Cowan JO, Herbison GP, Silva PA, Poulton R. A longitudinal, population-based, cohort study of childhood asthma followed to adulthood. N Engl J Med 2003; 349:1414–1422.

64. Currie GP, Jackson CM, Lee DK, Lipworth BJ. Determinants of airway hyperresponsiveness in mild asthma. Ann Allergy Asthma Immunol 2003; 90:560–563.

65. Demark JJ, Bennett GW. Adult German cockroach (Dictyoptera: Blattellidae) movement patterns and resource consumption in a laboratory arena. J Med Entomol 1995; 32:241–248.

66. Helm RM, Squillace DL, Jones RT, Brenner RJ. Shared allergenic activity in Asian (*Blattella asahinai*), German (*Blattella germanica*), American (*Periplaneta americana*), and Oriental (*Blatta orientalis*) cockroach species. Int Arch Allergy Appl Immunol 1990; 92:154–161.

67. Imamura S, Kita M, Yamaoka Y, Yamamoto T, Ishimaru A, Konishi H, Wakabayashi N, Mitsufuji S, Okanoue T, Imanishi J. Vector potential of cockroaches for *Helicobacter pylori* infection. Am J Gastroenterol 2003; 98:1500–1503.

68. Fischer OA, Matlova L, Dvorska L, Svastova P, Pavlik I. Nymphs of the Oriental cockroach (*Blatta orientalis*) as passive vectors of causal agents of avian tuberculosis and paratuberculosis. Med Vet Entomol 2003; 17:145–150.

69. Pai HH, Chen WC, Peng CF. Isolation of non-tuberculous mycobacteria from hospital cockroaches (*Periplaneta americana*). J Hosp Infect 2003; 53: 224–228.

70. Cotton MF, Wasserman E, Pieper CH, Theron DC, van Tubbergh D, Campbell G, Fang FC, Barnes J. Invasive disease due to extended spectrum beta-lactamase-producing *Klebsiella pneumoniae* in a neonatal unit: the possible role of cockroaches. J Hosp Infect 2000; 44:13–17.

71. Belanger K, Beckett W, Triche E, Bracken MB, Holford T, Ren P, McSharry JE, Gold DR, Platts-Mills TA, Leaderer BP. Symptoms of wheeze and persistent cough in the first year of life: associations with indoor allergens, air contaminants, and maternal history of asthma. Am J Epidemiol 2003; 158: 195–202.

72. Klinnert MD, Price MR, Liu AH, Robinson JL. Morbidity patterns among low- income wheezing infants. Pediatrics 2003; 112:49–57.

73. Rogers L, Cassino C, Berger KI, Goldring RM, Norman RG, Klugh T, Reibman J. Asthma in the elderly: cockroach sensitization and severity of airway obstruction in elderly nonsmokers. Chest 2002; 122:1580–1586.

74. Taylor PE, Flagan R, Miguel AG, Valenta R, Glovsky MM. Identification of birch pollen respirable particles. Chest 2003; 123:433S.

75. Knox RB, Suphioglu C, Taylor P, Desai R, Watson HC, Peng JL, Bursill LA. Major grass pollen allergen *Lol p* 1 binds to diesel exhaust particles: implications for asthma and air pollution. Clin Exp Allergy 1997; 27:246–251.

76. Solomon WR. Aerobiology of pollinosis. J Allergy Clin Immunol 1984; 74:449–461.

77. Burge HA, Solomon WR, Muilenberg ML. Evaluation of indoor plantings as allergen exposure sources. J Allergy Clin Immunol 1982; 70:101–108.

78. Lewis SA, Corden JM, Forster GE, Newlands M. Combined effects of aerobiological pollutants, chemical pollutants and meteorological conditions on asthma admissions and A & E attendances in Derbyshire UK, 1993–96. Clin Exp Allergy 2000; 30:1724–1732.

79. Tobias A, Galan I, Banegas JR, Aranguez E. Short term effects of airborne pollen concentrations on asthma epidemic. Thorax 2003; 58:708–710.

80. Lierl MB, Hornung RW. Relationship of outdoor air quality to pediatric asthma exacerbations. Ann Allergy Asthma Immunol 2003; 90:28–33.

81. Sutherland MF, Drew A, Rolland JM, Slater JE, Suphioglu C, O'Hehir RE. Specific monoclonal antibodies and human immunoglobulin E show that *Hev b* 5 is an abundant allergen in high protein powdered latex gloves. Clin Exp Allergy 2002; 32:583–589.

82. Wagner S, Sowka S, Mayer C, Crameri R, Focke M, Kurup VP, Scheiner O, Breiteneder H. Identification of a *Hevea brasiliensis* latex manganese superoxide dismutase (*Hev b* 10) as a cross-reactive allergen. Int Arch Allergy Immunol 2001; 125:120–127.

83. Banerjee B, Kanitpong K, Fink JN, Zussman M, Sussman GL, Kelly KJ, Kurup VP. Unique and shared IgE epitopes of *Hev b* 1 and *Hev b* 3 in latex allergy. Mol Immunol 2000; 37:789–798.

84. Beezhold D, Horton K, Hickey V, Daddona J, Kostyal D. Glove powder's carrying capacity for latex protein: analysis using the ASTM ELISA test. J Long Term Eff Med Implants 2003; 13:21–30.

85. Bernstein DI, Karnani R, Biagini RE, Bernstein CK, Murphy K, Berendts B, Bernstein JA, Bernstein L. Clinical and occupational outcomes in health care workers with natural rubber latex allergy. Ann Allergy Asthma Immunol 2003; 90:209–213.

86. Helbling A, Gayer F, Brander KA. Respiratory allergy to mushroom spores: not well recognized, but relevant. Ann Allergy Asthma Immunol 1999; 83: 17–19.

87. Chang CY, Chou H, Tarn MF, Tang RB, Lai HY, Shen HD. Characterization of enolase allergen from *Rhodotorula mucilaginosa*. J Biomed Sci 2002; 9: 645–655.

88. Green BJ, Mitakakis TZ, Tovey ER. Allergen detection from 11 fungal species before and after germination. J Allergy Clin Immunol 2003; 111: 285–289.

89. Park JH, Szponar B, Larsson L, Gold DR, Milton DK. Characterization of lipopolysaccharides present in settled house dust. Appl Environ Microbiol 2004; 70:262–267.

90. Michel O, Dentener M, Corazza F, Buurman W, Rylander R. Healthy subjects express differences in clinical responses to inhaled lipopolysaccharide that are related with inflammation and with atopy. J Allergy Clin Immunol 2001; 107:797–804.

91. Michel O, Nagy AM, Schroeven M, Duchateau J, Neve J, Fondu P, Sergysels R. Dose–response relationship to inhaled endotoxin in normal subjects. Am J Respir Crit CareMed 1997; 156:1157–1164.
92. Brass DM, Savov JD, Gavett SH, Haykal-Coates N, Schwartz DA. Subchronic endotoxin inhalation causes persistent airway disease. Am J Physiol Lung Cell Mol Physiol 2003; 285:L755–L761.
93. Lange JH, Mastrangelo G, Fedeli U, Fadda E, Rylander R, Lee E. Endotoxin exposure and lung cancer mortality by type of farming: is there a hidden dose–response relationship? Ann Agric Environ Med 2003; 10:229–232.
94. Rylander R. Endotoxin in the environment—exposure and effects. J Endotoxin Res 2002; 8:241–252.
95. Zhiping W, Malmberg P, Larsson BM, Larsson K, Larsson L, Saraf A. Exposure to bacteria in swine-house dust and acute inflammatory reactions in humans. Am J Respir Crit Care Med 1996; 154:1261–1266.
96. Wang XR, Eisen EA, Zhang HX, Sun BX, Dai HL, Pan LD, Wegman DH, Olenchock SA, Christiani DC. Respiratory symptoms and cotton dust exposure; results of a 15 year follow up observation. Occup Environ Med 2003; 60:935–941.
97. Kline JN, Jagielo PJ, Watt JL, Schwartz DA. Bronchial hyperreactivity is associated with enhanced grain dust-induced airflow obstruction. J Appl Physiol 2000; 89:1172–1178.
98. Roy CJ, Thorne PS. Exposure to particulates, microorganisms, beta(1–3)-glucans, and endotoxins during soybean harvesting. AIHA J (Fairfax, Va) 2003; 64:487–495.
99. Christiani DC, Wang XR, Pan LD, Zhang HX, Sun BX, Dai H, Eisen EA, Wegman DH, Olenchock SA. Longitudinal changes in pulmonary function and respiratory symptoms in cotton textile workers. A 15-yr follow-up study. Am J Respir CritCareMed 2001; 163:847–853.
100. Chattopadhyay BP, Saiyed HN, Mukherjee AK. Byssinosis among jute mill workers. Ind Health 2003; 41:265–272.
101. Hoffmann HJ, Iversen M, Brandslund I, Sigsgaard T, Omland O, Oxvig C, Holmskov U, Bjermer L, Jensenius JC, Dahl R. Plasma C3d levels of young farmers correlate with respirable dust exposure levels during normal work in swine confinement buildings. Ann Agric Environ Med 2003; 10:53–60.
102. Von Essen S, Donham K. Illness and injury in animal confinement workers. Occup Med 1999; 14:337–350.
103. Boehlecke B, Hazucha M, Alexis NE, Jacobs R, Reist P, Bromberg PA, Peden DB. Low-dose airborne endotoxin exposure enhances bronchial responsiveness to inhaled allergen in atopic asthmatics. J Allergy Clin Immunol 2003; 112:1241–1243.
104. Reed CE, Milton DK. Endotoxin-stimulated innate immunity: a contributing factor for asthma. J Allergy Clin Immunol 2001; 108:157–166.
105. Park JH, Gold DR, Spiegelman DL, Burge HA, Milton DK. House dust endotoxin and wheeze in the first year of life. Am J Respir Crit Care Med 2001; 163:322–328.

106. Pirie RS, Dixon PM, McGorum BC. Endotoxin contamination contributes to the pulmonary inflammatory and functional response to *Aspergillus fumigatus* extract inhalation in heaves horses. Clin Exp Allergy 2003; 33:1289–1296.
107. Gordon T. Acute respiratory effects of endotoxin-contaminated machining fluid aerosols in guinea pigs. Fundam Appl Toxicol 1992; 19:117–123.
108. Pitt JI, Basilico JC, Abarca ML, Lopez C. Mycotoxins and toxigenic fungi. Med Mycol 2000; 38(suppl 1):41–46.
109. Sylla A, Diallo MS, Castegnaro J, Wild CP. Interactions between hepatitis B virus infection and exposure to aflatoxins in the development of hepatocellular carcinoma: a molecular epidemiological approach. Mutat Res 1999; 428: 187–196.
110. Iavicoli I, Brera C, Carelli G, Caputi R, Marinaccio A, Miraglia M. External and internal dose in subjects occupationally exposed to ochratoxin A. Int Arch Occup Environ Health 2002; 75:381–386.
111. Eadie MJ. Convulsive ergotism: epidemics of the serotonin syndrome?. Lancet Neurol 2003; 2:429–434.
112. Todd BE, Buchan RM. Total dust, respirable dust, and microflora toxin concentrations in Colorado corn storage facilities. Appl Occup Environ Hyg 2002; 17:411–415.
113. Van Vleet TR, Mace K, Coulombe RA Jr. Comparative aflatoxin B(1) activation and cytotoxicity in human bronchial cells expressing cytochromes P450 1A2 and 3A4. Cancer Res 2002; 62:105–112.
114. Skaug MA, Eduard W, Stormer FC. Ochratoxin A in airborne dust and fungal conidia. Mycopathologia 2001; 151:93–98.
115. Acute pulmonary hemorrhage/hemosiderosis among infants—Cleveland, January 1993–November 1994. MMWR Morb Mortal Wkly Rep 1994; 43:881–883.
116. From the Centers for Disease Control and Prevention. Acute pulmonary hemorrhage/hemosiderosis among infants—Cleveland, January 1993–November 1994. JAMA 1995; 273:281–282.
117. Montana E, Etzel RA, Allan T, Horgan TE, Dearborn DG. Environmental risk factors associated with pediatric idiopathic pulmonary hemorrhage and hemosiderosis in a Cleveland community. Pediatrics 1997; 99:E5.
118. Update: Pulmonary hemorrhage/hemosiderosis among infants—Cleveland, Ohio, 1993–1996. MMWR Morb Mortal Wkly Rep 2000; 49:180–184.
119. Jarvis BB. Chemistry and toxicology of molds isolated from water-damaged buildings. Adv Exp Med Biol 2002; 504:43–52.
120. Rao CY, Burge HA, Brain JD. The time course of responses to intratracheally instilled toxic *Stachybotrys chartarum* spores in rats. Mycopathologia 2000; 149:27–34.
121. Rao CY, Brain JD, Burge HA. Reduction of pulmonary toxicity of *Stachybotrys chartarum* spores by methanol extraction of mycotoxins. Appl Environ Microbiol 2000; 66:2817–2821.
122. Wilkins CK, Larsen ST, Hammer M, Poulsen OM, Wolkoff P, Nielsen GD. Respiratory effects in mice exposed to airborne emissions from *Stachybotrys chartarum* and implications for risk assessment. Pharmacol Toxicol 1998; 83:112–119.

123. Investigation of a ricin-containing envelope at a postal facility—South Carolina, 2003. MMWR Morb Mortal Wkly Rep 2003; 52:1129–1131.

124. Bradberry SM, Dickers KJ, Rice P, Griffiths GD, Vale JA. Ricin poisoning. Toxicol Rev 2003; 22:65–70.

125. Feldman KA, Enscore RE, Lathrop SL, Matyas BT, McGuill M, Schriefer ME, Stiles-Enos D, Dennis DT, Petersen LR, Hayes EB. An outbreak of primary pneumonic tularemia on Martha's Vineyard. N Engl J Med 2001; 345: 1601–1606.

126. Bunger J, Antlauf-Lammers M, Westphal G, Muller M, Hallier E. [Immunological reactions and health complaints in biological refuse personnel and composting by biological aerosol exposure]. Schriftenr Ver Wasser Boden Lufthyg 1999; 104:141–148.

127. Predicala BZ, Urban JE, Maghirang RG, Jerez SB, Goodband RD. Assessment of bioaerosols in swine barns by filtration and impaction. Curr Microbiol 2002; 44:136–140.

128. Purdy CW, Straus DC, Parker DB, Wilson SC, Clark RN. Comparison of the type and number of microorganisms and concentration of endotoxin in the air of feedyards in the Southern High Plains. Am J Vet Res 2004; 65:45–52.

129. Seifert SA, Von Essen S, Jacobitz K, Crouch R, Lintner CP. Organic dust toxic syndrome: a review. J Toxicol Clin Toxicol 2003; 41:185–193.

130. Selim MI, Juchems AM, Popendorf W. Assessing airborne aflatoxin B1 during on-farm grain handling activities. Am In: Hyg Assoc J 1998; 59: 252–256.

131. Ryckeboer J, Mergaert J, Coosemans J, Deprins K, Swings J. Microbiological aspects of biowaste during composting in a monitored compost bin. J Appl Microbiol 2003; 94:127–137.

132. Fischer G, Muller T, Schwalbe R, Ostrowski R, Dott W. Exposure to airborne fungi, MVOC and mycotoxins in biowaste-handling facilities. Int J Hyg Environ Health 2000; 203:97–104.

133. Brown CM, Nuorti PJ, Breiman RF, Hathcock AL, Fields BS, Lipman HB, Llewellyn GC, Hofmann J, Cetron M. A community outbreak of Legionnaires' disease linked to hospital cooling towers: an epidemiological method to calculate dose of exposure. Int J Epidemiol 1999; 28:353–359.

134. Sethi KK, Brandis H. Direct demonstration and isolation of *Legionella pneumophila* (serogroup 1) from bathroom water specimens in a hotel. Zentralbl Bakteriol Mikrobiol Hyg [B] 1983; 177:402–405.

135. Kusnetsov J, Torvinen E, Perola O, Nousiainen T, Katila ML. Colonization of hospital water systems by legionellae, mycobacteria and other heterotrophic bacteria potentially hazardous to risk group patients. APMIS 2003; 111:546–556.

136. Oie S, Masumoto N, Hironaga K, Koshiro A, Kamiya A. Microbial contamination of ambient air by ultrasonic humidifier and preventive measures. Microbios 1992; 72:161–166.

137. Yamamoto Y, Osanai S, Fujiuchi S, Yamazaki K, Nakano H, Ohsaki Y, Kikuchi K. Extrinsic allergic alveolitis induced by the yeast *Debaryomyces hansenii*. Eur Respir J 2002; 20:1351–1353.

138. Alvarez-Fernandez JA, Quirce S, Calleja JL, Cuevas M, Losada E. Hypersensitivity pneumonitis due to an ultrasonic humidifier. Allergy 1998; 53: 210–212.

139. Topp R, Wimmer K, Fahlbusch B, Bischof W, Richter K, Wichmann HE, Heinrich J. Repeated measurements of allergens and endotoxin in settled house dust over a time period of 6 years. Clin Exp Allergy 2003; 33: 1659–1666.

140. Park JW, Kim CW, Kang DB, Lee IY, Choi SY, Yong TS, Shin DC, Kim KE, Hong CS. Low-flow, long-term air sampling under normal domestic activity to measure house dust mite and cockroach allergens. J Investig Auergol Clin Immunol 2002; 12:293–298.

141. Sawyer MH, Chamberlin CJ, Wu YN, Aintablian N, Wallace MR. Detection of varicella-zoster virus DNA in air samples from hospital rooms. J Infect Dis 1994; 169:91–94.

142. Warris A, Klaassen CH, Meis JF, De Ruiter MT, De Valk HA, Abrahamsen TG, Gaustad P, Verweij PE. Molecular epidemiology of *Aspergillus fumigatus* isolates recovered from water, air, and patients shows two clusters of genetically distinct strains. J Clin Microbiol 2003; 41:4101–4106.

143. Schmechel D, Gorny RL, Simpson JP, Reponen T, Grinshpun SA, Lewis DM. Limitations of monoclonal antibodies for monitoring of fungal aerosols using *Penicillium brevicompactum* as a model fungus. J Immunol Methods 2003; 283:235–245.

144. Hodgson MJ, Morey P, Leung WY, Morrow L, Miller D, Jarvis BB, Robbins H, Halsey JF, Storey E. Building-associated pulmonary disease from exposure to *Stachybotrys chartarum* and *Aspergillus versicolor*. J Occup Environ Med 1998; 40:241–249.

145. Patovirta RL, Reiman M, Husman T, Haverinen U, Toivola M, Nevalainen A. Mould specific IgG antibodies connected with sinusitis in teachers of mould damaged school: a two-year follow-up study. Int J Occup Med Environ Health 2003; 16:221–230.

146. Van Emon JM, Reed AW, Yike I, Vesper SJ. ELISA measurement of stachylysin in serum to quantify human exposures to the indoor mold *Stachybotrys chartarum*. J Occup Environ Med 2003; 45:582–591.

147. Hybl JD, Lithgow GA, Buckley SG. Laser-induced breakdown spectroscopy detection and classification of biological aerosols. Appl Spectrosc 2003; 57:1207–1215.

148. Andre FE. Vaccinology: past achievements, present roadblocks and future promises. Vaccine 2003; 21:593–595.

149. Nardell EA. Environmental infection control of tuberculosis. Semin Respir Infect 2003; 18:307–319.

150. Hall KK, Giannetta ET, Getchell-White SI, Durbin LJ, Fair BM. Ultraviolet light disinfection of hospital water for preventing nosocomial *Legionella* infection: a 13-year follow-up. Infect Control Hosp Epidemiol 2003; 24:580–583.

151. Sehulster L, Chirm RY. Guidelines for environmental infection control in health care facilities. Recommendations of CDC and the Healthcare Infection Control Practices Advisory Committee (HICPAC). MMWR Recomm Rep 2003; 52:1–42.

152. Anaissie EJ, Stratton SL, Dignani MC, Lee CK, Mahfouz TH, Rex JH, Summerbell RC, Walsh TJ. Cleaning patient shower facilities: a novel approach to reducing patient exposure to aerosolized *Aspergillus* species and other opportunistic molds. Clin Infect Dis 2002; 35:E86–E88.

153. Jarvis JQ, Morey PR. Allergic respiratory disease and fungal remediation in a building in a subtropical climate. Appl Occup Environ Hyg 2001; 16:380–388.

154. Foarde KK, Menetrez MY. Evaluating the potential efficacy of three antifungal sealants of duct liner and galvanized steel as used in HVAC systems. J Ind Microbiol Biotechnol 2002; 29:38–43.

155. Halken S, Host A, Niklassen U, Hansen LG, Nielsen F, Pedersen S, Osterballe O, Veggerby C, Poulsen LK. Effect of mattress and pillow encasings on children with asthma and house dust mite allergy. J Allergy Clin Immunol 2003; 111:169–176.

156. Arbes SJ Jr, Sever M, Mehta J, Gore JC, Schal C, Vaughn B, Mitchell H, Zeldin DC. Abatement of cockroach allergens (*Bla g* 1 and *Bla g* 2) in low-income, urban housing: month 12 continuation results. J Allergy Clin Immunol 2004; 113:109–114.

157. Bjornsdottir US, Jakobinudottir S, Runarsdottir V, Juliusson S. The effect of reducing levels of cat allergen (*Fel d* 1) on clinical symptoms in patients with cat allergy. Ann Allergy Asthma Immunol 2003; 91:189–194.

158. Gore RB, Durrell B, Bishop S, Curbishley L, Woodcock A, Custovic A. High-efficiency particulate arrest-filter vacuum cleaners increase personal cat allergen exposure in homes with cats. J Allergy Clin Immunol 2003; 111: 784–787.

159. Gore RB, Bishop S, Durrell B, Curbishley L, Woodcock A, Custovic A. Air filtration units in homes with cats: can they reduce personal exposure to cat allergen? Clin Exp Allergy 2003; 33:765–769.

11

Combustion Emissions: Contribution to Air Pollution, Human Exposure and Risk to Cancer, and Related Effects

JOELLEN LEWTAS

University of Washington, Seattle, Washington, U.S.A.

I. Introduction

Combustion products of coal tars and soot from chimneys were the first recognized chemical carcinogens in the early 1900s (1,2). Fractionation and animal bioassay of these combustion products resulted in the identification of fluorescent polycyclic aromatic hydrocarbons (PAH) as chemical carcinogens (1–4). The earliest experimental evidence that air pollution was carcinogenic in rodents was reported by Leiter et al. in the 1940s (5,6). These and more recent studies in the 1950s and 1960s (7,8) reported tumors were induced in animals treated with the organic matter extracted from urban air particles. The development of in vitro mutagenesis assays (9) advanced bioassay-directed fractionation and chemical identification studies of potential carcinogens in airborne particulate organic matter and combustion particles (10,11). In addition to confirming the importance of PAH, more polar nitro-polycyclic aromatic hydrocarbons (NO2-PAH) were discovered in diesel emissions and urban air. Initially identified as mutagens, these compounds were also carcinogenic in animals (12).

The role of air pollution in human lung cancer was reviewed by Samet and Cohen (13) in the first edition of this volume and several other major reviews were published in the 1990s (14,15). This chapter provides an overview of chemical, mechanistic, animal, and human evidence for a link between particulate air pollution from combustion sources, lung cancer, and other genotoxic and reproductive effects. There are several non-combustion related respiratory carcinogens found in air and linked to lung cancer through occupational studies that were reviewed earlier (13), including radon and asbestos. These and gaseous pollutants, such as those emitted from home furnishings, (e.g., formaldehyde) are not specifically considered in this review. Several comprehensive reviews of individual chemical air pollutants, their sources, and experimental evidence for carcinogenic activity are available (16–18).

II. Combustion Emissions: Source Characterization, Ambient Source Apportionment, and Exposure
A. Chemical and Toxicological Characterization of Combustion Particle Emissions

The complex incomplete combustion mixture emitted from combustion and related sources include particles, semi-volatile matter, and gases. The respirable particles less than 2.5 μm ($PM_{2.5}$), referred to as fine or respirable particles, are often referred to in older literature as soot particles if they have a high content of black elemental carbon. The polycyclic organic matter includes thousands of chemicals ranging from alkanes and aromatic compounds to polar substituted aromatics and carboxylic acids. Hundreds of individual organic compounds have been identified in the organic atmospheric aerosol (19); however, together these compounds constitute less than 10% of the organic carbon (OC) of urban and rural aerosol (20,21). The unresolved organic mass includes polar compounds (e.g., tetrols oxidation products of isoprene) difficult to identify by gas chromatography without derivitization (22), large insoluble polymeric molecules possibly of biogenic origin (23–26), humic acids (27,28) and humic-like substances (e.g., polycarboxylic acids). A number of substances of natural origin such as wood dust (29), some naturally occurring plant products, and substances (30,31) produced by molds such as mycotoxins (e.g., aflotoxin) have been shown to be carcinogenic to human; however, there is little evidence suggesting the biogenic mass in fine particles has been evaluated for mutagenic or carcinogenic activity.

The cancer risk from the particles is thought to arise primarily from the polycyclic organic aromatic compounds including PAH (4) and many diverse classes of hydrocarbons (e.g.,), substituted aromatic hydrocarbons such as nitroarenes (12), lactones, and other substituted aromatic hydrocarbons, and heterocyclic aromatic compounds (e.g., aza-arenes). The primary source of polycyclic aromatic compounds in air pollution is from combustion of fossil fuels (e.g., coal, oil, gasoline, and diesel fuel), vegetative matter (e.g., wood, tobacco, paper products, and biomass), and synthetic chemicals (e.g., from plastics and other chemical products in incinerated municipal, hospital, and hazardous wastes).

The organic extractable mass from carbonaceous soot particles emitted from several well-studied combustion sources (coal, diesel, and tobacco) induces tumors in animals, mutations in cells, and have been clearly implicated in epidemiological studies as human carcinogens (32–34). Incomplete combustion products, however, also contain gaseous chemicals that are carcinogenic, such as benzene, aldehydes, and alkenes (e.g., 1, 3-butadiene) and semi-volatile organic compounds that partition between the gas and particle phase (e.g., pyrene).

1. Coal-Related Sources

Coal tars and soots produced from coal through heating, combustion and related processes (e.g. pyrolysis and reductive distillation) emit organic pollutants in both the gaseous phase and in fine particles. Coal has been used for both residential heating and in industrial processes (e.g., steel mills, aluminum smelters, power plants) resulting in air pollution emissions containing organic pollutants. Coal tars and soot from chimneys were recognized in the early 1900s as causing scrotal and other skin cancers in chimney sweeps. In the 1980s, occupational exposures to emissions from coke production, coal gasification, aluminum production, and iron and steel founding were found by international panels of experts at the World Health Organization's International Agency for Research on Cancer to cause respiratory cancers in humans (32,33).

Historically, short-term episodes of high air pollution resulting from coal combustion have been associated with respiratory symptoms and mortality (34). The most famous of these episodes occurred in London in 1952 (37) but other episodes in areas predominantly impacted by coal combustion have occurred in the Meuse Valley in 1930, Belgium (38,39), in Donora, PA (40). In the 1990s, extensive studies were conducted in Northern Bohemia (Teplice, Czech Republic) on the health impact of air pollution from coal combustion including both coal-fired power plants and extensive use of residential burning of coal. These studies have documented a wide range of health effects (41) including respiratory effects in children (42), genetic damage (43,44), male and female reproductive effects (45,46), cardiopulmonary and cancer mortality (32,47). Lung cancer was found to be highly elevated in women exposed to indoor air pollution from cooking and heating with coal burned without venting to the outdoors in Xuan Wei, China (48).

Coal combustion emissions including coal tars and soots are the best documented complex chemical carcinogens (32,33). In the 1930s, coal soot (black particles) and the tars extracted from them were fractionated and applied to animal skin to identify the carcinogenic fractions that were ultimately identified as carcinogenic PAH (1). Although these mixtures are very complex, PAH are still considered to be the primary human cancer causative agents associated with coal combustion. These early studies have been reviewed by Kipling (2) and others (32,47). More recent comparative fractionation and in vitro bioassay have confirmed that the aromatic neutral fractions containing PAH and related compounds are responsible for a predominant fraction of the mutagenic and tumorigenic activity of coal tar and coal combustion emissions. In some reductive distillations of coal, such as the coking process found in coke ovens, in addition to PAH, aromatic amines and heterocyclic aromatic compounds (e.g., aza-arenes) are also formed (33). Coke oven emissions therefore have a significant basic fraction containing these aromatic nitrogen containing compounds (48) that include mutagenic and carcinogenic chemicals (49–51).

Source apportionment studies of ambient fine particles in northeastern United States (Vermont) identified coal-fired power plants located in the mid-west as a major source of fine particles in the northeast (52,53). Comparative source receptor analysis using the chemical composition of fine particles from three northeastern US locations (Washington, DC, Brigantine, NJ, and Underhill, VT) also found coal combustion was a major source of fine particles at all these sites; however, there were two separate coal source profiles characterized (54). The largest source contributing to the $PM_{2.5}$ mass was coal combustion with enhanced secondary sulfate. A second coal combustion source dominant in the winter exhibited a receptor modeling profile with significant organic and elemental carbon (54).

Although coal tars and emissions from residential coal burning and poorly combusted coal emissions are clearly carcinogenic to humans (32), the impact of modern coal-fired power plants on cancer risk of ambient fine particles is not clear. Studies in the 1980s of fly ash particles emitted from utility power plants (55,56) found the mutagenic activity of the extractable organic matter to be comparable in magnitude to other combustion sources (57). In a comparative assessment of the impact of coal powered utility plants on the potential cancer risk of various energy sources, these large plants had the lowest emission rates of particulate organic mass and mutagenicity per joule of energy (58); however, coal-fired power plants are the major energy source for many regions. Additional research is needed to investigate the impact of volatile and semi-volatile organic emissions from coal combustion sources and their atmospheric reaction products.

2. Petroleum Combustion Sources: Diesel, Fuel Oil, Gasoline, and Related Sources

Petroleum products include crude oil, residual oil, heating oil, diesel fuel, gasoline, jet fuel, kerosene, propane and liquefied gases. The consumption of petroleum products in the United States has increased 300% since 1950 with the average person consuming 3 gallons per day to meet their energy needs (59) including transportation and heating and other petroleum requiring products (e.g., such as plastics).

a. Fuel Oil Emissions

The heavier petroleum products, such residual fuel oils (no. 4–6 fuel oils), are carcinogenic on mouse skin and mutagenic both in vitro and in vivo (60). This category of residual (heavy) fuel oils has been classified by IARC as possibly carcinogenic to humans (Group 2B) (61). These fuel oils contain carcinogenic PAH in addition to relatively high sulfur, ash, carbon residue, and asphaltenes (aromatic and naphthenic ring compounds containing nitrogen, sulfur, and oxygen) (62). Combustion of residual oil in industrial or commercial boilers results in the emission of residual oil fly ash (ROFA). ROFA contains a relatively high content of toxic trace metals (e.g., soluble nickel and vanadium sulfate salts) and compared to coal fly ash was more highly toxic to pulmonary alveolar macrophages, in part due to the soluble toxic metals (63). Geneally, higher particle emissions are found with heavier petroleum products. Therefore, the emission rates would be expected to be greatest with residual oil (no. 6 fuel oil) > home heating oil (no. 2) that is often equivalent to the fuel used in diesel vehicles > kerosene > the "cleaner" and lighter petroleum products such as propane and liquefied gas fuels.

Toxicity and mutagenicity of combustion particles (fly ash) emitted from coal and petroleum combustion were first reported in the 1980s (64,65). Studies of inflammation and acute lung injury in rats when ROFA was administered by intratracheal instillation (66) stimulated an increased interest in ROFA as a model particle for ambient fine particles. The biological effects and potential mechanisms of ROFA toxicity associated with transition metals have been reviewed by Ghio et al. (67). Unfortunately, very little research has been reported on the mutagenicity or cancer risk of ROFA. Recently, however, an occupational repeated measure study of boilermakers exposed metal fumes and ROFA during repair of the boiler found evidence of exposure to PAH and metals in the urine and associations between these exposures and oxidative DNA injury (as measured by 8-hydroxy-2'-deoxyguanosine, 8-OH-dG, in urine) (68). This suggests that ROFA may induce both cancer and non-cancer health effects.

b. Diesel and Gasoline Emissions

One of the major sources of air pollution in urban areas is the combustion of diesel and gasoline fuels in cars, buses, trucks, and other on-road transportation sources (68). Additional particles and gases are emitted from numerous off-road sources (such as lawn mowers, tractors, snow mobiles, construction equipment, and marine vessels). Although emissions have been reduced through improved control technology, the number of vehicles and other sources utilizing diesel and gasoline fuels has continued to increase as indicated by EPA trend reports of vehicle miles traveled (69). Diesel vehicles emit as much as 100 times the elemental carbon (EC) and 20 times the OC per mile as compared with the newer low emitting gasoline vehicles (70). Recent source apportionment studies of fine particle mass (PM$_{2.5}$) across the United States and in many other urban locations, where motor vehicles are the primary mode of transportation, reported diesel and gasoline vehicles to be one of the major sources of particulate matter (71–73). These studies have primarily relied on EC as a source tracer for diesel. Vehicles are also the dominant source of ultrafine particles near streets and roadways (74). Diesel sources emit relatively high concentrations of both OC and EC whereas gasoline sources emit less EC and the OC temperature fractions for diesel vary from diesel sources (71–73,75).

The US EPA initiated diesel emission research in 1977 to evaluate the human health implications of a proposed increase in the diesel engines (76). In the wake of the energy crisis in the early 1970s, the US Congress enacted fuel economy standards in 1975 (77). It was estimated that by 1985 up to 10% of the new US passenger cars would be diesel powered due to their fuel efficiency. The first diesel characterization research led to the discovery that diesel particles contained relatively large quantities of mutagenic organic compounds (78). The diesel emission research program resulted in publications on the potential cancer risk of diesel particles based on comparative tumor-initiating activity on mouse skin (79–86) as well as inhalation toxicology studies (88,89). Diesel and gasoline particle extracts were compared to a series of organic extracts from coal tar, a coke oven, and cigarette smoke emissions with respect to their chemical composition (48,80), mutagenicity (49,86), and animal tumor potency (84,85) to assess the relative potential cancer risk (89,90). Mouse skin tumor potency comparisons for emission components are listed in Table 1. Bioassay-directed fractionation and chemical characterization studies were used to identify mutagenic PAH and nitro-PAH in the extractable organic matter from diesel particles (10,11,78,91). Animal tumor assays (7,92) have also been used to investigate the contribution of PAH and nitro-PAH to the carcinogenicity of diesel exhaust.

Cancer studies of diluted diesel exhaust, filtered exhaust, particles, and particle extracts have been documented in over 25 publications and reviewed in the latest EPA Health Assessment Document for Diesel Exhaust (70). Earlier reviews and assessment of the cancer risk of diesel exhaust were conducted by the International Agency for Research on Cancer (12), the International Program on Chemical Safety (93), and the California EPA (94). The animal cancer studies include inhalation, lung implantation, and skin application studies. Although Kotin et al. (7) reported in 1955 that diesel particle extracts induced tumors, this finding

Table 1 Comparative Tumor Initiation Potency of Particulate Organic Matter from Combustion Emissions and Ambient Air in the Sencar Mouse Skin Tumor Initiation Assay

Emission mixture/chemical	Pappilomas/mouse/mg
Smokey coal	2.10
Coke oven mains	2.10
Aluminum smelter	1.30
Roofing coal tar	0.61
Diesel car A	0.61
Ambient air (boise dominated by vehicles)	0.21
Gasoline (non-catalyst) vehicle	0.18
Diesel car B	0.16
Ambient air (boise dominated by wood smoke)	0.095
Gasoline catalyst vehicle	0.071
Diesel car C	0.046
Woodstove burning softwood	0.046
Residential oil (no. 2 fuel oil) heater	0.028
Woodstove burning hardwood	0.0087
Cigarette smoke condensate	0.0029

was not confirmed until the early 1980s (82–84). In the 1990s a relatively large number of animal inhalation studies were conducted in the United States, Japan, and Europe and are well summarized in a series of health assessment documents (12,70,93).

Cancer epidemiology studies of occupational exposures to diesel exhaust provide the largest body of evidence for the carcinogenicity in humans with the most recent assessment evaluating 22 key lung cancer studies in more detail (70). In addition to lung cancer, cancers of the bladder, and lymphatic tissue are the other most common cancers associated within populations with higher exposures to diesel exhaust than is found in the general environment. The occupational exposures in these studies include diesel exhaust from buses, taxis, trucks, trains, ships, and other diesel engines used for transportation. Exposures to diesel exhaust in mines have also been examined; however, they are often confounded by other exposures (e.g., coal dust and radon). The EPA assessment (76) found a persistent association of risk for lung cancer and diesel exhaust exposure in over 30 epidemiologic studies.

Meta-analyses of studies reporting the relationship between diesel exhaust exposure and lung cancer risk have been conducted by two groups. The first study by Bhatia et al. (95) analyzed 23 studies that met their criteria for inclusion in the analysis and found the pooled relative risk weighted by study precision was 1.33 (95% CI $= 1.24, 1.44$) indicating an increased relative risk for lung cancer from occupational exposure to diesel exhaust. Lipsett and Campleman (96) analyzed 30 studies that met their criteria. The pooled smoking-adjusted relative risk was 1.47 (95% CI = 1.29, 1.67). Both meta-analyses of lung cancer concluded that the data support a causal association between lung cancer and diesel exhaust exposure.

A special report of the Health Effects Institute (97) convened a diesel epidemiology expert panel to assess the relationship between diesel emissions and lung cancer. They reviewed 35 epidemiologic studies, including 19 case–control studies and 16 cohort studies of occupational exposure to diesel exhaust. This panel concluded that occupational exposure to diesel exhaust from diverse sources increases the rate of lung cancer by 20–40% in exposed workers, and with prolonged exposure, the lung cancer rate was greater. The results of these studies taken together were concluded to not be explicable by confounding due to cigarette smoking or other known sources of bias.

Since 1988, the human carcinogenic potential of diesel exhaust has been evaluated by six organizations including two international organizations affiliated with WHO including IARC (12) and BPCS (93), US agencies (NIOSH) (98), NTP (99), and EPA (70) as well as a state environmental agency, California EPA (94). Their evaluations are summarized in Table 2. As more research is reported, the strength and magnitude of evidence suggests that diesel exhaust is a carcinogenic risk to humans. The most recent assessment by US EPA (70) concludes diesel exhaust is "likely to be carcinogenic to humans by inhalation" and based on the evidence for a mutagenic mode of action "a cancer hazard is presumed at environmental exposure levels." The highest range of estimated environmental exposures to diesel particles is close to or overlapping with the lower range of occupational exposure for which lung cancer increases have been reported. However, the diesel exhaust exposure–response data were considered to be too uncertain in 2002 to derive a quantitative cancer unit risk with confidence (70).

In spite of the progress in understanding the potential hazards of diesel and gasoline exhaust, many questions still remain. Among those questions are the relationship between the source characteristics (engines, operating conditions, etc.), chemical characteristics of the toxic components, and mechanisms of toxicity. Recent publications (100–102) highlight the lack of a systematic approach to understanding the relationship between the source and toxic emission components as well as between cancer and non-cancer health effects. Comparison of two diesel particle samples used in many studies can result in very different chemical and toxicological profiles. One of these samples, a diesel forklift sample available as a standard reference material (SRM 2975) (103,104), has been studied with respect to genotoxicity and chemical composition such as PAH and nitro-PAH content. The other sample, automobile-derived diesel exhaust particle (A-DEP) from Japan (105,106), has been examined for effects on pulmonary

Table 2 Diesel Exhaust Assessments as a Human Carcinogen

Organization and year	Reference	Animal data	Human data	Overall evaluation
NIOSH, 1988	98	Confirmatory	Limited	Potential occupational carcinogen
IARC, 1989	12	Sufficient	Limited	Probably carcinogenic to humans
IPCS, 1996	93	Not evaluated	Not evaluated	Probably carcinogenic to humans
California EPA, 1998	94	"Demonstrated Carcinogenicity"	"Consistent evidence for a causal association"	Diesel particulate matter (DPM) classified as a "toxic air contaminant"
NTP, 2000	99	"Supporting animal and mechanistic data"	"Elevated lung cancer in occupationally exposed groups"	DPM-reasonable anticipated to be a carcinogen
US EPA, 2002	70	Adequate evidence for carcinogenicity	"Probable" human carcinogen"	Probably human carcinogen (Group B1) "Likely to be carcinogenic to humans by inhalation" and this evaluation applies to environmental exposures

inflammation and exacerbation of allergic asthma-like responses. The studies by DeMarini et al. (101) and Singh et al. (102) investigate both genotoxicity and pulmonary toxicity in both samples.

Gasoline vehicles, due to their relatively low particle emission rates compared to diesel, have received much less attention. Recent comparative studies by Mauderly and colleagues (107–109) highlight the variation in emissions and toxicity and mutagenicity of high emitting "white smoker" vehicles. The gaseous organic species from gasoline and diesel as well as the particle and semi-volatile toxic components need additional ongoing research to understand their impact on human health as engines and fuels continue to change. The US EPA assessment of motor vehicle-related air toxics (109) clearly implicates both the gaseous and particulate emissions as contributing to the air toxic risk.

Carcinogenic PAH emissions differ between gasoline and diesel emissions. Gasoline vehicles without catalytic converters have the highest PAH emission rate (6.6 μg/km) compared to gasoline vehicles with catalytic converters (0.3 μg/km) while diesel vehicles emitted less than 0.3 μg/km of PAH (110). The nitration of PAH in diesel emissions is thought to reduce the carcinogenic PAH through the formation of nitro-PAH (111,112) that have also been shown to be carcinogenic (12).

3. Vegetative and Biomass Combustion and Cooking Emissions

The combustion or burning of vegetative matter or other biomass, such as wood, paper and trash, forest fires, and agricultural burning all result in particle and gaseous emissions that are characterized by a high organic carbon composition compared to other sources (113–116). These sources all emit volatile, semi-volatile, and particulate organic matter. The particles emitted from vegetative burning have less elemental or black carbon emissions than diesel soot and higher extractable organic mass. Vegetative burning emissions contain levoglucosan and pimaric acid, that have been used as organic tracers (117,118) and cooking emissions are distinguished by the high fatty acid emissions (119).

a. Wood Smoke, Forest Fires, and Agricultural Burning

A major component of the emissions from wood and forest fires are derived from the combustion and pyrolysis of lignin and polysaccharides (e.g., cellulose) (117). The pyrolysis of wood lignins generates oxygenated organic compounds, including the semivolatile and reactive methoxyphenols (115–119) that can constitute up to 30% of the carbonaceous particle mass. The stability of the cellulose combustion product, levoglucosan, and evidence that it may be solely attributable to wood combustion has led to the recent development of microanalytical methods for measuring levoglucosan in personal exposure and source apportionment studies (120).

Ambient source apportionment studies using solvent-extractable organic compounds (referred to as molecular source markers) in chemical mass balance models in a winter study in California (121) and a study in eight locations in the southeastern US (122), all of the levoglucosan and pimaric acid were attributed to wood combustion. The pimaric acid is not a combustion product but a naturally occurring diterpenoid carboxylic acid referred to as a resin acid found in high concentrations in softwoods.

For many years, soil corrected potassium was used as a tracer for woodsmoke and was validated using carbon dating methods (123,124). In a recent $PM_{2.5}$ source apportionment study in Seattle, WA $PM_{2.5}$ arsenic (As) was highly correlated with the wood smoke component of ambient fine particles (71). It appears that even occasional use of some chromated copper arsenate treated wood burned in fireplaces, woodstoves, or trash is sufficient for arsenic to serve as a source tracer for wood smoke in source apportionment studies. Wood treated with metal containing preservatives results in the emission of arsenic during burning (125).

Vegetative combustion products also emit mutagenic and carcinogenic PAH (126,127) as do nearly all sources of incomplete combustion. Residential combustion of wood has been estimated to be the largest source of PAH in Sweden and the United States based on estimated emissions countrywide (110). In urban areas, however, mobile sources are generally the major source of exposure to PAH (110). The mutagenicity of wood stove emissions and relationship to PAH have been evaluated in emissions (128) and wood smoke impacted air (129,130). In addition, several studies of the influence of atmospheric transformation on the chemistry and mutagenicity of wood smoke provide evidence that the mutagenic products are further chemically modified in the air (131,132).

Forest fires (133,134) and prescribed forest burning (135,136) also result in many of the same emissions as residential wood fireplaces and stoves with differences dependent on the fuel (type and condition of the biomass) and burning conditions (e.g., oxygen availability to the combustion), dryness of the trees, and other atmospheric and environmental conditions. Agricultural burning including grasslands, crops (e.g., wheat stubble), rangelands is used in certain regions to dispose of crop debris and control weeds, and disease. The emissions from these agricultural burns can result in tons of increased air pollutants that may impact nearby communities. Biomass burning emits significant quantities of carbon monoxide (CO), carbon dioxide (CO_2), fine particulate matter ($PM_{2.5}$), and volatile hydrocarbons as well as nitrogen and sulfur oxides, and potentially toxic and carcinogenic organic emissions (136,137). Emission factors for PAH species have a wide range depending on the burning conditions; however, several studies have reported the highest emissions at greater than 2000 mg benz[a]anthracene per kg fuel (137–140). Air pollutant emissions associated with forest, grassland, and agricultural burning in Texas (141) and from fires in savanna ecosystems of Africa (142) have also been reported. Wheat stubble and grass burning have been used by farmers in the NW US including Washington, Oregon, and Idaho. A source apportionment study conducted over several years in Spokane, WA, was able to identify and apportion the agricultural burning using inorganic source tracers and wind directional analysis (143).

b. Cooking Emissions

Restaurants, home barbecues, kitchens, and other sources of meat cooking, charbroiling, and other forms of cooking food also emit fine particles and organic carbon species that make significant contributions to both indoor and outdoor air pollution (144–157). These emissions also have relatively high emission rates of organic mass. Saturated and unsaturated fatty acids (alkanoic and alkenoic acids) are the major organic compounds emitted during cooking. Rogge et al. (146–149) have reported emission rates for about 150 organic compounds emitted during residential cooking including *n*-alkanes, *n*-alkanoic acids, *n*-alkenoic acids, *n*-alkanols, *n*-alkanals, *n*-alkan-2-ones, dicarboxylic acids, furans, furanones, amides, steroids, PAH, and heterocyclic aromatic amines (HAA). Electric and natural gas powered ranges and ovens were compared and foods were cooked using pan-frying, stir-frying, sautéing, deep-frying, boiling, and oven cooking methods including baking, roasting, and broiling. In these studies, oven broiling with natural gas had emissions 10-fold higher than oven broiling with electricity. In general, pan-frying and oven broiling with natural gas stoves generally gave the highest overall emissions. Related studies have also examined highly polar compounds in meat smoke (150), charbroiling (151,152), and cooking oil fumes (153).

The residential cooking emissions have the largest impact on the quality of indoor air in the home (154,155). Characterization of the mutagenicity and mutagens present in fumes from cooking meats (156) and cooking oils (157) has also been investigated. The highest PAH emissions were reported for oven broiling steaks and the highest heterocyclic amine emissions were found during pan-frying bacon (149). Mutagenic and carcinogenic PAH and heterocyclic amines (e.g., methyl-IQ, IQ, PhiP) are the most likely cooking emissions to have an impact on cancer risk, although these constituents are also present in the foods. No studies have examined the human cancer risk to the combined exposures by inhalation during cooking and subsequent ingestion of PAH and heterocyclic amines from cooked foods.

Several outdoor air pollution source apportionment studies using organic compounds as molecular source tracers have quantified the contribution of cooking from restaurants or meat cooking to the $PM_{2.5}$ mass in a series of cities in the SE US and California (72,121,122). Zheng et al. (122) reported that meat cooking contributed from 5% to 12% of the $PM_{2.5}$ mass. In this study, the particle-phase nonanal was all attributed to the meat cooking, whereas only 65% of the 9-hexadecanoic acid was from cooking and the remainder was attributed to wood burning and road dust.

c. Tobacco Smoke

Tobacco smoking had been reported to be a lung cancer risk for many years prior to the 1986 evaluation by the International Agency for Research on Cancer (IARC) (158). In this IARC monograph (51), the chemistry, exposure, toxicology, and epidemiology are reviewed in detail and evaluated by an international panel of experts. This report concludes that tobacco smoke is carcinogenic to humans (Group 1). The health effects of environmental tobacco smoke or passive smoking were not evaluated until the US EPA's report in 1993 (159) and were then followed by the California EPA's report on the health effects of exposure to environmental tobacco smoke (ETS) (160). Recently, the California EPA has released a report proposing that ETS be classified for regulation as a toxic air contaminant (161) for regulation under the California environmental regulations. These reports and other reviews of air pollution and cancer (13–15) provide a comprehensive review of the chemistry, exposure, toxicology, and human health effects of tobacco smoking and exposures to environmental tobacco smoke. A review by Hecht (162) focuses on the chemical carcinogens in tobacco smoke and provides a clear mechanistic framework linking nicotine addiction with lung cancer through exposure to specific carcinogens.

Tobacco smoke is a vegetative burning source; however, the emissions are characterized with a much higher proportion of nitrogen containing nitrosamines (163) and other nitrogen containing organics found in the mutagenic basic fraction of cigarette smoke condensate (49) than is found in wood smoke or other biomass combustion products, except for charbroiling of meats. Over 50 carcinogens evaluated by IARC are present in tobacco smoke including PAH and the nitrogen containing aza-arenes, *N*-nitrosamines, aromatic amines, and heterocyclic aromatic amines (162). Hecht (162) reviews the evidence that among these carcinogens, the PAH, and the tobacco-specific nitrosamine, NNK (4-(methylnitrosamino)-1-(3-pyridyl)-1-butanone) are the most likely to play major role in human cancer. Among the many organic nitrogen containing compounds in tobacco smoke, nicotine is a sensitive tracer of human exposure to tobacco smoke exposure (164). Nicotine's metabolite, cotinine, is one of the best validated biomarkers of exposure to a specific combustion product (165). The wide use of this biomarker of exposure to tobacco in large population-based studies (166) has improved the quantification of human exposure to tobacco smoke in a wide range of classical and molecular epidemiology studies.

d. Cancer Risk of Vegetative Combustion Emissions

The best documented vegetative combustion source is tobacco smoke as discussed above. Quantitative assessments of the cancer potency (risk per unit of particle or organic carbon exposure) suggest that tobacco and other vegetative combustion emissions are less carcinogenic per unit of exposure in both animal and human studies as compared to fossil fuel emissions (e.g., coal or petroleum combustion emissions). Lung cancer mortality was significantly greater for women exposed indoors to smoky coal (low sulfur bituminous coal) as compared to smokeless coal (high sulfur coal) or wood combustion in different communes in Xuan Wei, China County (46). The smoky coal organic emissions were also higher in PAH content, mutagenic activity, mouse skin tumor initiation potency (167,168).

Comparative tumor studies conducted in both the United States and Germany of vegetative emissions (e.g., cigarette smoke and wood smoke) found vegetative emissions have both a lower content of PAH and a lower potency in a series of different animal tumor assays when compared to fossil fuel emissions. Studies by Grimmer et al. (169) using two animal tumor assays (rat lung implantation and mouse skin) showed that cigarette smoke condensate had a lower tumor response than fossil fuel combustion emissions (residential coal furnace emissions, diesel, and gasoline exhaust) and the tumor responses were related to the PAH content of the emissions. Studies conducted in the United States to compare the tumor initiation potency in the Sencar mouse skin assay to human lung cancer risk estimates from epidemiological data also found that fossil fuel emissions were more tumorigenic than cigarette smoke condensate or woodstove emissions (170). Ambient particles ($PM_{2.5}$) collected in Boise, ID during the winter heating season of 1986–1987 (a period of high use of woodstoves) were combined after chemical analysis and source apportionment to form two composite samples. The sample with the highest wood smoke content (78% wood smoke and 11% vehicle exhaust) was less tumorigenic ($\sim$50%) as compared to the composite with 55% wood smoke and 33% vehicle exhaust (171,172).

A new series of studies to compare the toxicology and carcinogenic potential for a series of combustion emissions from vegetative sources (wood smoke, tobacco smoke, cooking fumes) and fossil fuel emission sources (diesel, gasoline, and coal), and road dust are being conducted at the National Environmental Respiratory Center (173). The initial studies of wood combustion report on the exposure characterization and subchronic effects of exposures to wood smoke in rats (174,175).

4. Incineration, Waste Burning, and Combustion of Plastic, Chemical, Medical, and Other Waste

Plastics, chemicals, and other household, industrial, and medical wastes when combusted for disposal can lead to the formation of mutagenic and potentially hazardous air pollutants. Depending on the location and regulation of the waste material, the combustion can range from uncontrolled open burning to incineration in large-scale incinerators to smaller incinerators (e.g., rotary kiln incinerators), industrial furnaces, and boilers. The US EPA regulates hazardous chemical incineration through destruction and removal efficiency measures of the principal organic hazardous constituents; however, many plastic and chemical wastes may not considered hazardous and even those wastes that are regulated for removal efficiency are not controlled for the formation of new toxic compounds resulting from transient periods of incomplete combustion.

A series of chemical and biological characterization studies of emissions from chemical and plastic wastes incinerated in a rotary kiln were conducted to determine how the chemical nature of the waste and operating conditions impact the emitted mass, chemical composition, and mutagenic activity (176). The mutagenic emission factors (revertants/kilogram of fuel or /mega joule of heat) for the polyethylene and toluene were similar to those for municipal waste combustors. Bioassay-directed chemical analysis led to the identification of mutagenic PAH emitted from the polyethylene incineration emissions. PAH emissions also resulted from a batch-type contralled-air incinerator where the highest PAH emissions were from high-density polyethylene (HDPE) and less from polypropylene andpolyvinyl chloride (PVC), and plastic wastes (177).

Open burning of plastics (178–186), tires (181,182), and other chemical waste and mixed waste (183–185) were also evaluated. Emissions were analyzed for combustion gases; volatile, semi-volatile, and particulate organics; and toxic and mutagenic properties. Alkanes, alkenes, aromatic, and PAH were identified in the volatile, semi-volatile, and particulate fractions of these emissions. Organic extracts of the particle samples were mutagenic and similar to residential wood heating emissions. Mixed chemical wastes were combusted in furnaces and boilers to evaluate the use of such combustion systems for the disposal of the nitrogen-containing pesticide, dinoseb (2-sec-butyl-4, 6 dinitrophenol), in a fuel-oil/xylene solvent (179,183).

5. Atmospheric Transformation Products

Atmospheric transformation reactions may result in the formation or destruction of mutagenic chemicals in the air. Normal atmospheric processes increased the direct-acting mutagenicity wood smoke and automobile emissions in a smog chamber (129,186). The gas-phase mutagenic transformation products did not require an exogenous activation system suggesting they were either nitrated organic compounds (e.g., peroxyacetyl nitrate) which may be activated by enzymes present in the bacteria or are reactive species which do not require any activation, In winter field studies in Boise, ID, mutagenic nitro-aromatic and hydroxy-nitro-aromatic species, previously shown to occur primarily from atmospheric transformation reactions, were found in ambient air in the (130).

Nitro-PAH lactones have been found in smog chambers as irradiation products of phenanthrene under conditions similar to those found in ambient air in southern California (187). These nitro lactones account for a major fraction of the mutagenic activity of the reaction products that are in the particle phase. Vapor-phase PAH were converted to nitro-PAH, accounting for major fraction of the mutagenic activity of the reaction products that are in the vapor phase (188). Chemical analyses of the smog chamber products showed that most of the mutagenicity was due to products derived from acenaphthalene, retene, and pyrene; somewhat less important precursors are 2-methylphenanthrene and benz[a]anthracene (189). The most mutagenic fractions of the irradiation products of the eight remaining PAH were those containing simple nitro-derivatives. By considering both the extent to which particular PAH reacted to yield mutagenic products in the smog chamber, and the ambient concentrations of these PAH, the most important contributors to ambient mutagenicity are naphthalene, 1-and 2-methylnaphthalene, fluorene, dibenzothiophene, phenanthrene, fluoranthene, and pyrene. Approximately half of ambient mutagenicity can be ascribed to atmospheric reaction products of two-to-four-ring PAH. Not all of the mutagenicity can be ascribed to particular compounds, but much of it is due to nitro-PAH lactones and to simpler nitro-PAH (188–191). Atmospheric reaction products of naphthalene and phenanthrene have recently been shown to be genotoxic in human lymphoblasts and appear to undergo oxidative metabolism (192–195).

B. Source Apportionment: Estimating the Contribution of Sources to Exposure and Risk

1. Source Apportionment Methods and Application to Ambient Air

The initial tools used for source apportionment were either dispersion modeling, receptor modeling (196) or a hybrid method (197). Dispersion modeling relies on emission factors which are used as input data for atmospheric dispersion models using meteorological and geographical information. Receptor modeling uses ambient measurements of the parameter being apportioned (e.g., particle mass) with simultaneously measured tracer analysis. The tracers used are generally individual chemical species, or other measures of components of $PM_{2.5}$ (e.g., inorganic ions, trace metals, organic and elemental carbon) whose presence in the atmosphere is primarily due to its emission from a single source category. The chemical mass balance (CMB) receptor model has been used in conjunction with emission inventories for making source apportionment estimates (198,199). Other receptor modeling approaches use a mathematical method (e.g., multiple linear regression analysis) to separate contributions from individual sources or source categories and estimate source emission profiles.

Due to an increased focus on understanding and controlling the sources of fine particle particles ($PM_{2.5}$), there has been an effort in the 1990s to develop and apply improved receptor models to apportion the sources of $PM_{2.5}$ (200). Several alternative multivariate models, positive matrix factorization (PMF) (201,202), and UNMIX (203,204) have been applied to this problem in a number of urban areas (50–52,204–206). As direct comparison the multivariate receptor models PMF and UNMIX to EPA's Chemical Mass Balance model using the traditional chemical species from the visibility (IMPROVE) network at a central urban site in Seattle, WA (71), Recently, more sophisticated and powerful models for source apportionment, such as the multilinear engine (ME), are being evaluated (207–209).

2. Contribution of Combustion Sources to Indoor and Personal Exposure

Indoor exposures to $PM_{2.5}$ and its combustion components are expected to differ from outdoor due to many factors including infiltration efficiency, indoor sources, and human activities. The sources that contribute to personal $PM_{2.5}$ exposures are also impacted by time spent in different environments and personal activities. Understanding the sources contributing to these exposures is important to interpreting health studies and also to setting relevant control policies. The source apportionment techniques used above have had limited application to indoor, personal, or total human exposure assessment (210–212). In a recent study of $PM_{2.5}$, PMF was found to be a useful approach apportioning the sources of personal exposure to $PM_{2.5}$ using personal, indoor, and outdoor, filter-based particle measurements of both trace elements as well as light absorption coefficient to simultaneously apportion the sources of indoor, outdoor and personal air (213). Several other recent studies have applied receptor modeling to assessment of personal exposure to $PM_{2.5}$ (214,215).

An individual's exposure to PM derives from indoor and outdoor source emissions as well as PM generated by personal activities. The identification of sources and the assessment of their relative contribution to total indoor and personal exposures can provide valuable information for epidemiologists and regulatory agencies. Only recently have researchers possessed the tools and technologies to be able to examine the health effects of individual PM components (216–225) and source types (226–231). These efforts have been based on either traditional factor analysis or a priori source profiles.

Assessment of human exposure to various PM sources is important to understanding how specific outdoor PM components or sources contribute to the observed associations between PM concentrations as measured at an outdoor monitoring site and adverse health effects. An early indoor and outdoor source apportionment study of exposures to wood smoke and mobile sources in Boise, ID is estimated in the winter of 1986–1987 when wood stoves were a common source of heating (172). The ambient concentrations averaged $15.3 \, \mu g/m^3$ of the particulate extractable particulate organic matter (EOM) from wood smoke fine particles and $4.2 \, \mu g/m^3$ of EOM from mobile sources. Human exposures for the same period are estimated to average $9.5 \, \mu g/m^3$ EOM for wood smoke and $2.1 \, \mu g/m^3$ EOM from mobile sources. Annual estimates for exposure to EOM from wood smoke and auto exhaust are 3.4 and $1.2 (\mu g/m^3$, respectively. Thus, wood smoke accounted for about 73% of the annual exposure to EOM.

Simple physical models were used by Koutrakis et al. (232) to estimate the relative contribution of indoor and outdoor aerosol sources to indoor concentrations of particles. The PM characterization data from a large study of total exposure to particles in Riverside, CA (1991 Particle Total Exposure Assessment Methodology study) was the first analysis to identify and estimate the contribution of major PM sources to personal exposure (212). This study used positive matrix factorization in the simultaneous analysis of indoor, outdoor, and personal data. Later, Hopke et al. (214) simultaneously analyzed indoor, outdoor, and personal data from EPA's 1998 Baltimore exposure panel study using the multilinear engine. Recently, Larson et al. (213) used positive matrix factorization (both PMF2 and PMF3) to apportion $PM_{2.5}$ sources for a central site, outdoor, indoor, and personal PM samples collected from the Seattle exposure and health effects panel study of high-risk subpopulations (215). In this study, the attenuation of various sources from outdoor to indoor and personal environments is evaluated in the context of total exposure to $PM_{2.5}$.

Larson et al. (213) examined the attenuation of various sources from outdoor to indoor and personal environments in the context of total exposure to $PM_{2.5}$. This report, as well as others, has recently reported on the effects of personal activities on the personal $PM_{2.5}$ source estimates (214,215). There appear to be robust features in the outdoor particle data that provide information on outdoor source contributions to indoor concentrations and personal exposures (213). Larson et al. (213) found that both positive matrix factorization methods (PMF2 and PMF3) were able to resolve the indoor and personal exposures after excluding indoor and personal samples whose mass concentration was $> 120\%$ of the corresponding outdoor sample. In this Seattle study, vegetative burning contributed more $PM_{2.5}$ mass on average than any other source in all microenvironments.

3. Source Apportionment Applications to Health Risk

An early source apportionment study combining a biological endpoint, mutagenicity, with air quality monitoring data was conducted by Lewis et al. (123) to better understand the potential impact of wood smoke in a relatively simple winter study in Boise, ID where the only other major combustion sources were from traffic of automobiles and trucks. The ambient concentrations of unique tracers were measured simultaneously with the pollutant of interest (e.g., mass of POM and mutagenicity) (233). The key chemical tracer species that were used were fine particle lead and potassium which are tracers of motor vehicle emissions and wood smoke, respectively. The resulting regression analysis with the two tracers was consistent with emission inventories, showing that, on average, 90% of the measured ambient EOM was contributed by these two sources. The wood smoke contribution dominated during both day and night periods, but made its greatest impact during night-time periods. The contribution from motor vehicle emissions was greater at the roadway site than at the residential site (123). This study, part of the Integrated Air Cancer Project (234) to characterize exposure and potential cancer risk of combustion sources, also collected sufficient ambient $PM_{2.5}$ mass to evaluate the tumorigenic activity of the source apportioned composites (171) constructed to maximize the contribution of wood smoke while minimizing the motor vehicle contribution for one sample and a second sample with the maximum motor vehicle contribution. Motor vehicle emissions and ambient air dominated by vehicle emissions were more mutagenic and more tumorigenic than wood smoke emissions or ambient $PM_{2.5}$ dominated by wood smoke domination of EOM mass (172,235). Quantitatively, this can be expressed in terms of potency: approximately 1 and 3 revertants per microgram (rev/mg) were found for ambient EOM originating from wood smoke and motor vehicle emissions, respectively. Thus, the greater potency of EOM from motor vehicle emissions outweighs the smaller amount of motor vehicle EOM, in comparison with wood smoke. Within experimental uncertainties (approximately 30%), the two potency values are completely consistent with results found in two other studies to apportion airborne mutagenicity in airsheds containing wood smoke and auto exhaust (123,233).

III. Biomarkers of Exposure, Dose, Susceptibility, and Risk to Air Pollution and Combustion Emissions

A. Exposure Biomarkers

Exposure biomarkers provide a key tool to relate health outcomes to individual personal exposures. Human exposures to environmental chemicals have been routinely analyzed in blood and urine samples (236) as part of the US National Health and Nutrition Examination Survey (NHANES). This continuous annual survey uses a stratified, multistage, probability-cluster design to select a representative sample of the population. Recent advances in the analytical measurements of environmental chemicals or their metabolites in whole blood, serum, or urine have increased the reporting of chemical exposures from 27 to 116 chemicals. The latest report (236) includes several categories of chemicals related to air pollution and combustion source exposures including a series of PAH metabolites of both semi-volatile and particulate associated PAH and serum cotinine, a well-established biomarker of smoking and exposure to environmental tobacco smoke in non-smokers. Other chemicals relevant to air pollution exposures are lead and mercury in blood and urine. Previous studies demonstrating the decrease of blood lead levels as lead was removed from gasoline have demonstrated the utility of these exposure biomarkers. In addition to providing a valuable research tool, NHANES provides reference levels of exposure enabling recognition of unusually high levels of exposure in workers and patients.

1. Environmental Tobacco Smoke: Cotinine as a Model Biomarker of Exposure

The validation and accepted use of cotinine as a biomarker of environmental exposure to tobacco smoke (ETS) is a useful example for the development of exposure biomarkers for other air pollution sources (237). Nicotine is a relatively unique source tracer of tobacco smoke and dietary sources of nicotine are very minor since few individuals ingest sufficient nicotine-containing foods and beverages to compromise the validity of cotinine as an estimator of exposure to nicotine in ETS (238,239). A workshop on exposure assessment of ETS in the workplace (237) concluded that the relationship between ETS, nicotine, and cotinine was relatively robust under current smoking conditions. Cotinine measured in blood, saliva, or urine is the most specific and sensitive biomarker of exposure to ETS meets the criteria for a valid marker of ETS exposure using the criteria for validity used by an NRC panel on ETS exposure and health effects (238–240).

The use of cotinine as a biomarker for tobacco smoke exposure is one of the most successful applications of exposure biomarkers in international and national scale studies. Cotinine analyses of approximately 12,000 blood samples from NHANES HI collected from 1988 to 1991 were used to estimate the US population exposures to ETS and to examine the contribution of the home and workplace environment to exposure (241). This study found measurable levels of cotinine in 88% of the population including a high proportion of non-smokers. They reported ETS exposure (based on cotinine levels) was higher among children, non-Hispanic blacks, and men. New results from NHANES III Phase 2 (1991–1994) and the most recent NHANES 1999 document a continuing decline in exposures of the US population to ETS indicating that public health measures taken to reduce ETS exposures have been successful (236).

More than 50 studies of lung cancer risk in non-smokers exposed to ETS (e.g., spouses of smokers) have been published during the last 25 years and recently reviewed by IARC (242). The IARC evaluation considered cotinine a highly specific marker of exposure to ETS and the most suitable biomarker for assessing recent exposure to secondhand tobacco smoke uptake and metabolism in adults, children, and newborns. Cotinine, and its parent compound nicotine are highly specific for exposure to second-hand smoke. Because of its favorable biological half-life and the sensitivity of techniques for quantifying it (165,166), cotinine is currently the most suitable biomarker for assessing recent exposure to secondhand tobacco smoke uptake and metabolism in adults, children, and newborns (246–248)

The cancer evaluation of ETS as well as other combustion source mixtures or ambient air particles require data on human exposure, dose, and mechanistic evidence to link exposure to the health outcomes. Hecht, in a series of papers, has presented biochemical data on carcinogen uptake in non-smokers, including children, as well as the mechanisms and steps that link ETS exposure to cancer from tobacco smoke carcinogens (162,243–245). An adaptation of this scheme for tobacco smoke carcinogens to other combustion emissions and air pollution is shown in Fig. 1.

2. Polycyclic Aromatic Hydrocarbons (PAH) Exposure and Biomarkers

Polycyclic aromatic hydrocarbons are emitted from a wide range of combustion sources and are present both in the gas phase and particle phase, dependent on the molecular size, vapor pressure, and atmospheric conditions. Polycyclic aromatic hydrocarbons are found in urban and rural air,

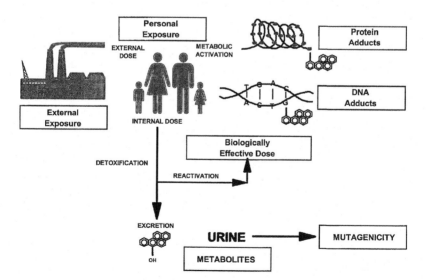

Figure 1   Scheme showing human exposure to combustion emissions and air pollution.

soot particles, and in a wide range of combustion, pyrolysis, and reductive distillation emissions (4,32,33,50,249). Other sources of PAH exposure in the general population are food, including smoked, charcoal-broiled, and roasted foods and plant foods that are contaminated by atmospheric deposition or processing (e.g., drying of cereal grains).

Dipple (256) reviewed PAH carcinogens starting with Percival Pott's postulation in 1775 that chimney sweep's scrotal cancer was due to soot exposures (251). By 1933, Cook et al. (252) had used large-scale isolation to identify a fluorescent carcinogenic constituent, benzo(a)pyrene. This was a key step leading to the discovery that benzo(a)pyrene (BaP) in coal soot was a causative agent in human cancer, including respiratory or lung cancer (3). Since that time, over 500 PAH have been detected in air samples. The carcinogenicity of BaP and its association with soot (or particulate matter), most of the air monitoring data were focused on benzo(a) pyrene up through the 1990s (4). As the sampling and analytical measurement methods advanced, the range of PAH in both the gas and particle phase expanded. In addition, research on the atmospheric reactions of PAH has led to the discovery of mutagenic and carcinogenic nitro-PAH (253), nitro-lactones, and other nitroarenes (254). Since the advancement of air monitoring methods and development of major air monitoring programs for PAH, it has become clear that the gaseous and semi-volatile PAH are present in the atmosphere at higher concentrations than the more carcinogenic 4–5 ring PAH.

Canada recently reported data from approximately 2200 daily PAH samples collected at 35 sites (255). Although this study was conducted over a 10-year period (1987–1997), most of the data were collected between 1995 and 1997. The PAH monitored included benzo(a)pyrene (BaP), benzo(b)-fluoranthene, benzo(j)fluoranthene, benzo(k)fluoranthene, and indeno(1,2,3-(cd)pyrene) as well as acenapthene, fluorene, phenanthrene, anthracene, fluoranthene, pyrene, benz(a)anthracene, and naphthalene. Mean PAH concentrations varied by more than three orders of magnitude from the rural-remote sites to an industrial site.

Urinary PAH metabolites have been widely used as biomarkers of PAH exposure in occupational studies (256). PAH urinary metabolites in general and more commonly the hydroxylated metabolite of pyrene, 1-hydroxypyrene (1-OHP) have been used as biomarkers of exposure to PAH (256–266). The urinary PAH metabolites have been used in both occupational (256–259) and ambient air pollution studies in the general population (260–264) and in children (265,266). Pyrene is a semi-volatile non-carcinogenic PAH that is distributed between the gas and particle phase in the ambient air and human exposure samples (267). The literature indicates conflicting evidence on the utility of 1-OHP as a biomarker of exposure to carcinogenic PAH or PAH DNA adducts. A lack of association between DNA adducts and urinary 1-HOP has been reported in garage workers exposed to automobile exhaust (268), but the adduct level correlated with urinary 1-HOP in foundry workers (269). In a study of human exposure to ambient air pollution, no correlations were observed between 1-OHP and either DNA adducts or PAH-albumin adduct levels (270).

The hydroxylated metabolites of the PAHs are excreted in human urine both as free hydroxylated metabolites and as hydroxylated metabolites conjugated to glucuronic acid and sulfate. In many of the studies cited above, the PAH are deconjugated to release free hydroxylated metabolites for analysis. Methods are also available for quantifying the glucuronides (e.g., 1-hydroxypyrene-glucuronide). Lee et al. (271) compared three analytical methods for 1-hydroxypyrene-glucuronide in urine after non-occupational exposure to polycyclic aromatic hydrocarbons; and urinary PAH metabolites were measured in the NHANES study US National Health and Nutrition Examination Survey (NHANES) using an isotope-dilution gas chromatography–high resolution mass spectroscopy method (272).

Measurement of PAH metabolites is thought to reflect exposure to PAH that has occurred within the previous few days; however, more studies of the urinary half-lives of PAH metabolites are needed. Geometric mean levels of the demographic groups were compared after adjustment for race/ethnicity, age, gender, urinary creatinine, and log serum cotinine. Children aged 6–11 years had about a two times higher urinary 1-OHP adjusted geometric means than did people in the two other age groups. This age-related difference also has been found by other investigators (265,273). The urinary 1-OHP levels for children in the CDC Report were similar to levels measured in other studies cited here. No differences were observed for race/ethnicity or gender in the CDC study as has been reported consistent with previous studies (260,264,266). Since pyrene is present in the environment at much higher concentrations than the 4–5-ring carcinogenic PAH, it is not surprising that it was detected in 99% of the NHANES 1999–2000 subsample. CDC found the geometric mean level for the overall population to be similar to that of other general populations residing in an urban setting (260–266). People who work in certain occupations (e.g., carbon electrode production) can have urinary 1-hydroxypyrene levels 100 times higher than the geometric mean level reported for the general US population (257,258). An additional source of PAH exposure for children is the ingestion of PAH-contaminated soil (265).

3. Combustion Source-Specific Exposure Biomarkers

Other organic species emitted from combustion emissions have been investigated as potential exposure biomarkers including aromatic amines from coke ovens, heterocyclic amines from cooking meats (146–149), nitrosamines from tobacco smoke (243–245), and methoxyphenols from wood smoke (115–118). These are discussed in Sec. II above on each combustion emission source category. It is beyond the scope of this review to discuss all of the possible exposure biomarkers for each of these source-specific organic species.

A method has recently been reported for determining methoxyphenols in human urine as a biomarker of exposure to wood smoke (265). Specific chemicals quantified were guaiacol, 4-methylguaiacol, 4-ethylguaiacol, 4-propylguaiacol, syringol, 4-methylsyringol, 4-ethylsyringol, vanillin, eugenol, and syringaldehyde. Wood smoke exposures for a relatively short period (2.5 hr) resulted in excretion rates of methoxyphenols reflecting the period of wood smoke exposure. Although this study did not determine inhalation elimination half-lives for the urinary methoxyphenols, they estimated them to be relatively short (2–3 hr) and suggest that short episodic exposures would be detectable for only 1–2 days after an exposure (274). The development of a method to measure personal exposures to levoglucosan (275) is facilitating the evaluation of urinary methoxyphenols as a biomarker for wood smoke exposure a large panel study in Seattle, WA (276). In this study, questionnaires were used to account for dietary sources of the methoxyphenols. Methoxyphenols were detected in all urine samples analyzed and a wide dynamic range of metabolite concentrations (1000-fold) was observed (267).

B. Biomarkers of Genetic Susceptibility, Dose, and DNA Damage

The role of genetic susceptibility (or genotype) as it may influence the uptake, metabolism, excretion, and binding of metabolites to DNA or protein plays an important role in modern molecular epidemiology studies (277–286). The interaction of genetic susceptibility and air pollutant exposures in the risk for cancer, adverse reproductive outcomes, and cardiovascular disease has become an important area of biomarker research since the development of genotyping methods and molecular epidemiology. Among the benefits of studying gene–environment interactions are the possibility of increasing the characterization of relatively low population risks, if a substantial proportion of the population's cancer burden is attributed to high risk among a smaller group of genetically susceptible members. Gene–environment interaction studies also provide insight into the mechanism of carcinogenesis and other diseases caused by environmental exposures. Understanding these interactions can help establish the biologic plausibility of an exposure–cancer relationship (281–283).

Genetic differences in metabolism, as measured by genotype, have been shown to influence the exposure–dose relationship for PAH, nitro-PAH, aromatic amines, and other combustion organics and risk of a variety of health outcomes from air pollution and combustion emissions. Until recently, most gene–environment studies relied on surrogate exposure measures. In community air pollution studies, these estimates were initially based on home or work locations (e.g., industrial urban location vs. a rural location) (284) or in occupational settings the exposures were estimated by job category (285). This approach led to a number of studies demonstrating the importance of genotype on biomarkers and potential health outcomes (286–288); however, it was not possible to determine if the genotype was altering the effective exposure, dose, or genetic damage. The use of gene–environment studies becomes more powerful when exposures are measured at the individual level using personal exposure monitoring (289) and both exposure biomarkers (e.g., urinary metabolites) and biomarkers of dose (e.g., DNA adducts or protein adducts) are deployed together in the same subjects.

Many of the organic species associated with fine particles or present in the gas phase are metabolized by polymorphic enzymes that activate and detoxify organic pollutants using certain P450 enzymes such as glutathione-*S*-transferase Ml (GSTM1) (290,291) involved in PAH metabolism and *N*-acetyltransferase (NAT2) (292,293) involved in nitro-PAH and aromatic amine metabolism. When urinary metabolites or other biomarkers are used as an exposure measure in a study, knowledge of the impact of genotype on the biomarker is very useful in the final interpretation of the exposure data. Genotype (e.g., GSTM1 and NAT2), as expected, does influence the relationship between personal exposure to PAH and the formation DNA adducts as well as the excretion of urinary PAH metabolites (289). Other gene–environment studies in this Czech population used exposure, dose, and measures of genetic damage in reproductive outcome studies (41,294–301) where biomarker measurements were made in urine and blood, and in the reproductive studies were measured in placental tissue (299–301) and sperm (42,298,301). Reproductive studies in Poland have also measured biomarkers as part of a study of the impact of air pollution on reproductive outcomes (284,302,303).

DNA and protein adducts are also molecular biomarkers of exposure and dose. DNA adduct biomarkers are particularly relevant to cancer risk since they are linked mechanistically to the induction of cancer (304,305) and are viewed as reflecting the dose to DNA. DNA adducts, however, may be repaired and therefore have a shorter half-life than protein adducts that are not repaired and the half-life is related to the turnover of the protein used in the assay (e.g., hemoglobin or albumin). DNA and protein adducts of PAH and related aromatic compounds have been applied to a number of occupational and environmental study populations (306–310).

IV. Summary

The complex emissions associated with incomplete combustion include complex PM of varied composition, semi-volatile organic and inorganic materials and vapors, as well as an array of gases, largely oxidant products.

Smaller respirable particles $< 2.5\,\mu m$ ($PM_{2.5}$) have previously been considered as soot in the older literature if there was a high content of elemental carbon. Often, embedded in these PM is a wide range of organic matter from simple alkanes to polycyclic organic matter, including a myriad of complex aromatic compounds, to polar substituted aromatics and carboxylic acids. The cancer risk from PM is generally believed to arise primarily from the polycyclic organics, including polycyclic aromatic hydrocarbons (PAH), and their derivatives. The primary source of PAHs in air pollution is from combustion of fossil fuels, vegetative matter, and synthetic chemicals. The major fraction of the emissions from wood and forest fires is derived from the combustion and pyrolysis of lignin and polysaccharides, of which 30% of them are carbonaceous mass comprises oxygenated organic compounds.

Atmospheric transformation reactions among the many components of combustion emissions may undergo photolytic transformation in the air resulting in the formation or destruction of the mutagenic potency of the air (actually its content). For example, controlled studies with smog chambers have demonstrated that normal atmospheric processes can increase the direct-acting mutagenicity of wood smoke and automobile emissions. Due to an increased focus on understanding and controlling the sources of $PM_{2.5}$, there has been an effort over the last decade to develop and apply improved receptor models to apportion the sources of $PM_{2.5}$. Several alternative multivariate models, positive matrix factorization, and UNMIX have been applied to this problem in a number of urban areas.

As summarized, airborne PM is a mixture of many different chemical species and elevated morbidity and mortality have been associated with outdoor PM mass concentrations in many epidemiologic studies. However, an individual's exposure to PM derives from indoor and outdoor source emissions as well as PM generated by personal activities. Investigation based studies relating outdoor air pollutants to indoor air and personal exposure will further our understanding of the relationship of ambient measurements to human exposure and risk. Exposure biomarkers can provide a key tool to relate health outcomes to individual personal exposures. The continued identification of sources and the assessments of their relative contribution to total indoor and personal exposures can provide valuable information for epidemiologists and regulatory agencies.

References

1. Cook JW, Kennaway EL. Chemical compounds as carcinogenic agents. Am J Cancer 1938; 33:50.
2. Kipling MD. Soots, tars, and oils as causes of occupational cancer. In: Searle CE, ed. Chemical Carcinogens. Washington, DC, American Chemical Society, 1976:315–323.

3. Hoffman D, Wynder EL. Environmental respiratory carcinogenesis. In: Searle CE, ed. Chemical Carcinogens. Washington, DC, American Chemical Society, 1976:334–365.
4. IARC. World Health Organization. Polynuclear Aromatic Compounds. Part 1. Chemical, Environmental and Experimental Data (Monograph 32). Geneva, Switzerland, International Agency for Research on cancer. IARC Monographs on the Evaluation of the Carcinogenic Risk of Chemicals to Humans, 1984.
5. Leiter J, Shimkin MB, Shear MJ. Production of subcutaneous sarcomas in mice with tars extracted from atmospheric dusts. J Nat Cancer Inst 1942; 3: 155–165.
6. Leiter J, Shear MJ. Production of tumors in mice with tars from city air dusts. J Natl Cancer Inst 1942; 3:167–174.
7. Kotin P, Falk HL, Mader P, Thomas M. Aromatic hydrocarbons: presence in the Los Angeles atmosphere and the carcinogenicity of atmospheric extracts. Arch Indust Hyg 1954; 9:153–163.
8. Hueper WC, Kotin P, Tabor EC, Payne W, Falk HL, Sawiciki E. Carcinogenic bioassays on air pollutants. Arch Pathol 1962; 74:89–116.
9. Ames BN, McCann J, Yamasaki E. Methods for detecting carcinogens and mutagens with the Salmonella/mammalian microsome mutagenicity test. Mutat Res 1975; 31:347–364.
10. Schuetzle D, Lewtas J. Bioassay-directed chemical analysis in environmental research. Anal Chem 1986; 58:1060A–1075A.
11. Lewtas J. Genotoxicity of complex mixtures: strategies for the identification and comparative assessment of airborne mutagens and carcinogens from combustion sources. Fundam Appl Toxicol 1988; 10:571–589.
12. IARC. World Health Organization. Diesel and Gasoline Engine Exhausts and Some Nitroarenes (Monograph 46). Geneva, Switzerland, International Agency for Research on cancer. IARC Monographs on the Evaluation of the Carcinogenic Risk of Chemicals to Humans, 1989.
13. Samet JM, Cohen AJ. Air pollution and lung cancer. In: Swift DL, Foster WM, eds. Air Pollutants and the Respiratory Tract. New York: Marcel Dekker, 1999:181–217.
14. Tomatis L. Indoor and Outdoor Air Pollution and Human Cancer. New York: Springer-Verlag, European School of Oncology Monographs, 1993.
15. Samet JM. Epidemiology of Lung Cancer. New York: Marcel Dekker, 1994.
16. Graedel TE, Hawkins DT, Claxton LD. . Atmospheric Chemical Compounds: Sources, Occurrence, and Bioassay. Orlando: Academic Press, 1986.
17. Fishbein L. Sources nature and levels of air pollutants. In: Tomatis L, ed. Indoor and Outdoor Air Pollution and Human Cancer. New York: Springer-Verlag, 1993:17–87.
18. Lewtas J. Experimental evidence for the carcinogenicity of indoor and outdoor air pollutants. In: Tomatis L, ed. Indoor and Outdoor Air Pollution and Human Cancer. New York: Springer-Verlag, 1993:103–118.
19. Saxena P, Hildemann LM. Water-soluble organics in atmospheric particles: a critical review of the literature and application of thermodynamics to identify candidate compounds. J Atmos Chem 1996; 24:57–109.

20. Rogge WF, Mazurek MA, Hildemann LM, Cass GR, Simoneit BRT. Quantification of urban organic aerosols at a molecular level: identification, abundance and seasonal variation. Atmos Environ 1993; 27A:1309–1330.

21. Puxbaum H, Rendl J, Allabashi R, Otter L, Scholes MC. Mass balance of atmospheric aerosol in a South-African subtropical savanna (Nylsvley, May 1997). J Geophys Res 2000; 105:20697–20706.

22. Zappoli S, Andracchio A, Fuzzi S, Facchini MC, Gelencser A, Kiss G, Krivacsy Z, Molnar A, Meszaros E, Hansson H-C, Rosman K, Zebühr Y. Inorganic, organic and macromolecular components of fine aerosol in different areas of Europe in relation to their water solubility. Atmos Environ 1999; 33:2733–2743.

23. Claeys M, Graham B, Vas G, Wang W, Vermeylen R, Pashynska V, Cafmeyer J, Guyon P, Andreae MO, Artaxo P, Maenhaut W. Formation of secondary organic aerosol through photooxidation of isoprene. Science 2004; 303: 1173–1176.

24. Havers N, Burba P, Lambert J, Klockow D. Spectroscopic characterisation of humic-like substances in airborne particulate matter. J Atmos Chem 1998; 29:45–54.

25. Jang M, Czoschke N, Lee S, Kamens RM. Heterogeneous atmospheric aerosol formation by acid catalysed particle-phase reactions. Science 2002; 298:814–817.

26. Kalberer M, Paulsen D, Sax M, Steinbacher M, Dommen J, Prevot ASH, Fisseha R, Weingartner E, Frankevich V, Zenobi R, Baltensperger U. Identification of polymers as major components of atmospheric organic aerosols. Science 2004; 303:1659–1662.

27. Simoneit BRT. Organic matter in eolian dusts over the Atlantic Ocean. Mar Chem 1977; 5:443–464.

28. Simoneit BRT, Mazurek MA. Organic matter of the troposphere, II. Natural background of biogenic lipid matter in aerosols over the rural western United States. Atmos Environ 1982; 16:2139–2215.

29. IARC. World Health Organization. Wood dust and formaldehyde (Monograph 62). Geneva, Switzerland, International Agency for Research on cancer. IARC Monographs on the Evaluation of the Carcinogenic Risk of Chemicals to Humans, 1995.

30. IARC. World Health Organization. Some Naturally Occurring Substances (Monograph 10). Geneva, Switzerland, International Agency for Research on cancer. IARC Monographs on the Evaluation of the Carcinogenic Risk of Chemicals to Humans, 1976.

31. IARC. World Health Organization. Some Naturally Occurring Substances: Food Items and Constituents, Heterocyclic Aromatic Amines and Mycotoxins (Monograph 56). Geneva, Switzerland, International Agency for Research on cancer. IARC Monographs on the Evaluation of the Carcinogenic Risk of Chemicals to Humans, 1993.

32. IARC. World Health Organization. Polynuclear Aromatic compounds. Part 4 Bitumens, Coal-tars and Derived Products, Shale-oils and Soot (Monograph 35). Geneva, Switzerland, International Agency for Research on cancer.

IARC Monographs on the Evaluation of the Carcinogenic Risk of Chemicals to Humans, 1985.

33. IARC. IARC Monograph on the Evaluation of the Carcinogenic Risk of Chemicals to Humans. Polynuclear Aromatic compounds. Part 3. Industrial Exposures in Aluminum Production, Coal Gasification, Coke Production, and Iron and Steel Founding. Vol. 34. Lyon, France: IARC, 1984.

34. Bates DV. Environmental Health Risks and Public Policy. Seattle, London: University of Washington Press, 1994.

35. Logan WPD, Glasg MD. Mortality in the London fog incident. Lancet 1953; 14:336–338.

36. Firket J. Fog along the Meuse Valley. Trans Faraday Soc 1936; 32:1192–1197.

37. Nemery BN, Hoet PHM, Nemmar A. The Meuse Valley fog of 1930: an air pollution disaster. Lancet 2001; 357(9257):704–708.

38. Schrenk HH, Heimann H, Clayton GD, Gafafer WM, Wexler H. Air Pollution in Donora, PA: Epidemiology of the Unusual Smog Episode of October 1948, Preliminary Report. Public Health Bulletin No 306. Washington, DC: U.S. Public Health Service, 1949.

39. Šrám R, Beneŝ I, Binková B, Dejmek J, Horstman D, Kotešovec F, Otto D, Perreault S, Rubeš J, Selevan S, Skalík I, Stevens R, Lewtas J. Teplice Program—the impact of air pollution on human health. Environ Health Perspect 1996; 104:699–714.

40. Horstman D, Kotesovec F, Nozicka J, Šrám R. Pulmonary functions of school children in highly polluted Northern Bohemia. Arch Environ Health 1997; 52:56–62.

41. Binková B, Lewtas J, Míšková I, Rössner P, Cerná M, Mracková G, Peterková K, Mumford J, Meyer J, Šrám RJ. Biomarkers studies in the Northern Bohemia. Bohemia, Environ Health Perspect 1996; 104:591–597.

42. Binková B, Lewtas J, Míšková I, Lenícek J, Šrám RJ. DNA adducts and personal air monitoring of carcinogenic polycyclic aromatic hydrocarbons in an environmentally exposed population. Carcinogenesis 1995; 16:1037–1046.

43. Dejmek J, Selevan SG, Benes I, Solansky I, Sram, RJ. Fetal growth and maternal exposure to particulate matter during pregnancy. Environ Health Perspect 1999; 107:475–480.

44. Selevan SG, Borkovec L, Slott VL, Zudova Z, Rubes J, Evenson DP, Perreault, SD. Semen quality and reproductive health of young Czech men exposed to seasonal air pollution. Environ Health Perspect 2000; 108:887–894.

45. Peters A, Skorkovsky J, Kotesovec F, Brynda J, Spix C, Wichmann HE, Heinrich J. Associations between mortality and air pollution in Central Europe. Environ Health Perspect 2000; 108:283–287.

46. Mumford JL, He XZ, Chapman RS, et al. Lung cancer and indoor air pollution in Xuan Wei, China. Science 1987; 235:217–220.

47. Searle CE. Chemical Carcinogens. Washington, DC: American Chemical Society, 1976.

48. Williams R, Sparacino C, Petersen B, Bumgarner J, Jungers RH, Lewtas J. Comparative characterization of organic emissions from diesel particles, coke oven mains, roofing tar vapors, and cigarette smoke condensate. Int J Environ Anal Chem 1986; 26:27–49.

49. Austin AC, Claxton LD, Lewtas J. Mutagenicity of the fractionated organic emissions from diesel, cigarette smoke condensate, coke oven and roofing tar in the Ames Assay. Environ Mutagen 1985; 7:471–487.

50. IARC. World Health Organization. Certain polycyclic Aromatic Hydrocarbons and Heterocyclic Compounds (Monograph 3). Geneva, Switzerland, International Agency for Research on cancer. IARC Monographs on the Evaluation of the Carcinogenic Risk of Chemicals to Humans, 1973.

51. IARC. World Health Organization. Overall Evaluations of Carcinogenicity: An Updating of IARC Monographs Volumes 1 to 42 (Supplement 7). Geneva, Switzerland, International Agency for Research on cancer. IARC Monographs on the Evaluation of the Carcinogenic Risk of Chemicals to Humans, 1987.

52. Polissar AV, Hopke PK, Poirot RL. Atmospheric aerosol over Vermont: chemical composition and sources. Environ Sci Technol 2001; 35:4604–4621.

53. Poirot RL, Wishinski PR, Hopke PK, Polissar AV. Comparative application of multiple receptor methods to identify aerosol sources in northern Vermont. Environ Sci Technol 2001; 35:4622–4636.

54. Song X-H, Polissar AV, Hopke PK. Sources of fine particle composition in the Northeast. Atmos Environ 2001; 35:5277–5286.

55. Mumford JL, Lewtas J. Mutagenicity and cytotoxicity of coal fly ash from fluidized-bed and conventional combustion. J Toxicol Environ Health 1982; 10:565–586.

56. Mumford JL, Lewtas J. Evaluation of fly ash collection methods for short-term bioassay studies of fluidized-bed coal combustion. Environ Sci Technol 1984; 18:765–768.

57. Lewtas J. Combustion emissions: characterization and comparison of their mutagenic and carcinogenic activity. In: Stich HF, ed. Carcinogens and Mutagens in the Environment. Vol. IV. The Workplace, Boca Raton, FL: CRC Press, 1985:59–74.

58. Lewtas J. Development of a comparative potency method for cancer risk assessment of complex mixtures using short-term in vivo and in vitro bioassays. Toxicol Indust Health 1985; 1:193–203.

59. American Petroleum Institute, 1220 L Street, NW, Washington DC, USA (www.api.org).

60. ConocoPhillips, Material Safety Data Sheet #724290:1–8, 2003, http://sewebl.phillips66.com/hes%5CMSDS.nsf/MSDSID/US724290/$file/30017426.pdf.

61. IARC. IARC Monograph on the Evaluation of the Carcinogenic Risk of Chemicals to Humans. Vol. 45. Occupational Exposures in Petroleum Refining; Crude Oil and Major Petroleum Fuels, IARC, Lyon, France, 1989:322.

62. Groenzin H, Mullins OC. Molecular size and structure of asphaltenes from various sources. Energy Fuels 2000; 14:677–684.

63. Fisher GL, McNeill KL, Prentice BA, McFarland AR. Physical and biological studies of coal and oil fly ash. Environ Health Perspect 1983; 51:181–186.

64. Hatch GE, Boykin E, Graham JA, Lewtas J, Pott F, Loud K, Mumford JL. Inhalable particles and pulmonary host defense: in vivo and in vitro effects of ambient air and combustion particles. Environ Res 1985; 36:67–80.

65. Lewtas J. Impact of fuel choice on comparative cancer risk of emissions. Energy Fuels 1992; 7:4–6.
66. Costa DL, Dreher KL. Bioavailable transition metals in particulate matter mediate cardiopulmonary injury in healthy and compromised animal models. Environ Health Perspect 1997; 105(suppl 5):1053–1060.
67. Ghio AJ, Silbajoris R, Carson JL, Samet JM. Biological effects of oil fly ash. Environ Health Perspect 2002; 110(suppl 1):89–102.
68. US EPA. Air quality criteria for particulate matter (Fourth External Review Draft VI & VII). EPA/600/P-99/002 2003. U.S. Environmental Protection Agency, Office of Research and Development, National Center For Environmental Assessment, Research Triangle Park Office, Research Triangle Park, NC.
69. US EPA. Brochure on National Air Quality: Status and Trends Report. EPA/454/F-98-006 August 1998. US Environmental Protection Agency, Office of Air Quality Planning and Standards, Research Triangle Park Office, Research Triangle Park, NC.
70. US EPA. Health Assessment Document for Diesel Engine Exhaust. EPA/600/8-90/057F May 2002. US Environmental Protection Agency, Office of Research and Development, National Center For Environmental Assessment, Washington, DC.
71. Maykut NN, Lewtas J, Kim E, Larson TV. Source apportionment of PM2.5 at an Urban IMPROVE site in Seattle, WA. Environ Sci Technol 2003; 37: 5135–5142.
72. Schauer JJ, Rogge WF, Hildemann LM, Mazurek MA, Cass GR, Simoneit BRT. Source apportionment of airborne particulate matter using organic compounds as tracers. Atmos Environ 1996; 30:3837–3855.
73. Watson JG, Chow JC. Source characterization of major emission sources in the Imperial and Mexicali Valleys along the US/Mexico border. Sci Total Environ 2001; 276:33–47.
74. Palmgren F, Wahlin P, Kildeso J, Afshari A, Fogh C. Characterisation of particle emissions from the driving care fleet and the contribution to ambient and indoor particle concentrations. Phys Chem Earth 2003; 28:327–334.
75. Watson JG, Chow JC, Lowenthal DH, Pritchett LC, Frazier CA, Neuroth GR, Robbins R. Differences in the carbon composition of source profiles for diesel-and asoline-powered vehicles. Atmos Environ 1994; 28:2493–2505.
76. US EPA. The Diesel Emissions Research Program. EPA/625/9-79–004, US Environmental Protection Agency, Office of Research and Development, Center for Environmental Research Information, Cincinnati, OH, December 1979. 44 pp.
77. US CRS. Automobile and Light Duty Truck Fuel Economy: The CAFÉ Standards. CRS-IB90122. June 2003. US Library of Congress. Congressional Research Service, Washington, DC.
78. Huisingh J, Bradow R, Jungers R, Claxton L, Zweidinger R, et al. Application of bioassay to the characterization of diesel particle emissions. In: Waters MD, Nesnow S, Huisingh JL, et al. eds. Application of Short-term Bioassays in the Fractionation and Analysis of Complex Environmental Mixtures. New York: Plenum Press, 1979:383–418.

79. Lewtas Huisingh J. Short-term carcinogenesis and mutagenesis bioassays of unregulated automotive emissions. Bull NY Acad Med 1981; 57:251–261.

80. Lewtas J, Bradow RL, Jungers RH, Harris BD, Zweidinger RB, Cushing KM, Gill BE, Albert RE. Mutagenic and carcinogenic potency of extracts of diesel and related environmental emissions: study design, sample generation, collection, and preparation. Environ Int 1981; 5:383–387.

81. Casto BC, Hatch GG, Huang SL, Lewtas J, Nesnow S, Waters MD. Mutagenic and carcinogenic potency of extracts of diesel and related environmental emissions: in vitro mutagenesis and oncogenic transformation. Environ Int 1981; 5:403–409.

82. Nesnow S, Lewtas J. Mutagenic and carcinogenic potency of extracts of diesel and related environmental emissions: summary and discussion of the results. Environ Int 1981; 5:425–429.

83. Lewtas J. Toxicological Effects of Emissions from Diesel Engines. New York: Elsevier, 1982.

84. Nesnow S, Evans C, Stead A, et al. Skin carcinogenesis studies of emission extracts. In: Lewtas J, ed. Toxicological Effects of Emissions from Diesel Engines. Amsterdam: Elsevier, 1982:295–320.

85. Nesnow S, Triplett LL, Slaga TJ. Comparative tumor-initiating activity of complex mixtures from environmental particulate emissions on SENCAR mouse skin. J Natl Cancer Inst 1982; 68:829–834.

86. Lewtas J. Evaluation of the mutagenicity and carcinogenicity of motor vehicle emissions in short-term bioassays. Environ Health Perspect 1983; 47:141–152.

87. Pepelko WE. EPA studies on the toxicological effects of inhaled diesel engine emissions. In: Lewtas J, ed. Toxicological Effects of Emissions from Diesel Engines. Amsterdam: Elsevier, 1982:121–142.

88. Pepelko WE, Peirano WB. Health effects of exposure to diesel engine emissions. J Am Coll Toxicol 1983; 2:253–306.

89. Albert RE, Lewtas J, Nesnow S, Thorslund T, Anderson E. Comparative potency method for cancer risk assessment: application to diesel particulate emissions. Risk Anal 1983; 3:101–117.

90. Lewtas J, Nesnow S, Albert RE. A comparative potency method for cancer risk assessment: clarification of the rationale, theoretical basis, and application to diesel particulate emissions. Risk Anal 1983; 3:133–137.

91. Claxton LD. Characterization of automotive emissions by bacterial mutagenesis bioassay: a review. Environ Mutagen 1983; 5:609–631.

92. Grimmer G, Brune H, Deutsch-Wenzel R, et al. Contribution of polycyclic aromatic hydrocarbons and nitro-derivatives to the carcinogenic impact of diesel engine exhaust condensate evaluated by implantation into the lungs of rats. Cancer Lett 1987; 37:173–180.

93. World Health Organization (WHO-IPCS). Diesel fuel and exhaust emissions. Environmental Health Criteria 171, WHO-IPCS, Geneva, Switzerland, 1996.

94. California Environmental rotection Agency. (CAL-EPA, OEHHA) Health risk assessment for diesel exhaust. Public and Scientific Review Draft. Feb 1998.

95. Bhatia R, Lopipero P, Smith A. Diesel exhaust exposure and lung cancer. Epidemiology 1998; 9(1):84–91.

96. Lipsett M, Campleman S. Occupational exposure to diesel exhaust and lung cancer: a meta-analysis. Am J Public Health 80(7):1009–1017.

97. Health Effects Institute (HEI). Diesel Emissions and Lung Cancer: Epidemiology and Quantitative Risk Assessment. A Special Report of the Diesel Epidemiology Expert Panel. Cambridge, MA: Health Effects Institute (HEI), June 1999.

98. National Institute for Occupational Safety and Health (NIOSH). Carcinogenic effects of exposure to DE. NIOSH Current Intelligence Bulletin 50. DHHS (NIOSH) Publication No. 88–116. Atlanta, GA: Centers for Disease Control, 1988.

99. National Toxicology Program (NTP). 9th report on carcinogens. Public Health Service, US Department of Health and Human Services, Research Triangle Park, NC, 2000. Available from: http://ntp-server.niehs.nih.gov.

100. Arey J. A tale of two diesels. Environ Health Perspect 2004; 112:812–813.

101. DeMarini DM, Brooks LR, Warren SH, Kobayashi T, Gilmour MI, Singh P. Bioassay-directed fractionation and Salmonella mutogenecity of automobile and forklift diesel exhaust particles. Environ Health Perspect 2004; 112:814–819.

102. Singh P, DeMarini DM, CAJ Dick, Tabor DG, Ryan JV, Linak WP, Kobayashi TK, Gilmour MI. Sample characterization of automobile and forklift diesel exhaust particles and comparative pulmonary toxicity in mice. Environ Health Perspect 2004; 112:820–825.

103. NIST. 2000. Certificate of Analysis, Standard Reference Material 2975. Gaithersburg, MD: National Institute of Standards & Technology. Available: http://patapsco.nist.gov/srmcatalog/certificates/2975.pdf.

104. Hughes TJ, Lewtas J, Claxton LD. Development of a standard reference material for diesel mutagenicity in the Salmonella plate incorporation assay. Mutat Res 1997; 391:243–258.

105. Kobayashi T, Ito T. Diesel exhaust particulates induce nasal mucosal hyperresponsiveness to inhaled histamine aerosol. Fundam Appl Toxicol 1995; 27:195–202.

106. Sagai M, Saito H, Ichinose T, Kodama M, Mori Y. Biological effects of diesel exhaust particles. I. In vitro production of superoxide and in vivo toxicity in mouse. Free Radic Biol Med 1993; 14:37–47.

107. Seagrave JC, McDonald JD, Gigliotti AP, Nikula KJ, Seilkop SK, Gurevich M, Mauderly JL. Mutagenicity and in vivo toxicity of combined particulate and semi-volatile organic fractions of gasoline and diesel engine emissions. Toxicol Sci 2002; 70:212–226.

108. Seagrave J, Mauderly JL, Seilkop SK. In vitro relative toxicity screening of combined particulate and semivolatile organic fractions of gasoline and diesel engine emissions. J Toxicol Environ Health A 2003; 66:1113–1132.

109. US EPA. Motor vehicle-related air toxics study. Ann Arbor, MI: Office of Mobile Sources. EPA/420/R-93/005. Available from National Technical Information Service, Springfield, VA, PB93–182590/XA, 1993.

110. Bostrom C-E, Gerde P, Hanberg A, Jernstrom B, Johansson C, Kyrklund T, Rannug A, Tornqvist M, Victorin K, Westerholm R. Cancer risk assessment,

indicators, and guidelines for polycyclic aromatic hydrocarbons in the ambient air. Environ Health Perspect 2002; 119:451–489.

111. Lewtas J, Nishioka MG. Nitroarenes: their detection, mutagenicity and occurrence in the environment. In: Howard P, ed. Nitroarenes: Occurence, Metabolism and Biological Impact. New York: Plenum Press, 1990:61–72.

112. Gallagher J, Heinrich U, George M, Hendee L, Phillips DH, Lewtas J. Formation of DNA adducts in rat lung following chronic inhalation of diesel emissions, carbon black and titanium dioxide particles. Carcinogenesis 1994; 15:1291–1299.

113. Cooper JA, Malek D. . Residential Solid Fuels, Environmental Impacts and Solutions. Oregon, USA: Oregon Graduate Center, 1981.

114. Purvis CR, McCrillis RC, Kariher PH. Fine particulate matter (PM) and organic speciation of fire place emissions. Environ Sci Technol 2000; 34:1653–6158.

115. Hawthorne SB, Miller DJ, Barkley RM, Krieger MS. Identification of methoxylated phenols as candidate tracers for atmospheric wood smoke pollution. Environ Sci Technol 1988; 22:1191–1196.

116. Edye LA, Richards GN. Analysis of condensates from wood smoke: components derived from polysaccharides and lignins. Environ Sci Technol 1991; 25:1133–1137.

117. Hawthorne SB, Miller DJ, Langenfeld JJ, Krieger MS. PM-10 high-volume collection and quantitation of semi-and nonvolatile phenols, methoxylated phenols, alkanes, and polycyclic aromatic hydrocarbons from winter urban air and their relationship to wood smoke emissions. Environ Sci Technol 1992; 26:2251–2262.

118. Simoneit BRT, Rogge WF, Mazurek MA, Standley LJ, Hildemann LM, Cass GR. Lignin pyrolysis products, lignins, and resin acids as specific tracers of plant classes in emissions from biomass combustion. Environ Sci Technol 1993; 27:2533–2541.

119. Rogge WF, Hildemann LM, Mazurek MA, Cass GR, Simoneit BRT. Sources of fine organic aerosol: 9. Pine, oak, and synthetic log combustion in residential fireplaces. Environ Sci Technol 1998; 32:13–22.

120. Simpson C, Dills R, Katz B, Kalman D, Determination of levoglucosan in atmopheric fine particulate matter. J. Air Waste Manage June 2004. In press.

121. Schauer JJ, Cass GR. Source apportionment of wintertime gas-phase and particle-phase air pollutants using organic compounds as tracers. Environ Sci Technol 2000; 34:1821–1832.

122. Zheng M, Cass GR, Schauer JJ, Edgerton ES. Source apportionment of PM2.5 in the southeastern United States using solvent-extractable organic compounds as tracers. Environ Sci Technol 2002; 36:2361–2371.

123. Lewis CW, Baumgardner RE, Claxton LD, Lewtas J, Stevens RK. The contribution of wood smoke and motor vehicle emissions to ambient aerosol mutagenicity. Environ Sci Technol 1988; 22:968–971.

124. Lewis CW, Einfeld W. Origins of carbonaceous aerosol in Denver and Albuquerque during winter. Environ Int 1985; 11:243–247.

125. McMahon, CK, Bush, PB, Woolson EA. Release of copper, chromium, and arsenic from burning wood treated with preservatives. APCA 1985; 4:56–72.

126. Zeedij IH. Polycyclic aromatic hydrocarbon concentrations in smoke aerosol of domestic stoves burning wood and coal. J Aerosol Sci 1986; 17:635–638.

127. Freeman DJ, Cattell FC. Woodburning as a source of atmospheric polycyclic aromatic hydrocarbons. Environ Sci Technol 1990; 24:1581–1585.

128. McCrillis RC, Watts RR, Warren SH. Effects of operating variables on PAH emissions and mutagenicity of emissions from woodstoves. JAWMA 1992; 42:691–694.

129. Moeller M, Ramdahl T, Alfheim I, Schjoldager J. Mutagenic activity and PAH-analysis of airborne particles from a woodheating community in Norway. Environ Int 1985; 11:189–195.

130. Watts RR, Drago RJ, Merrill RG, Williams RW, Perry E, Lewtas J. Wood smoke impacted air: mutagenicity and chemical analysis of ambient air in a residential area of Juneau, Alaska. JAPCA 1988; 38:652–660.

131. Kleindienst TE, Shepson PB, Edney EO, Claxton LD, Cupitt LT. Wood smoke: measurement of the mutagenic activities of its gas and particulate phase photoxidation products. Environ Sci Technol 1986; 20:493–501.

132. Nishioka MG, Lewtas J. Quantification of nitro-and hydroxylated nitro-aromatic/poly-cyclic aromatic hydrocarbons in selected ambient air daytime winter samples. Atmos Environ 1992; 26A:2077–2087.

133. Ward DE, Hardy CC. Smoke emissions from wildland fires. Environ Int 1991; 17:117–134.

134. Susott R, Ward D, Babbitt R, Latham D. Fire dynamics and chemistry of large fires. In: Levine JS, ed. Global Biomass Burning: Atmospheric Climate and Biospheric Implications. Cambridge, MA: MIT Press 1991.

135. Chi CT, Horn DA, Reznik RB, et al. Source assessment: prescribed burning, state of the art. EPA 600/2-79–019h US Environmental Protection Agency, Office of Research and Development, Research Triangle Park, NC, 1979:106.

136. US EPA. Prescribed burning background document and technical information document for prescribed burning best available control measures. EPA-450/2-92–003. 1992 Research Triangle Park, NC: Office of Air Quality Planning and Standards, 317.

137. US EPA 1998. Compilation of Air Pollutant Emission Factors (AP-42). Vol. I: Stationary Point and Area Sources. 5th ed. 1998 US EPA. Table 2.5-5 (Headfire burning of wheat refuse).

138. Ramdahl T, Moller M. Chemical and biological characterization of emissions from a cereal straw burning furnace. Chemosphere 1983; 12:23–34.

139. Jenkins BM, Jones AD, Turn SQ, Williams RB. Emission factors for polycyclic aromatic hydrocarbons from biomass burning. Environ Sci Technol 1996; 30:2462–2469.

140. Jenkins BM, Jones AD, Turn SQ, Williams RB. Particle concentrations, gas-particle partitioning, and species intercorrelations for polycyclic aromatic hydrocarbons (PAH) emitted during biomass burning. Atmos Environ 1996; 30:3825–3835.

141. Dennis A, Fraser M, Anderson A, Allen D. Air pollutant emissions associated with forest, grassland and agricultural burning in Texas. Atmos Environ 2002; 36:3779–3792.

142. Shea RW, Shea BW, Kaufmann JB, Ward DE, Haskins CI, Scholes MC. Fuel biomass and combustion factors associated with fires in savanna ecosystems of South Africa and Zambia. J Geophys Res 1996; 101(D19):23551–23568.

143. Kim E, Larson TV, Hopke PK, Slaughter C, Sheppard LE, Claiborn C. Source identification of PM2.5 in an arid Northwest US City by positive matrix factorization. Atmos Res 2003; 66:291–305.

144. Maga JA. Polycyclic aromatic hydrocarbon (PAH) composition of mesquite (Prosopis Fuliflora) smoke and grilled beef. J Agric Food Chem-ACS 1986; 34:249.

145. Ross DI, Upton SL, Hall DJ, Bennett IP. Preliminary measurement of ultra-fine aerosol emissions from gas cooking. Proc Indoor Air 1999; 4:1043–1048.

146. Rogge WF, Hildemann LM, Mazuerk MA, Cass GR, Simoneit BRT. Sources of fine organic aerosol 1. Charbroilers and meat cooking operations. Environ Sci Technol 1991; 25:1112–1125.

147. Rogge WF, Hildemann LM, Mazurek MA, Cass GR, Simoneit BRT. Sources of fine organic aerosol. 5. Natural Gas Home Appl. Environ Sci Technol 1993; 27:2736–2744.

148. Rogge WF, Cui W, Zhang Z, Yan Y, Sit S. Characterizations of gaseous and particulate emissions from natural gas cooking flames on a molecular level. In: Proceedings of Symposium on Engineering Solutions to Indoor Air Quality Problems, Research Triangle Park, NC, July 1997:128–136.

149. Rogge WG, Cui W, Yan Y, Zhang Z, Sit S. Organic PM2.5 emissions from residential cooking, Proceedings of the International State of the Science Workshop on Organic Speciation in Atmos Aerosols Res, April, 2004; available at: http://ocs.fortlewis.edu/Aerosols/SPECIATION/default.htm.

150. Nolte CG, Schauer JJ, Cass GR, Simoneit BRT. Highly polar organic compounds present in meat smoke. Environ Sci Technol 1999; 33:3313–3316.

151. Schauer JJ, Kleeman MJ, Cass GR, Simoneit BRT. Measurement of emissions from air pollution sources Cl through C29 organic compounds from meat charbroiling. Environ Sci Technol 1999; 33:1566–1577.

152. Kleeman MJ, Schauer JJ, Cass GR. Size and composition distribution of fine particulate matter emitted from wood burning, meat charbroiling, and cigarettes. Environ Sci Technol 1999; 33(20):3516–3523.

153. Shuguang L, Dinhua P, Guoxiong W. Analysis of polycyclic aromatic hydrocarbons in cooking oil fumes. Arch Environ Health 1994; 49:119–122.

154. Raiyani CV, Shah SH, Desai NM, Venkaiah K, Patel JS, Parikh DJ, Kashyap SK. Characterization and problems of indoor pollution due to cooking stove smoke. Atmos Environ 1993; 27A:1643–1655.

155. Brauer M, Hirtle R, Lang B, Ott W. Assessment of indoor fine aerosol contributions from environmental tobacco smoke and cooking with a portable nephelometer. J Exp Anal Enviroon Epi 2000; 10:136–144.

156. Thiebaud HP, Knize MG, Kuzmicky PA, et al. Mutagenicity and chemical analysis of fumes from cooking meat. J Agric Food Chem 1994; 42:1502–1510.

157. Shields PG, Xu GX, Blot WJ, Fraumeni JF Jr, Trivers GE, Pellizzari ED, Qu YH, Gao YT, Harris CC. Mutagens from Heated Chinese and U.S. Cooking Oils J NCI 1995; 87:836–841.

158. IARC. World Health Organization. Tobacco smoking (Monograph 38). Geneva, Switzerland, International Agency for Research on cancer. IARC Monographs on the Evaluation of the Carcinogenic Risk of Chemicals to Humans, 1986.

159. US EPA Respiratory Health Effects of Passive Smoking: Lung Cancer and Other Disorders. 1993 EPA/600/6-90/006F available at: http://cfpub 1. epa. gov/ncea/cfm/smoking. cfm? ActType=default.

160. California Environmental Protection Agency. (CAL-EPA, OEHHA) Health Effects of Exposure to Environmental Tobacco Smoke. 1997 http://www.oehha.org/air/environmental_tobacco/finalets.html.

161. California Environmental Protection Agency. (CAL-EPA, OEHHA) Proposed Identication of Environmental Tobacco Smoke as a Toxic Air Contaminant. 2003 http: //www.arb.ca.gov/toxics/ets/dreport/dreport.htm.

162. Hecht SS. Tobacco smoke carcinogens and lung cancer. J Natl Cancer Inst, 1999; 91(14):1194–1210.

163. Brunnemann KD, Hoffmann D. Analytical studies on tobacco-specific *N*-nitrosamines in tobacco and tobacco smoke. Crit Rev Toxicol 1991; 21(4):235–240.

164. Lofroth G, Burton RM, Forehand L, Hammond SK, Seila RL, Zweidinger RB, Lewtas J. Characterization of environmental tobacco smoke. Environ Sci Technol 1989; 23:610–614.

165. Watts RR, Langone JJ, Knight GJ, Lewtas J. Cotinine analytical workshop report: consideration of analytical methods for determining cotinine in human body fluids as a measure of passive exposure to tobacco smoke. Environ Health Perspect 1990; 84:173–182.

166. CDC. First National Report on Human Exposure to Environmental Chemicals, NCEH, Dept. Health & Human Services, March 2001 Atlanta GA (http://www.cdc.gov/exposurereport/).

167. Mumford JL, Chapman RS, Harris DB. Indoor air exposure to coal and wood combustion emissions associated with a high lung cancer rate in Xuan Wei, China. Environ Int 1989; 15:315–320.

168. Mumford JL, Chapman RS, Nesnow S, Helmes CT, Li X. Mutagenicity, carcinogenicity, and human cancer risk from indoor exposure to coal and wood combustion in Xuan Wei, China. In: Waters MD, Daniel FB, Lewtas J, Moore MM, Nesnow S, eds. Genetic Toxicology of Complex Mixtures. New York: Plenum Press, 1990:157–164.

169. Grimmer G, Brune H, Dettbarn G, Jacob J, Misfeld J, Mohr, U, Naujack K-W, Timm J, Wenzel-Hartung R. Contribution of polycyclic aromatic hydrocarbons and other polycyclic aromatic compounds to the carcinogenicity of combustion source and air pollution. In: Waters MD, Daniel FB, Lewtas J, Moore MM, Nesnow S, eds. Genetic Toxicology of Complex Mixtures. New York: Plenum Press, 1990:127–140.

170. Lewtas J. Complex mixtures of air pollutants: characterizing the cancer risk of polycyclic organic matter (POM). Environ Health Perspect 1993; 100:211–218.

171. Lewtas J, Zweidinger RB, Cupitt L. Mutagenicity, tumorigenicity and estimation of cancer risk from ambient aerosol and source emissions from woodsmoke and motor vehicles. AWMA 1991; 91–131.6:1–12.

172. Cupitt L, Glen WG, Lewtas J. Exposure and risk from ambient particle-bound pollution in an airshed dominated by residential wood combustion and mobile sources. Environ Health Perspect 1994; 102:75–84.

173. Lovelace Respiratory Research Institute. Final Technical Report for US EPA Assistance Agreement CR5826442–01-0, National Environmental Respiratory Center. November 2003, 29 pp. http://www.nercenter.org/EPAFinalRpt.pdf.

174. McDonald JD, Zielinska B, Fujita EM, Sagebiel JC, Chow JC, Watson JG. Fine particle and gaseous emission rates from residential wood combustion. Environ Sci Technol 2000; 34:2080–2091.

175. Tesfaigzi Y, Singh SP, Foster JE, Kubatko J, Barr EB, Fine PM, McDonald JD, Hahn FF, Mauderly JL. Health effects of subchronic exposure to low levels of wood smoke in rats. Toxicol Sci 2002; 65:115–125.

176. DeMarini DM, Williams RW, Perry E, Lemieux PM, Linak WP. Bioassay-directed chemical analysis of organic extracts of emissions from a laboratory-scale incinerator: combustion of surrogate compounds. Combust Sci Technol 1992; 85:437–453.

177. Li C-T, Zhuang H-K, Hsieh L-T, Lee W-J, Tsao M-C. PAH emission from the incineration of three plastic wastes. Environ Int 2001; 27:61–67.

178. Linak WP, Ryan TV, Perry E, Williams RW, DeMarini DM. Chemical and biological characterization of products of incomplete combustion from the simulated field burning of agricultural plastic. J Air Pollut Control Assoc 1989; 39:836–846.

179. Linak WP, McSorley JA, Hall RE, Srivastava RK, Ryan JV, Mulholland JA, Nishioka MG, Lewtas J, DeMarini DM. Application of staged combustion and reburning to the co-firing of nitrogen-containing wastes. Haz Waste Haz Matls 1991; 8:1–15.

180. Watts RR, Lemieux PM, Grote RA, Lowans RW, Williams RW, Brooks LR, Warren SH, DeMarini DM, Bell DA, Lewtas J. Development of source testing, analytical, and mutagenicity bioassay procedures for evaluating emissions from municipal and hospital waste combustors. Environ Health Perspect 1992; 98:227–234.

181. DeMarini DM, Lemieux PM, Ryan JV, Brooks LR, Williams RW. Mutagenicity and chemical analysis of emissions from the open burning of scrap rubber tires. Environ Sci Technol 1994; 28:136–141.

182. Lemieux PM, Ryan JV, DeMarini DM, Bryant DW, McCarry BE. Tires, open burning. In: Meyers RA, ed. Encyclopedia of Environmental Analysis and Remediation. New York: Wiley & Sons Inc., 1998:4813–4832.

183. DeMarini DM, Houk VS, Lewtas J, Williams RW, Nishioka MG, Srivastava RK, Ryan JV, McSorley JA, Hall RE, Linak WP. Measurement of mutagenic emissions from the incineration of the pesticide dinoseb during the application of combustion modifications. Environ Sci Technol 1991; 25: 910–913.

184. DeMarini DM, Williams RW, Brooks LR, Taylor MS. Use of cyanopropyl-bonded HPLC column for bioassay-directed fractionation of organic extracts from incinerator emissions. Int J Environ Anal Chem 1992; 48:187–199.

185. Linak WP, Mulholland JA, McSorley JA, Hall RE, Srivastava RK, Ryan JV, Nishioka MG, Lewtas J, DeMarini DM. Application of staged combustion

and reburning to the co-firing of nitrogen-containing wastes. Haz Waste Haz Matls 1991; 8:1–15.

186. Shepson PB, Kleindienst TE, Edney EO. The Production of Mutagenic Compounds as a Result of Urban Photochemistry, EPA 600/3-87/020, NTIS PB87–199675, 1987.

187. Arey J. Atmospheric reactions of PAHs including formation of nitroarenes. In: Neilson AH, ed. PAHs and Related Compounds—Chemistry. The Handbook of Environmental Chemistry. Vol. 3. Hutzinger O, Series Ed. Anthropogenic Compound Part I. Berlin, Heidelberg: New York, Springer-Verlag 1998: 347–385.

188. Gupta P, Harger WP, Arey J. The contribution of nitro-and methylnitro-naphthalenes to the vapor-phase mutagenicity of ambient air samples. Atmos Environ 1996; 30:3157–3166.

189. Arey J, Atkinson R. Formation of mutagens from the atmospheric photo-oxidations of PAH and their occurrence in ambient air. 1994. Research Note 94-22 NTIS Report NTIS No. PB95–104931.

190. Arey J, Atkinson R. Photochemical reactions of PAHs in the atmosphere. In: Douben PET, ed. PAHs: An Ecotoxicological Perspective. West Sussex, UK: Wiley, 47–63.

191. Phousongphouang PT, Arey J. Sources of the atmospheric contaminants, 2-nitrobenzanthrone and 3-nitrobenzanthrone. Atmos Environ :3189–3199.

192. Sasaki J, Arey J, Harger WP. Formation of mutagens from the photooxidations of 2-4-ring PAH. Environ Sci Technol :1324–1335.

193. Sasaki J, Aschmann SM, Kwok ESC, Atkinson R, Arey J. Products of the gas-phase OH and NO_3 radical-initiated reactions of naphthalene. Environ Sci Technol 31:3173–3179.

194. Sasaki JC, Arey J, Eastmond DA, Parks KK, Grosovsky AJ. Genotoxicity induced in human lymphoblasts by atmospheric reaction products of naphthalene and phenanthrene. Mutat Res 1997; 393:23–35.

195. Sasaki JC, Arey J, Eastmond DA, Parks KK, Phousongphouang PT, Grosovsky AJ. Evidence for oxidative metabolism in the genotoxicity of the atmospheric reaction product 2-nitronaphthalene in human lymphoblastoid cell lines. Mutat Res 1999; 445:113–125.

196. Henry, RC. Current factor-analysis receptor models are iii-posed. Atmos Environ 1987; 21:1815–1820.

197. Gordon G. Receptor models. Environ Sci Technol 1988; 22:1132–1142.

198. Miller MS, Friedlander SK, Hidy GM. A chemical element balance for the Pasadena aerosol. J Colloid Interface Sci 1972; 39:165–176.

199. Watson JG, Robinson NF, Chow JC, Henry RC, Kim BM, Pace TG, Meyer EL, Nguyen Q. . Environ Software 1990; 5:38–49.

200. Hopke PK. Receptor Modeling for Air Quality Management. Amsterdam: Elsevier, 1991.

201. Paatero, P. Least squares formulation of robust non-negative factor analysis. Chemom Intell Lab Sys. 1997; 37:23–35.

202. Ramadan Z, Song XH, Hopke PK. Identification of sources of Phoenix aerosol by positive matrix factorization. J Air Waste Manage Assoc 2000; 50:1308–1320.

203. Henry RC. Chemometrics Intell Lab Syst 1997; 37:37–42.
204. Lewis CW, Norris GA, Conner TL, Henry RC. Source apportionment of phoenix PM2.5 aerosol with the Unmix receptor model. J Air Waste Manage Assoc 2003; 53(3):325–338.
205. Kim E, Claiborn C, Sheppard L, Larson T. Source identification of $PM_{2.5}$ in an arid northwest US city by positive matrix factorization. Atmos Res 2003; 66:291–305.
206. Kim E, Hopke PK, Paatero P, Edgerton ES. Incorporation of parametric factors into multilinear receptor model studies of Atlanta aerosol. Atmos Environ 2003; 37:5009–5021.
207. Paatero, P. The multilinear engine—a table-driven least squares program for solving multilinear problems, including the *n*-way parallel factor analysis model. J Comput Graphical Stat 1999; 8:854–888.
208. Kim E, Hopke PK, Larson TV, Maykut NN, and Lewtas J. Factor analysis of seattle fine particles. Aerosol Sci Technol 2004, In press.
209. Ramadan Z, Eickhout B, Song XH, Buydens L, Hopke PK. Comparison of positive matrix factorization (PMF) and multilinear engine (ME-2) for the source apportionment of particulate pollutants. Chemom Intell Lab Syst 2003; 66:15–28.
210. Lewis CW. Sources of air pollutants indoors: VOC and fine particulate species. J Exposure Anal Environ Epidemiol 1991; 1:31–44.
211. Lewis CW and Zweidinger RB. Apportionment of residential indoor aerosol, VOC, and aldehyde species to indoor and outdoor sources, and their source strengths. Atmos Environ 1992; 26:521–527.
212. Yakovleva E, Hopke P, Wallace L. Receptor modeling assessment of particle total exposure assessment methodology data. Environ Sci Technol 1999; 33:3645–3652.
213. Larson T, Gould T, Simpson C, Claiborn C, Lewtas J, Liu L-J S. Source apportionment of indoor, outdoor and personal PM2.5 in Seattle, WA using positive matrix factorization. J Air Waste Manage 2004, In press.
214. Hopke P, Ramadan Z, Paatero P, Norris G, Landis MS, Williams R, Lewis, C. Receptor modeling of ambient and personal exposure samples: 1998 Baltimore Particulate Matter Epidemiology-Exposure Study. Atmos Environ 2003; 37:3289–3302.
215. Liu L-JS, Box M, Kalman D, Kaufman J, Koenig J, Larson T, Lumley T, Sheppard L, Wallace L. Exposure assessment of particulate matter for susceptible populations in Seattle, WA. Environ Health Perspect 2003; 111(7):909–918.
216. Burnett RT, Brook J, Dann T, Delocla C, Philips O, Cakmak S, Vincent R, Goldberg MS, Krewski D. Association between particulate- and gas-phase components of urban air pollution and daily mortality in eight Canadian cities. In: Grant LD, ed. PM2000: Particulate Matter and Health. Inhalation Toxicol 2000; 12(suppl 4):15–39.
217. Burnett RT, Goldberg MS. Size-fractionated particulate mass and daily mortality in eight Canadian cities. In: Revised Analyses of Time-Series Studies of Air Pollution and Health. Special Report. Boston, MA: Health Effects Institute, 2003:85–90.

218. Fairley D. Mortality and air pollution for Santa Clara County, California, 1989-1996. In: Revised Analyses of Time-Series Studies of Air Pollution and Health. Special Report. Boston, MA: Health Effects Institute, 2003:97–106.

219. Goldberg MS, Bailar JC III, Burnett RT, Brook JR, Tamblyn R, Bonvalot Y, Ernst P, Flegel KM, Singh RK, Valois M-F. Identifying Subgroups of the General Population that May Be Susceptible to Short-Term Increases in Particulate Air Pollution: A Time-series Study in Montreal, Quebec. Cambridge, MA: Health Effects Institute, 2000, Research Report 97.

220. Ito K. Associations of particulate matter components with daily mortality and morbidity in Detroit, Michigan. In: Revised Analyses of Time-Series Studies of Air Pollution and Health. Special Report. Boston, MA: Health Effects Institute, 2003:143–156.

221. Lipfert FW, Morris SC, Wyzga RE. Daily mortality in the Philadelphia metropolitan area and size-classified particulate matter. J Air Waste Manage Assoc 2000; 50:1501–1513.

222. Lippmann M, Ito K, Nadas A, Burnett RT. Association of Particulate Matter Components with Daily Mortality and Morbidity in Urban Populations. Cambridge, MA: Health Effects Institute, 2000, Research report no. 95.

223. Klemm RJ, Mason RM Jr. Aerosol research and inhalation epidemiological study (ARIES): air quality and daily mortality statistical modeling—interim results. J. Air Waste Manage Assoc 2000; 50:1433–1439.

224. Hoek G, Brunekreef B, Verhoeff A, van Wijnen J, Fischer, P. Daily mortality and air pollution in the Netherlands. J Air Waste Manage Assoc 2000; 50:1380–1389.

225. Hoek, G. Daily mortality and air pollution in The Netherlands. In: Revised Analyses of Time-Series Studies of Air Pollution and Health. Special Report. Boston, MA: Health Effects Institute, 2003:133–142.

226. Laden F, Neas LM, Dockery DW, Schwartz, J. Association of fine particulate matter from different sources with daily mortality in six U.S. cities. Environ Health Perspect 2000; 108:941–947.

227. Schwartz, J. Daily deaths associated with air pollution in six US cities and short-term mortality displacement in Boston. In: Revised Analyses of Time-Series Studies of Air Pollution and Health. Special Report. Boston, MA: Health Effects Institute, 2003:219–226.

228. Mar TF, Norris GA, Koenig JQ, Larson TV. Associations between air pollution and mortality in Phoenix, 1995–1997. Environ Health Perspect 2000; 108:347–353.

229. Mar TF, Norris GA, Larson TV, Wilson WE, Koenig JQ. Air pollution and cardiovascular mortality in Phoenix, 1995–1997. In: Revised Analyses of Timeseries Studies of Air Pollution and Health. Special Report. Boston, MA: Health Effects Institute, 2003:177–182.

230. Tsai FC, Apte MG, Daisey JM. An exploratory analysis of the relationship between mortality and the chemical composition of airborne particulate matter. Inhalation Toxicol 2000; 12(suppl):121–135.

231. Özkaynak H, Xue J, Zhou H, Raizenne, M. Associations Between Daily Mortality and Motor Vehicle Pollution in Toronto, Canada. Boston, MA: Harvard

University School of Public Health, Department of Environmental Health, 1996, March 25.

232. Koutrakis P, Briggs S, Leaderer B. Source apportionment of indoor aerosols in Suffolk and Onondaga Counties, New York. Environ Sci Technol 1992; 26:521–527.

233. Stevens RK, Lewis CW, Dzubay TG, Cupitt LT, Lewtas J. Sources of mutagenic activity in urban fine particles. Toxicol Indust Health 1990; 6(5):81–94.

234. Lewtas J. Emerging methodologies for assessment of complex mixtures: application of bioassays in the Integrated Air Cancer Project. Toxicol Indust Health 5:81–94.

235. Lewtas, J. Complex mixtures of air pollutants: characterizing the cancer risk of poly cyclic organic matter (POM). Environ Health Perspect 1993; 100:211–218.

236. CDC. Second National Report on Human Exposure to Environmental Chemicals, NCEH, Dept Health & Human Services, Pub No. 02-0716 March 2003, Atlanta, GA (http: //www.cdc.gov/exposurereport/).

237. Samet JM. Workshop summary: assessing exposure to environmental tobacco smoke in the workplace. Environ Health Perspect 1999; 107S2:309–312.

238. Benowitz NL. Cotinine as a biomarker of environmental tobacco smoke exposure. Epidemiol Rev 1996; 18:188–204.

239. Benowitz NL. Biomarkers of environmental tobacco smoke exposure. Environ Health Perspect 1999; 107(suppl 2):349–355.

240. National Research Council. Environmental Tobacco Smoke. Measuring Exposures and Assessing Health Effects. Washington: National Academy Press, 1986.

241. Pirkle JL, Flegal KM, Bernert JT, Brody DJ, Etzel RA, Maurer KR. Exposure of the US population to environmental tobacco smoke. The Third National Health and Nutrition Examination Survey, 1988 to 1991. JAMA 1996; 275:1233–1240.

242. IARC. World Health Organization. Tobacco Smoke and Involuntary Smoking (Monograph 83). Geneva, Switzerland, International Agency for Research on Cancer. IARC Monographs on the Evaluation of the Carcinogenic Risk of Chemicals to Humans, 2004.

243. Hecht SS. Human urinary carcinogen metabolites: biomarkers for investigating tobacco and cancer. Carcinogenesis 2002; 23:907–922.

244. Hecht SS. Carcinogen derived biomarkers: applications in studies of human exposure to secondhand tobacco smoke. Tobacco Control 2003; 13(suppl I): i48–i56.

245. Hecht SS, Ye M, Carmella SG, Fredrickson A, Adgate JL, Greaves IA, Church TR, Ryan AD, Mongin SJ, Sexton K. Metabolites of a tobacco-specific lung carcinogen in the urine of elementary school-aged children. Cancer Epidemiol Biomarkers Prev 2001; 10:1109–1116.

246. Mattson ME, Boyd G, Byar D, Brown C, Callahan CF, Corle D, Cullen JW, Greenblatt J, Haley NJ, Hammond SK, Lewtas J, Reeves W. Passive smoking on commercial airline flights. J Am Med Assoc 1989; 261(6):867–872.

247. Henderson FW, Reid HF, Morris R, O-L, Wang O-L, Hu PC, Helms RW, Forehand L, Mumford J, Lewtas J, Haley NJ, Hammond SK. Home air

nicotine levels and urinary continine excretion in preschool children. Am Rev Resp Dis 1989; 140:197–201.

248. Collier AM, Goldstein GM, Shrewsbury RP, Davis SM, Koch GG, Zhang C, Benowitz NL, Williams RW, Lewtas J. Cotinine elimination following ETS exposure in young children as a function of age, sex, and race. Indoor Environ 1994; 3:353–359.

249. National Academy of Sciences. Polycyclic Aromatic Hydrocarbons: Evaluation of Sources and Effects. Washington, DC, National Research Council, 1983.

250. Dipple A. Polynuclear aromatic carcinogens. In: Searle CE, ed. Chemical Carcinogens. Washington, DC, American Chemical Society, 1976:245–314.

251. Pott P. "Chimrgical Observations" (1775) Reprinted in Natl Cancer Inst Monograph 1963; 10:7.

252. Cook JW, Hewett CL, Hieger I. J Chem Soc 1933; 395.

253. Pitts JN Jr. Nitration of gaseous polyaromatic hydrocarbons in simulated and ambient urban atmospheres: a source of mutagenic nitroarenes. Atmos Environ 1987; 21:2531–2547.

254. Arey J. Atmospheric reactions of PAHs including formation of nitroarenes. In: Neilson AH, Hutzinger O, Series ed. PAHs and Related Compounds. The Handbook of Environmental Chemistry. Vol. 3. Berlin: Springer-Verlag, 1998:347–385.

255. Environment Canada. Ambient Air Measurements of Polycyclic Aromatic Hydrocarbons (PAH), Polychlorinated Dibenzo-p-Dioxins (PCDD) and Polychlorinated Dibenzofurans in Canada (1987–1997), Environmental Technology Center Report, available at: http ://www.etc-cte.ec.gc.ca/publications/recent/pah_report_e.html.

256. Jongeneelen FJ, Bos RP, Anzion RBM, Theuws JLG, Henderson PT. Biological monitoring of polycyclic aromatic hydrocarbons. Metabolites in urine. Scand J Work Environ Health 1986; 12:137–143.

257. Goen T, Gundel J, Schaller KH, Angerer J. The elimination of 1-hydroxypyrene in the urine of the general population and workers with different occupational exposures to PAH. Sci Total Environ 1995; 163(1–3):195–201.

258. Cho SH, Kang JW, Ju YS, Sung JH, Lee CK, Lee YS, Strickland PT, Kang DH. Use of urinary PAH metabolites to assess PAH exposure intervention among coke oven workers. J Occup Health 2000; 42:138–143.

259. Szaniszlo J, Ungvary G. Polycyclic aromatic hydrocarbon exposure and burden of outdoor workers in Budapest. J Toxicol Environ Health A 2001; 62(5):297–306.

260. Roggi C, Minoia C, Sciarra GF, Apostoli P, Maccarini L, Magnaghi S. Urinary 1-hydroxypyrene as a marker of exposure to pyrene: an epidemiological survey on a general population group. Sci Total Environ 1997; 199(3): 247–254.

261. Strickland PT, Kang DH. Urinary 1-hydroxypyrene and other PAH metabolites as biomarkers of exposure to environmental PAH in air particulate matter. Toxicol Lett 1999; 108:191–199.

262. Gundel J, Mannschreck C, Buttner K, Ewers U, Angerer J. Urinary levels of 1-hydroxypyrene, 1-, 2-, 3-, and 4-hydroxyphenanthrene in females living in

an industrial area of Germany. Arch Environ Contam Toxicol 1996; 31(4):585–590.

263. Jongeneelen FJ. Biological monitoring of environmental exposure to polycyclic aromatic hydrocarbons; 1-hydroxypyrene in urine of people. Toxicol Lett 1994; 72(l–3):205–2ll.

264. Kanoh T, Fukuda M, Onozuka H, Kinouchi T, Ohnishi Y. Urinary 1-hydroxypyrene as a marker of exposure to polycyclic aromatic hydrocarbons in environment. Environ Res 1993; 62(2):230–241.

265. Chuang JC, Callahan PJ, Lyu CW, Wilson NK. Polycyclic aromatic hydrocarbon exposures of children in low-income families. J Expo Anal Environ Epidemiol 1999; 9:85–98.

266. van Wijnen JH, Slob R, Jongmans-Liedekerken G, van de Weerdt RH, Woudenberg F. Exposure to polycyclic aromatic hydrocarbons among Dutch children. Environ Health Perspect 1996; 104(5):530–534.

267. Williams RW, Watts RR, Stevens RK, Stone CL, Lewtas J. Evaluation of a personal air sampler for twenty-four hour collection of fine particles and semivolatile organics. J Expos Anal Environ Epidemiol 1999; 2:158–166.

268. Nielsen PS, Andreassen Å, Farmer PB, Øvrebø S, Autrap H. Biomonitoring of diesel exhaust-exposed workers. DNA and hemoglobin adducts and urinary 1-hydroxypyrene as markers of exposure.. Toxicol Lett 1996; 86:27–37.

269. Hemminki K, Dickey C, Karlsson S, Bell D, Hsu Y, Tsai W-Y, Mooney LA, Savela K, Perera FP. Aromatic DNA adducts in foundry workers in relation to exposure, life style and CYP1A1 and glutathione transferase Ml genotype. Carcinogenesis 1997; 18:345–350.

270. Autrup H, Daneshvar B, Dragsted LO, Gamborg M, Hansen AM, Loft S, Okkels H, Nielsen F, Nielsen PS, Raffn E, Wallin H, Knudsen LE. Biomarkers for exposure to ambient air pollution—comparison of carcinogen-DNA adduct levels with other exposure markers and markers for oxidative stress. Environ Health Perspect 1999; 107:233–238.

271. Lee CK, Cho SH, Kang JW, Lee SJ, Ju YS, Sung JH, Strickland PT, Kang DH. Comparison of three analytical methods for 1-hydroxypyrene-glucuronide in urine after non-occupational exposure to poly cyclic aromatic hydrocarbons. Toxicol Lett 1999; 108:209–215.

272. Smith CJ, Huang WL, Walcott CJ, Turner W, Grainger J, Patterson DG Jr. Quantification of monohydroxy-PAH metabolites in urine by solid-phase extraction with isotope dilution GC-HRMS. Anal Bioanal Chem 2002; 372:216–220.

273. Heudorf U, Angerer J. Internal exposure to PAHs of children and adults living in homes with parquet flooring containing high levels of PAHs in the parquet glue. Int Arch Occup Environ Health 2001; 74:91–101.

274. Dills RL, Zhu X, Kalman DA. Measurement of urinary methoxyphenols and their use for biological monitoring of wood smoke exposure. Environ Res 2001; 85:145–158.

275. Simpson, CD, Dills RL, Katz BS, Kalman DA. Determination of levoglucosan in atmospheric fine particulate matter. JAWMA 2004; 54:689–694.

276. Simpson CD. Contributions from Outdoor PM Sources to Indoor and Personal PM Exposures, International Workshop on Organic Speciation in

Atmospheric Aerosol Research, http://ocs.fortlewis.edu/Aerosols/ SPE-CIATION /Synopsis_topic7.htm.

277. Harris CC, Weston A, Willey JC, Trivers GE, Mann DL. Biochemical and molecular epidemiology of human cancer: indicators of carcinogen exposure, DNA damage, and genetic predisposition. Environ Health Perspect 1987; 75:109–119.

278. Bell DA, Taylor JA, Paulson DF, Robertson CN, Mohler JL, Lucier GW. Genetic risk and carcinogen exposure: a common inherited defect of the carcinogen-metabolism gene glutathione-*S*-transferase M1 (GSTM1) that increases susceptibility to bladder cancer. J Natl Cancer Inst 1993; 85(14):1159–1164.

279. Perera FP, Mooney LA, Dickey CP, Santella RM, Bell D, Blaner W, Tang D, Whyatt RM. Molecular epidemiology in environmental carcinogenesis. Environ Health Perspect. 1996; 104S3:441–443.

280. Perera F. Environment and cancer: who are susceptible? Science 1997; 278: 1066–1073.

281. Rothman N, Hayes RB. Environ Health Perspect 1995; 103(suppl 8):00–00.

282. Harris CC. Molecular epidemiology: overview of biochemical and molecular basis. In: Groopman JD, Skipper PL, eds. Molecular Dosimetry and Human Cancer: Analytical Epidemiological and Social Considerations. Boca Raton, FL: CRC Press, 1991:15–26.

283. Perera FP, Whyatt RM. Biomarkers and molecular epidemiology in mutation/cancer research. Mutat Res 1994; 313(2–3):117–129.

284. Perera FP, Hemminki K, Grzybowska E, Motykiewicz G, Michalska J, Santella RM, Young TL, Dickey C, Brandt-Rauf P, De Vivo I, Blaner W, Tsai WY, Chorazy M. Molecular and genetic damage in humans from environmental pollution in Poland. Nature 1992; 360:256–258.

285. Binkova B, Topinka J, Mrackova G, Gajdosova D, Vidova P, Stavkova Z, Peterka V,Pilcik T, Rimar V, Dobias L, Farmer PB, Sram RJ. Coke oven workers study: the effect of exposure and GSTM1 and NAT2 genotypes on DNA adduct levels in white blood cells and lymphocytes as determined by 32P-postlabelling. Mutat Res 1998; 416(1–2):67–84.

286. Perera FP. Molecular epidemiology and prevention of cancer. Environ Health Perspect 1995; 103(suppl 8):233–236.

287. Schulte PA, Rothman N, Perera FP, Talaska G. Biomarkers of exposure in cancer epidemiology. Epidemiology 1995; 6:637–638.

288. Vineis P, Martone T. Genetic–environmental interaction and low-level exposure to carcinogens. Epidemiology 1995; 6:455–457.

289. Costa DJ, Slott V, Binkova, B, Myers SR, Lewtas J. Influence of GSTM1 and NAT2 genotypes on the relationship between personal exposure to PAH and biomarkers of internal dose. Biomarkers 1998; 3:411–424.

290. Hayes JD, Pulford DJ. The glutathione-*S*-transferase supergene family: regulation of GST and the contribution of isoenzymes to cancer chemoprotection and drug resistance. Crit Rev Biochem Mol Biol 1995; 30:445–600.

291. Seidegard J, Ekstrom G. The role of human glutathione transferases and epoxide hydrolases in the metabolism of xenobiotics. Environ Health Perspect 1997; 105:791–799.

292. Kadlubar FF, Badawi AF. Genetic susceptibility and carcinogen-DNA adduct formation in human urinary bladder carcinogenesis. Toxicol Lett 1995; 82/83:627–632.

293. Culp SJ, Roberts DW, Talaska G, Lang NP, Fu PP, Lay JO, Teital CH, Snawder JE, VonTungeln LS, Kadlubar FF. Immunochemical, ^{32}P-postlabeling, and GC/MS detection of 4-aminobiphenyl-DNA adducts in human peripheral lung in relation to metabolic activation pathways involving pulmonary N-oxidation, conjugation, and peroxidation. Mutat Res 1997; 378:97–112.

294. Sram RJ. Future research directions to characterize environmental mutagens in highly polluted areas. Environ Health Perspect 1996; 104S3:603–607.

295. Lewtas J. Biomarkers of exposure and dose: case study of complex air pollution exposures in the Czech Republic. In: Kirk E, ed. Mixed Environmental Hazards and Health Washington, DC: American Association for the Advancement of Science, 2003:33–46.

296. Sram RJ, Binkova B. Molecular epidemiology studies on occupational and environmental exposure to mutagens and carcinogens, 1997–1999. Environ Health Perspect 2000; 108Sl:57–70.

297. Sram RJ. Teplice Program: Impact of Air Pollution on Human Health. Praha: Academia, 2001.

298. Robbins WA, Rubeš, J, Selevan, SG, Perreault, SD. Air pollution and sperm aneuploidy in healthy young men. Environ Epidemiol Toxicol 1999; 1:125–131.

299. Topinka J, Binková B, Mracková G, Stávková Z, Peterka V, Beneš I, Dejmek J, Leníek J, Pilík T, Šrám RJ. Influence of GSTM1 and NAT2 genotypes on placental DNA adducts in an environmentally exposed population. Environ Mol Mutagen 1997; 30:184–195.

300. Topinka J, Binková B, Dejmek J, Srám RJ. DNA adducts induced by environmental pollution in human placenta. Epidemiology 1995; 6:84.

301. Sram, RJ, Binkova, B, Rössner, P, Rubes, J, Topinka, J, Dejmek, J. Adverse reproductive outcomes from exposure to environmental mutagens. Mutat Res 1999; 428:203–215.

302. Perera FP, Whyatt RM, Jedrychowski W, Rauh V, Manchester D, Santella RM, et al. Recent developments in molecular epidemiology: a study of the effects of environmental polycylic aromatic hydrocarbons on birth outcomes in Poland. Am J Epidemiol 1998; 147:309–314.

303. Whyatt RM, Jedrychowski W, Hemminki K, Santella RM, Tsai WY, Yang K, et al. Biomarkers of polycyclic aromatic hydrocarbon-DNA damage and cigarette smoke exposures in paired maternal and newborn blood samples as a measure of differential susceptibility. Cancer Epidemiol Biomarker Prev 2001; 10:581–588.

304. Beland FA, Poirier MC. Significance of DNA adduct studies in animal models for cancer molecular dosimetry and risk assessment. Environ Health Perspect 1993; 99:5–10.

305. Farmer PB. Carcinogen adducts: use in diagnosis and risk assessment. Clin Chem 1994; 40(7):1438–1443.

306. Phillips DH, Farmer PB. Protein and DNA adducts as biomarkers of exposure to environmental mutagens. In: Phillips DH, Venitt S, eds. Environ Mutagen. Oxford: Bios: , 1995:367–395.

307. Farmer PB, Singh R, Kaur B, Sram RJ, Binkova B, Kalina I, Popov TA, Garte S, Taioli E, Gabelova A, Cebulska-Wasilewska A. Molecular epidemiology studies of carcinogenic environmental pollutants. Effects of polycyclic aromatic hydrocarbons (PAHs) in environmental pollution on exogenous and oxidative DNA damage. Mutat Res 2003; 544:397–402.

308. Farmer PB, Sepai O, Lawrence R, Autrup H, Sabro Nielsen P, et al. Biomonitoring human exposure to environmental carcinogenic chemicals. Mutagenesis 1996; 11:363–381.

309. Phillips DH. ^{32}P-Postlabelling: Special Issue of Mutation Research. Amsterdam: Elsevier, 1997:149.

310. Phillips DH. Detection of DNA modifications by the ^{32}P-postlabelling assay. Mutat Res 1997; 378:1–12.

12

Air Pollution, Public Health, and Regulatory Considerations

MORTON LIPPMANN

Nelson Institute of Environmental Medicine, School of Medicine,
New York University, Tuxedo, New York, U.S.A.

I. Historical Background
A. Community Air Contamination and Health

Community air contamination arising from the combustion of fossil fuels first received official recognition at the end of the 13th century, when Edward I of England issued an edict to the effect that, during sessions of Parliament, there should be no burning of sea coal or channel coal, so-called because it was brought from Newcastle to London by sea transport via ports on the English Channel. Despite a succession of further royal edicts, taxes, and even occasional prison confinements and torture, the use of coal for producing heat continued in London, especially as the increase in population led to a depletion in the availability of wood for fuel. The first scholarly report on the problem: "Fumifugium or the Inconvenience of Air and Smoke of London Dissipated, together with some Remedies Humbly Proposed" by John Evelyn, was published by the royal command of Charles II in 1661 (1). He recognized and discussed the problem in terms of the sources, effects, and feasibility of controls.

Unfortunately, no effective controls were instituted until after the report of the Royal Commission (2) on the effects of the "killer fog" of

December 1952, which attributed approximately 4000 excess deaths in London to that pollution episode. The report's retrospective examinations of vital statistics demonstrated that there had been numerous prior episodes involving excess deaths during periods of air stagnation in London and other British cities. The reductions in smoke levels achieved in Britain since the mid-1950s have eliminated readily observable excess deaths attributable to fossil fuel combustion, and have led to major beneficial changes in visibility and microclimate as well as health. Excess deaths attributable to coal smoke had also occurred elsewhere prior to 1952, but fortunately involved smaller populations. The most notable of these were in the Meuse Valley in Belgium in 1930 (3), and at Donora in Pennsylvania in 1948 (4).

By the 1990s, it became evident that fine particles in the ambient air were capable of producing excess mortality and morbidity at contemporary levels of air pollution. In response, a major research effort began to determine the causal components and biological mechanisms for such effects (5). Also, by the 1990s, the international aspects of air pollution had gained widespread recognition. This included not only conventional pollutant transport over the borders between the United States, Canada, and Mexico, but also stratospheric O_3 depletion in the polar regions caused by fluorocarbon emissions and global climate change caused by secular rises in carbon dioxide and methane releases associated with human economic activities. International agreements have drastically reduced fluorocarbon emissions.

While the focus of this chapter is on contaminants that are routinely encountered, mention should be made that occasional industrial accidents can be expected to occur. One of the world's worst industrial accidents occurred on December 2, 1984 at the Union Carbide Plant in Bhopal, India, where a release of a gas cloud of methyl isocyanate (MIC) killed over 3800 people. Among the more than 200,000 persons exposed to the gas, the initial death toll within a week following the accident was over 2000. By 1990, the Directorate of Claims in Bhopal had prepared medical folders for 361,966 of the exposed persons. Of these, 173,382 had temporary injuries and 18,922 had permanent injuries, with the recorded deaths totaling 3828 (6).

II. Public Perceptions of Air Pollution

Up to and through the beginning of the 20th century, there were two major categories of sources of air pollution. One was the combustion of biomass and/or coal. Combustion effluents from small sources caused obvious smoke and odor problems. The other category was industrial emissions from a relatively limited number of mining, refining, and manufacturing facilities. However, the industrial facilities were often concentrated in river valleys to take advantage of accessibility to water for plant operations and transport of raw materials and supplies and products, and river valleys were often both relatively densely populated and subject to temperature inversions and could experience fumigation events with noxious industrial air pollutants. By contrast, the dominant air pollution sources of the second half of the 20th century, i.e., motor vehicles and electric power generation were in their infancy in the first few decades, and more than 80% of the population lived in rural areas that were not influenced by city or industrial valley-based pollution.

Noxious odors and smoke from fuel combustion were traditionally tolerated because the heat they provided for cooking and warming occupied spaces was deemed to be essential, and few people had options for cleaner fuels. Also, industrial smokestacks were often viewed as an index of economic progress and opportunity for better paying and more secure jobs than those available in rural areas, and there was a continuing migration into the cities. This created a cycle in which the cities became both more populated and more polluted. However, the health effects of community air pollution were not always recognized because the migrants were mostly young adults and their children who did not exhibit readily detectable pollution-related health effects.

By 1930, air pollution resulting from coal combustion was getting noticeably worse, but the Great Depression and World War II were greater problems in the public's view, and it was not until mid-century that public perceptions and economic prosperity created opportunities to seriously address the growing problem of community air pollution from coal combustion and industrial operations. The Donora disaster of 1948 (4), and the London, England pollution episode of December 1952 (2) demonstrated to the public that significant mortality could follow peak levels of smoke pollution.

By mid-century, awareness of air pollution of an entirely different nature became evident. Whereas coal smoke pollution was black, oily, acidic, and reducing in character, pollution in Southern California, which began to cause substantial visibility reduction and damage to ornamental crops and rubber products, was whitish, and strongly oxidizing. While its demonstrated health effects were initially limited to reduced lung function and athletic performance, these effects were of some concern to residents of sunny California who greatly valued outdoor activity.

In the last few decades of the 20th century, it was demonstrated that it was possible to have both effective air pollution control and further economic growth and prosperity. In the United States, urban air pollution was substantially reduced in the 1960s by several factors. One was local law, most notably in California through the control of emissions of photochemical reaction precursors, and in northeastern urban centers in terms of restrictions on fuels and combustion processes. Another was the extension of natural gas pipelines from the states near the Gulf of Mexico to urban centers in the midwest and northeast states, providing a much cleaner burning fuel. Further reductions in pollution can be attributed to the actions taken by the states to implement the National Ambient Air Quality Standards (NAAQS) promulgated by the newly established U.S. Environmental Protection Agency (EPA) in 1971.

The NAAQS implementation plans were focussed on reducing ground level pollution and, in effect, encouraged power plants and smelters to erect taller smokestacks. Furthermore, the increasing amount of SO_2 emitted from these stacks had a greater residence time in the atmosphere, which resulted in a wider spread of both SO_2 and its atmospheric conversion products, sulfuric acid (H_2SO_4) and its ammonium salts, creating widespread regional visibility reductions and more acidic precipitation. The acid rain phenomenon and its effects on vegetation and aquatic life created more public awareness of air pollution and its public health as well as its ecological and economic impacts. Thus when, beginning in the mid-1980s, there were the first of an ever growing number of time-series studies linking daily mortality rates in urban centers with peak levels of particulate matter (PM) on the day of, or in the few days preceding the excess mortality, they helped re-establish the public's concern about the health effects of air pollution. This concern has been reinforced by emerging flood of further epidemiological studies that have shown not only increased rates of acute mortality in relation to pollution peaks, but also emergency department and hospital admissions, functional deficits, and lost-time from school and work. Recent reports documenting lifespan reductions from both cardiopulmonary and lung cancer causes in association with annual average concentrations of PM have further raised public concerns about current levels of ambient air pollution.

III. Measured Impacts of Airborne Particulate Matter on Public Health

Of all of the criteria pollutants, the greatest economic impacts on public health in terms of excess mortality have been attributed to PM, through its effects on the cardiovascular system. This section of the chapter on public health impacts is focussed on PM. The section that follows, on benefit–cost analyses for air pollution, briefly summarizes the established effects of the other criteria pollutants, such as ozone, which has been associated with effects on pulmonary function decrements and increased rates of hospital admissions for respiratory diseases.

This overview on quantitation of airborne PM on public health is limited to the past 130 years, when usable mortality data could be used to determine health impacts. A landmark event was the London smog of December 9–11, 1873, which produced a significant excess of human mortality, as well as mortality and pathological changes in show cattle that were on exhibit at that time. A similar smog episode of December 5–9, 1952 caused similar responses, and led to remedial action in the United Kingdom during the 1950s and 1960s that greatly reduced both black smoke (BS) concentrations and their public health impacts.

A summation of bronchitis mortality during and following the December 9–11, 1873 fog episode was tabulated in the Ministry of Health report (2) of the December 5–9, 1952 episode. As shown in Table 1, various 19th century fog episodes produced excesses in bronchitis deaths that were comparable to that reported for the more famous 1952 episode. Also, it is important to note the higher baseline bronchitis mortality for London in the late 19th century, when the population was below 3 million (compared to about 8 million in 1952), and at a time when that cigarette smoking could not have been a contributory cause.

The first scientific literature citation on the health effects of London smog was also related to the December 1873 episode. Some excerpts from this paper follow: excerpts from: The Veterinarian XL VII (7) follow.

THE EFFECTS OF THE LONDON FOG ON CATTLE IN LONDON

Our readers will have heard a good deal already about the terrible disturbance which was caused at the last show of the Smithfield Club by the sudden occurrence of a dense fog during a sharp frost.... The atmosphere became dense and pungent on the second day of the Show of 1873.... Before the fog had continued for many hours some of the cattle in the Agricultural Hall evinced palpable signs of distress. On Tuesday, the first day of the fog, as early as eleven o'clock in the morning several animals were marked as affected with difficult breathing. No abatement of the fog took place during the day; on the contrary, towards evening it became rather worse, and the majority of the cattle in the Hall showed evidence of suffering from its influence.... Sheep and pigs did not however experience any ill effect from the state of the atmosphere either then or during the remaining time of the Show.... During Wednesday night ninety-one cattle were removed from the Hall for slaughter. On Thursday the atmospheric conditions were improved, and no fresh attacks were recorded. On Friday, the air was comparatively clear, and all the animals which remained in the Hall were in good sanitary condition.... The post-mortem appearance were indicative of bronchitis; the mucous membrane of the smaller bronchial tubes was inflamed, and there was also present the lobular congestion and emphysema which belong to that disease.

While we have no air concentration data for the late 19th century episodes, we do have some visual impressions of air quality of that era. Figure 1 is a Gustave Dore woodblock print of 1872 of a downtown London F1 street showing a plume from a coal-fired locomotive, as well as horse drawn traffic and smoke from domestic furnaces. Claude Monet was so entranced

Table 1   Excess Bronchitis Deaths Associated with Historic London Fogs

Dates of fog	Average weekly bronchitis mortality in previous 10 years	Excess bronchitis deaths in 1st week of fog and during succeeding 3 weeks				Total 4-week excess in bronchitis deaths
9–11 December 1873	228	7–13 December, 133	14–20 December, 424	21–27 December, 129	28 December–3 January, 102	788
26–29 January 1880	294	25–31 January, 258	1–7 Februrray, 939	8–14 February, 453	15–21 February, 167	1817
2–7 February 1882	357	29 January–4 February, 14	5–11 February, 324	12–18 February, 186	19–25 February, 31	555
21–24 December 1891	375	20–26 December, 35	27 December–2 January, 583	3–9 January, 333	10–16 January, 437	1388
28–30 December 1892	451	25–31 December, −55	1–7 January, 208	8–14 January, 154	15–21 January, 2	309
26 November–1 December 1948	65	21–27 November, 14	28 November–4 December, 84	5–11 December, 33	12–18 December, 20	151
5–9 December 1952	86	1–6 December, −3	7–13 December, 621	14–20 December, 308	21–27 December, 92	1018

Source: Ref. 2, Report no. 95 on Public Health and Medical Subjects.

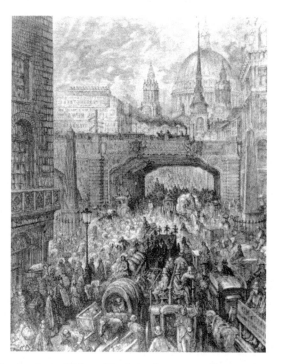

Figure 1   Ludgate Hill—a block in the street. Gustave Dore—1872.

by the varying colors of the coal smoke that he encountered during his residence in London in the early 1870s that he returned for a 3-year visit at the turn of the century and produced about 100 oil paintings of London and vicinity.

As shown in Fig. 2, the daily death rate rose rapidly with the onset of the fog on December 5, 1952, and peaked 1 day after the peak of pollution, as it was indexed by SO_2. There was also a rise in hospital emergency bed admissions, which peaked 2 days after the pollutant peaks. Both the deaths and hospital bed admissions remained elevated for several weeks after the fog lifted. Hospital admissions exhibited declines on Sundays, a finding consistent with the known practices for hospital admissions.

While the Ministry of Health report (2) attributed an excess of ~4000 deaths from all causes to the exposures during the 4 weeks following the 1952 episode, a recent re-examination of the data by Bell and Davis (8) concluded that the interim report of the Committee on Air Pollution that total mortality attributed 12,000 excess deaths to the December 1952 episode in the 12 weeks that followed was correct. Deaths peaked in the first full week, but were still above baseline levels for many weeks after that. The specific cause with the greatest number of excess deaths over the first 4 weeks was bronchitis (1156 excess deaths) and it had the greatest relative risk

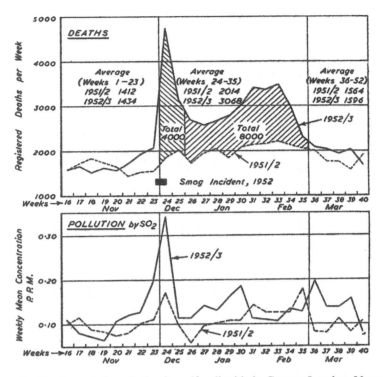

Figure 2   Deaths and air pollution by sulfur dioxide in Greater London, November 1952 to March 1953.

(RR = 6.67). The next greatest increase, for heart disease (737 excess deaths), had an RR of only 1.82. Overall, the excess mortality was concentrated among the elderly with pre-existing disease. It is of particular interest to current concerns that while recent daily mortality studies show much lower absolute risk levels from the much lower peaks in PM pollution, the elevated relative risks among the very young and oldest cohorts and the risk rankings among causes of death are quite similar today to those of December 1952.

The Ministry of Health report (2) also noted that there was a clear association between chronic air pollution and the incidence of bronchitis and other respiratory diseases. The death rate from bronchitis in England and Wales (where coal smoke pollution was very high) was much higher than in other northern European countries (with much lower levels of coal smoke pollution). The very high chronic coal smoke exposure in the United Kingdom, associated with a high prevalence of chronic bronchitis, appears to have created a large pool of individuals susceptible to "harvesting" by an acute pollution episode.

The December 1962 London fog episode followed a substantial reduction in airborne BS, and was the last to produce a clearly evident acute harvest of excess deaths, albeit a much smaller one than that of December 1952. Commins and Waller (9) developed a technique to measure H_2SO_4 in urban air, and made daily measurements at St. Bartholomew's Hospital in central London during the 1962 episode. As shown in Fig. 3, the airborne H_2SO_4 rose rapidly during the 1962 episode, with a greater relative increase than that for BS.

The U.K. Clean Air Act of 1954 had led to the mandated use of smokeless fuels and, as shown in Fig. 3, annual mean smoke levels had declined by 1962, to about one-half of the 1958 level. The annual average SO_2 concentrations had not declined by 1962, but dropped off markedly thereafter, along with a further marked decline in BS levels. For the period between 1964 and 1972, the measured levels of H_2SO_4 followed a similar pattern of decline.

During the later part of the coal smoke era in the United Kingdom, researchers begin to study the associations between long-term daily records of mortality and morbidity and ambient air pollution. In the first major time-series analysis of daily London mortality for the winter of 1958–1959, Martin and Bradley (10) and Lawther (11) used the readily available BS and SO_2 data. They estimated that both pollutants were associated with excess daily mortality when their concentrations exceeded about $750 \, \mu g/m^3$. However, additional analyses of this data set led to different conclusions. For example, Ware et al. (12) concluded that there was no demonstrable lower threshold for excess mortality down to the lowest range of observation (BS $\approx$ 150 $\mu g/m^3$), as illustrated in Fig. 4. Although $150 \, \mu g/m^3$ is now near the upper end of observed concentrations rather than at the lower end, time-series analyses indicate an increasing slope as concentrations decrease.

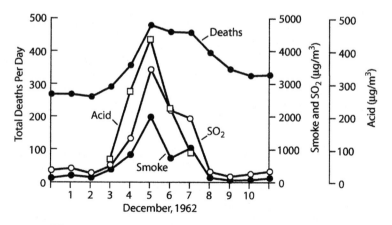

Figure 3 December 1962, London pollution episode.

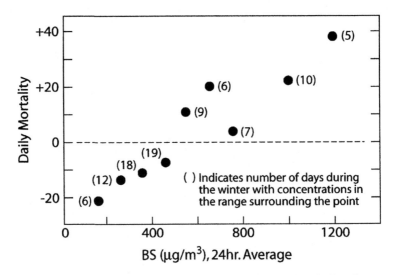

Figure 4 Martin and Bradley's data for winter of 1958–1959 in London as summarized by Ware et al. showing average deviations of daily mortality from 15-day moving average by concentration of black smoke (BS). (From Ref. 12.)

In terms of time-series analyses of morbidity, a study by Lawther et al. (13) reported the daily symptom scores of a panel of patients with chronic bronchitis in relation to the daily concentrations of BS and SO_2. As shown in Fig. 5, there was a close correspondence between symptom scores and both pollutant indices.

Chronic coal smoke exposure also affected baseline lung function. Holland and Reid (14) analyzed spirometric data collected on British postal workers in 1965. By that time, pollution levels were well below their peaks, but the postal workers had been exposed out of doors for many years when pollution levels were higher. As shown in Fig. 6, the London postal workers had lower forced expiratory volumes in 1 sec (FEV_1) and peak expiratory flow rates (PEFR) than their country town counterparts. As indicated in Fig. 6, the deleterious effects of smoking were accounted for in these analyses. Within each smoking category, the differences between the London and country town means were attributed to pollution on the basis that pollution levels were, on average, twice as high in London as in the country towns.

The marked reduction in U.K. smoke pollution levels during the 1960s was shown to be associated with a marked reduction in annual mortality in County Boroughs by Chinn et al. (15). As shown in Table 2, mortality rates in middle-aged and elderly men and women for the 1969–1973 period were no longer associated with an index of smoke pollution. By contrast, for both the 1948–1954 and 1958–1964 periods, the index of smoke exposure

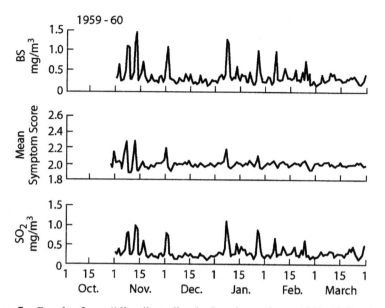

Figure 5 Results from "diary" studies in London, winter 1959–1960, showing day-to-day variations in the illness score for bronchitic subjects together with mean daily concentrations of black smoke (BS) and sulfur dioxide (SO_2).

correlated strongly with annual mortality rates for both chronic bronchitis and respiratory tract cancers. On the basis of such evidence of improved health status, our U.K. colleagues considered air pollution to be a problem solved, and essentially halted further investigations for the next several decades.

When dealing with lower levels of exposure that are closer to those of current concern, interpretation of human experience becomes more problematic. As discussed in Chapter 1, epidemiologic analyses are beset with inherent difficulties. One major problem is separation of the effects of a specific contaminant from the possible mediating effects of other factors that affect health, such as concurrent disease, diet, living conditions, cultural factors, and occupational exposures. The isolation of the effect of only one factor upon health requires data from large populations that ideally differ only with respect to exposure to the contaminant in question. Because of the many unknown factors, assumptions are often made that these factors are identical for all groups, or vary randomly with respect to levels of the contaminant. Other problems in epidemiologic studies involve: (a) possible synergism, antagonism, and other interaction between individual contaminants, especially since most communities are exposed to combinations that often make isolation of any one contaminant as the primary culprit of observed effects quite difficult; (b) the accuracy of the classification and reliability of the records of symptoms during the period under study; and

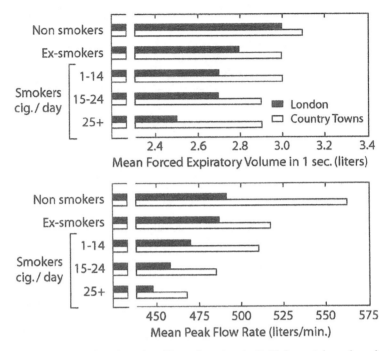

Figure 6   Cross-sectional study of lung function in British postal workers in 1965 standardized to age 40. SO$_2$ and smoke levels in the country towns were about half those in London. (Adapted from Ref. 14.)

(c) reliability and accuracy of the measurements of ambient levels in the area under study and the relationship between these levels and actual personal exposures to the population(s) of concern.

In recent years, there has been a growing sophistication in the methods used to determine rates of daily mortality and hospital admissions for pulmonary and cardiovascular causes, as well as of total nontraumatic mortality in large populations in relation to daily levels of ambient air pollution. These studies, known as "time series", are not significantly confounded by variations in smoking, diet, climate, and lifestyle, since the same population is at risk each day. Such studies have consistently indicated significant associations between daily, area-wide concentrations of fine particles, and both daily mortality and hospital admission rates. However, similar associations can often be seen with other regularly measured ambient air pollutants, such as O$_3$, SO$_2$, NO$_2$ and CO, making it difficult to assign a causal role for the short-term health effects of any of the specific constituents within ambient PM, or for copollutant gases.

For epidemiologic studies of the effects of chronic or cumulative exposures, it is usually necessary to rely on cross-sectional (intercommunity)

Table 2 Standardized Annual Mortality Rate Regression Coefficients on Smoke[a] for 64 U.K. Country Boroughs

Sex	Ages	Mortality in	Cancer of trachea, bronchus and lung	Chronic bronchitis
Males	45–64	1969–1973	0.07	0.02
		1958–1964	0.53**	0.32**
		1948–1954	0.71***	0.48***
	65–74	1969–1973	0.15	−0.06
		1958–1964	0.68***	0.31
		1948–1954	0.87***	0.37**
Females	45–64	1969–1973	−0.02	−0.02
		1958–1964	−0.64**	0.33**
		1948–1954	0.49**	0.49**
	65–74	1969–1973	0.07	0.03
		1958–1964	0.25	0.40**
		1948–1954	0.61**	0.31

[a]Based on index of black smoke pollution 20 years before death of Daly (Br J Prev Soc Med 1959; 13:14–27).
*$p < 0.05$.
**$p < 0.01$.
***$p < 0.001$.
Source: From Ref. 15.

differences in exposures and responses, or on prospective cohort studies based on individual risk-factor data for large numbers of subjects. The former are confounded by intercommunity differences in smoking and other influential factors, while the latter require large and long-term commitments of resources that have seldom been available.

Recent time-series analyses in the United States, where PM concentrations are much lower, have shown significant excesses of daily total nonaccidental mortality associated with thoracic PM, which refers to particles less than $10\,\mu m$ in aerodynamic diameter (PM_{10}) and/or fine particulate matter ($PM_{2.5}$). Figure 7 shows summary data for relative risk ($\pm 95\%$ confidence intervals) for a change of $50\,\mu g/m^3$ of PM_{10} in various U.S. communities in relation to the concentrations of the regulated gaseous air pollutants. This figure indicates that the association of daily total mortality with PM_{10} is not materially confounded by gaseous copollutants.

Figure 8 provides data that support a causal role for the PM association with total mortality. If total morbidity is increased, one would expect that mortality for respiratory causes would have a greater relative rise, with cardiovascular causes at an intermediate rate. One would also expect a larger increase in people needing acute medical attention, and that is also evident in Fig. 8. Still higher rates of cough and respiratory symptoms would be expected, and the data in Fig. 8 show such increased rates as well.

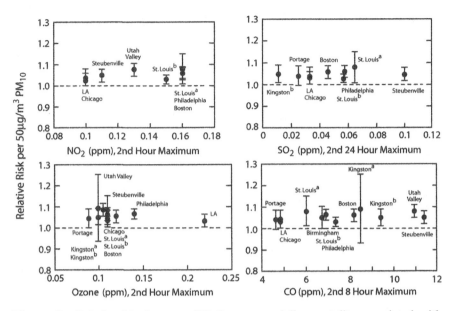

Figure 7 Relationship between RR for excess daily mortality associated with PM$_{10}$ and peak daily levels of other criteria pollutants. (Adapted from PM Staff Paper; U.S. EPA, 1996.)

The relative risks indicated in Figs. 7 and 8 are quite small, but since the entire population is at risk, the public health impacts can be substantial.

The most frequently cited PM chronic health effect studies are the Harvard Six Cities Study (16) and American Cancer Society (ACS) Cohort Study (17). They found increased mortality rates (decreased life expectancy) in cities with higher average ambient PM$_{2.5}$ and sulfate concentrations. Differences in city-specific mortality rates were not explained by data on personal risk factors.

In addition to mortality in adults, increased respiratory effects in children associated with long-term PM exposures were reported. The Harvard Six and Twenty-four Cities cross-sectional studies observed higher rates of respiratory symptoms (18) and lower lung function (19) for children in cities with higher average PM$_{2.5}$ and acidic sulfate concentrations.

Because of the high visibility of the Six Cities and ACS cohort studies and their major influence in the standard setting process, the Health Effects Institute (HEI) undertook sponsorship of a comprehensive independent validation and reanalysis of these studies. The HEI project (20) validated the quality of the original annual mortality study data, replicated the original findings, and demonstrated the validity and robustness of Six Cities and ACS mortality studies findings. For both of the cohorts studied, PM-associated mortality risk was highest for individuals with less than high school educations.

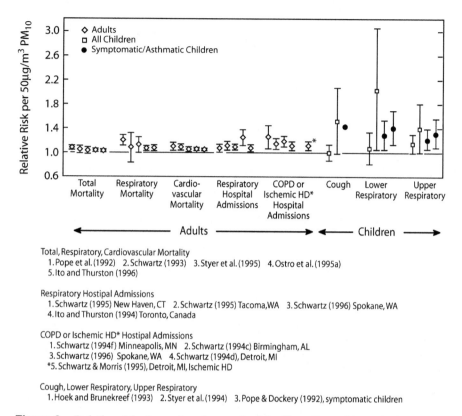

Total, Respiratory, Cardiovascular Mortality
  1. Pope et al. (1992) 2. Schwartz (1993) 3. Styer et al. (1995) 4. Ostro et al. (1995a)
  5. Ito and Thurston (1996)

Respiratory Hostipal Admissions
  1. Schwartz (1995) New Haven, CT 2. Schwartz (1995) Tacoma, WA 3. Schwartz (1996) Spokane, WA
  4. Ito and Thurston (1994) Toronto, Canada

COPD or Ischemic HD* Hostipal Admissions
  1. Schwartz (1994f) Minneapolis, MN 2. Schwartz (1994c) Birmingham, AL
  3. Schwartz (1996) Spokane, WA 4. Schwartz (1994d), Detroit, MI
  *5. Schwartz & Morris (1995), Detroit, MI, Ischemic HD

Cough, Lower Respiratory, Upper Respiratory
  1. Hoek and Brunekreef (1993) 2. Styer et al. (1994) 3. Pope & Dockery (1992), symptomatic children

Figure 8 Relative risks for various human health effects for ambient air PM_{10} concentration difference of $50\,\mu g/m^3$. (From US EPA.)

Data from other chronic exposure mortality studies have been limited. Survival analyses of male nonsmokers in California (the Adventist Health and Smog Study) reported increased mortality associated with $PM_{2.5}$ concentrations (21). Preliminary analyses of male veterans being treated for hypertension reported no statistically significant increased mortality associated with fine particle concentrations (22).

    Continued follow-up of the original Six Cities and ACS cohorts, respectively, for an additional 9 years has yielded findings illustrated in Fig. 9. The updated ACS study involved the analysis of more extensive $PM_{2.5}$, sulfate, and gaseous copollutant data. For the Six Cities cohort, $PM_{2.5}$ and sulfate concentrations continued to be associated with decreased survival and with increased mortality from cardiovascular and pulmonary causes (23). In addition, increased lung cancer deaths were significantly associated with $PM_{2.5}$ and sulfates in the extended follow-up. For the ACS cohort, $PM_{2.5}$ and sulfate also continued to be associated with increased cardiovascular

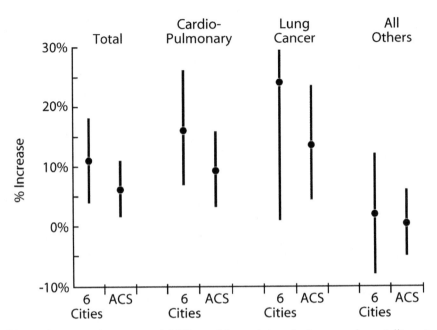

Figure 9 Mean increase and 95% confidence intervals for annual mortality rate increases per $10 \, \mu g/m^3$ increment of $PM_{2.5}$ for the Six Cities and ACS cohorts based on 16 years of mortality data.

and pulmonary mortality, and there was also an excess of lung cancer (24). The excess risks in the ACS cohort were seen only among individuals with less than high school educations in these extended analyses.

Recent analyses have attempted to bridge the time spans for health effects observed in studies of acute daily exposures vs. long-term chronic exposures. Analyses of the association between daily mortality and hospital admissions with PM concentrations during the preceding weeks to months have highlighted the importance of subchronic exposures. In Boston, for example, an increase in the 2-day average $PM_{2.5}$ of $10 \, \mu g/m^3$ was associated with an increase in mortality by 2.1%, while for the same increase in monthly average, mortality increased by 3.8% (25). In the ACS cohort study, this same increase in annual average $PM_{2.5}$ was associated with a 6.8% increase in mortality.

The Children's Health Study (CHS) in southern California showed that $PM_{2.5}$ is significantly associated with slower growth of lung function in children residing in communities with higher than average annual $PM_{2.5}$ concentrations (26). Furthermore, children who have moved from the high PM areas into areas with lower PM did not recover their lost lung function but had subsequent rates of lung function growth equal to that of the children in their new communities. Children who moved from low PM areas to communities with higher PM levels had less lung function growth than children who remained in the low PM areas (27).

A. Lack of Quantitative Knowledge on Effects of Air Toxics

In order to determine the extent of any health risk existing among the members of the population resulting from the inhalation of airborne chemicals from point sources, we need to know: (1) the concentrations of the agents in the air (and, for PM, the particle sizes) and (2) the unit risk factor, i.e., the number of cases and/or the extent of the adverse effects associated with a unit of exposure. We may also need to know more about the population of concern, such as the distribution of ages, pre-existing diseases, predisposing factors for illness, such as cigarette smoking, dietary deficiencies or excesses, etc. While such direct comparisons can, in practice, be made with some quantitative reality for the so-called criteria pollutants, whose ambient air levels are routinely monitored, and for whom human exposure-response relationships are known, comparable comparisons cannot be made for hundreds of other airborne chemicals, known collectively as hazardous air pollutants (HAPs), a.k.a. air toxics. For them, there are neither extensive ambient air concentration data nor unit risk factors that do not heavily err on the side of safety. This disparity has resulted from the different control philosophies built into the Clean Air Act (CAA) and maintained by the EPA as a part of its regulatory strategy.

Most HAPs are considered to originate from definable point sources at fixed locations. Downwind concentrations are highly variable, and generally drop rapidly with distance from the source, due to dilution into cleaner, background air. The National Emission Standards for Hazardous Air Pollutants (NESHAPs) rely on technologically based source controls and are intended to limit facility fenceline air concentrations to those that would not cause an adverse health effect to the (most exposed) individual (living at the fenceline). Also, until quite recently, there has been no program for routine measurements of air toxics in ambient air.

Most of the unit risk factors for air toxics are based on cancer as the health effect of primary concern. In these studies, and in studies to assess noncancer effects, the data are derived from controlled exposures in laboratory animals at maximally tolerated levels of exposure. The translation of the results of these studies to unit risk factors relevant to humans exposed at much, much lower levels in the environment is inherently uncertain, and is approached conservatively. The resulting unit risk factors are generally based on an assumption of no threshold and a linear extrapolation to zero risk at zero dose. They are generally described in terms of being 95% upper bound confidence limits, but this descriptor is undoubtedly conservative in itself. When these conservative unit risk factors are used for the prediction of the consequences of human exposures, they are multiplied by estimates of predicted ambient air concentrations which are, themselves, in the almost universal absence of air concentration measurements, almost certainly upper bound estimates from pollutant dispersion models that apply to the most highly exposed individuals in the community.

The resulting estimates of health risk are therefore highly conservative upper bound levels. Thus, they are inherently incompatible with the more realistic population impacts estimated for the more widely dispersed criteria pollutants. The margins of safety for criteria pollutants are generally less than a factor of two, rather than the multiple orders of magnitude of safety factors built into the risk assessments for air toxics.

The highly conservative nature of unit risk factors for air toxics was well illustrated by a calculation made during work done for EPA during the preparation of the congressionally mandated report on the benefits and costs of the Clean Air Act: 1970–1990, which is discussed later in this chapter. It was concluded that the imposition of the vinyl chloride NESHAP had prevented 6000 cases of cancer (angiosarcoma). Since the calculated cancer incidence reduction was considered larger than the historic incidence level for this cancer, it was obvious that the benefit claimed for the imposition of the NESHAP was grossly exaggerated. As a result, air toxics benefits were not included in the final report.

IV. Standards and Guidelines to Protect Ambient Air Quality

In broad terms, guidelines are nonbinding recommendations prepared by knowledgeable professionals to assist other professionals and public health authorities in evaluating the nature and extend of health risks associated with exposures. They are an essential part of the process that has become known in recent years as risk assessment. By contrast, concentration limits or emission limits having the force of law behind their enforcement are commonly known as standards. Such standards are generally established and enforced by regulatory agencies in national governments. However, there are also "Consensus Standards" established by the International Standards Organization (ISO) and/or affiliated National Standards Organizations that only have the force of law behind them when they are also adopted by regulatory authorities.

In terms of ambient air quality limits on the international level, the lead agency is the World Health Organization (WHO), which has, through its worldwide headquarters office in Geneva, established Air Quality Guidelines. The purpose of WHO guidelines is to provide a basis for protecting public health from adverse effects of pollution and for eliminating, or reducing to a minimum, those contaminants that are known or likely to be hazardous to human health and well being. In moving from guidelines to standards, prevailing exposure levels and environmental, social, economic, and cultural conditions can be taken into account. For example, WHO explicitly acknowledges that, in certain circumstances, there may be valid reasons to pursue policies that will result in pollutant concentrations above or below the guideline values.

At its simplest, an environmental quality standard should be defined in terms of one or more concentrations and associated averaging times. In addition, information on the form of exposure and monitoring, as well as methods of data analysis and quality assurance and quality control requirements, should be parts of a standard. In some countries, a standard is further qualified by defining an acceptable level of attainment or compliance. Levels of attainment may be defined in terms of the fundamental units of definition of the standard. Percentiles have been used: for example, if the unit defined by the standard is the day, then a requirement for 99% compliance allows 3 days exceedance of the standard in the year. The cost of meeting any standard is likely to critically depend on the degree of compliance required. It is important to remember that the development of standards is only a part of an adequate environmental quality management strategy. Legislation, identification of authorities responsible for enforcement of emission standards, and penalties for exceedances are all also necessary.

The process by which contamination criteria and exposure limits are established and subsequently modified is inherently difficult, slow, and contentious. There are generally conflicting forces at play, with major economic interests, public health and environmental quality concerns, and professional reputations at stake. The available effects data are always inadequate, sometimes pathetically so. Criteria and limits are, therefore, heavily dependent upon "informed judgment."

A. Bases for Establishing Air Contamination Criteria and Exposure Limits

There are many possible bases for the establishment of air contamination criteria and the setting of exposure limits. These include: (a) epidemiological studies of populations exposed in their occupations, or through community air. Such studies can provide statistically significant associations between contaminant levels and reported effects; (b) toxicologic studies, i.e., studies of groups of animals intentionally exposed in controlled laboratory experiments where it is possible to define the exposures. Such studies can provide more complete information on metabolic pathways, storage depots, and the types and degrees of biological damage that the agents produce, including information on whole body effects; and (c) extrapolation of available epidemiological and toxicological data on other related materials to the material in question, based on their similarities in chemical structure and metabolism, and perhaps their effects in simplified biological test systems, such as bacteria and cell or organ tissue cultures.

Excessive exposures can be controlled by enforcing concentration limits in environmental media (air, water, and foods), by enforcing emission limits (into ambient air and surface waters and onto land) or a combination of both. Concentration limits are generally most appropriate for monitoring exposures to chemicals arising from multiple and widespread sources (often including natural background sources), while emission limits are generally most appropriate for identifiable point sources that can produce important local impacts downwind or downstream.

When ambient air concentration limits are exceeded, control agencies generally will need to conduct an emissions inventory in order to determine which specific sources or source categories are causing the elevated exposures, and then to impose emission restrictions on those sources or source categories that are responsible for the excesses. Concentration limits established by EPA to control atmosphere contamination that are directly related to human health are known as "primary standards." Those that are based upon recognized adverse effects on animals, vegetation, or building materials, economic losses, or evidence of aesthetic degradation of surface air or water are considered to be effects upon "public welfare," and are known as "secondary standards."

B. Bases for Establishing Emission Limits and Source Controls

The attainment of reduced exposure levels through effective control of emissions requires the establishment of rational and enforceable emission limits. The first step is generally an inventory of sources and their strengths. It is also important to know the location of the discharge point and the temporal pattern of emissions, since the latter affects contaminant dispersion. Other important factors are the technological and economic feasibility of the application of controls. Finally, it is important that there will be some positive incentives for the installation and maintenance of controls and/or penalties for not installing them or maintaining their effectiveness. For example, the effectiveness of the manufacturer-supplied motor-vehicle emission controls has often been considerably less than their potential because of improper maintenance and some deliberate disconnections and alterations of the system components. In some states, there are no requirements for mandatory inspection or maintenance of auto-emission controls. Other types of emission controls have been, predictably, more effective. These include those for lead, achieved through the phased elimination of the lead content of gasoline, and SO_2, achieved through reductions in the sulfur content of fossil fuels used in boilers and motor vehicles.

C. Development of Federal Standards for Ambient Air and Pollutant Emissions

Air contamination was long considered to be a local problem in the United States, and standards for contaminant levels that did exist were established for local jurisdictions such as cities, counties, and states. Different jurisdictions regulated different air contaminants and often had different standards for the same contaminants. These disparities led to the establishment of national standards.

The U.S. Air Quality Act of 1967 required: (a) the establishment of the President's Air Quality Advisory Board, the Advisory Committee on Criteria, and the Advisory Committees for the various contaminants, comprised of experts from industry, academia, and other agencies outside the federal government, to assist in developing criteria and control documents; (b) the conducting of comprehensive cost studies to assess the economic impact of air standards on industry; (c) the expansion of research and development programs for air pollution control; (d) the study of emissions from aircraft and national emission standards; and (e) the registration of fuel additives.

Criteria and control documents were issued in 1969 and 1970 for PM, SO_X, CO, photochemical oxidants, hydrocarbons, and NO_X, the chemicals that were designated as criteria air pollutants. These documents were relied upon in 1971 by the newly established EPA in setting the initial suite of NAAQS.

The 1970 CAA amendments were also concerned with: (a) controlling existing mobile or stationary sources of contaminants to bring air quality to levels defined by the NAAQS; (b) setting national emission standards for new or existing HAPs for which ambient air quality standards were not applicable; and (c) setting nationwide performance standards for new or modified stationary air contaminant sources. A primary purpose of the 1970 CAA amendments was to prevent the general occurrence of new air contamination problems by requiring the installation of the best available controls during initial construction, when the installation of such controls is least expensive. The new standards were not, however, to be applied to existing sources. Examples of the source categories for which EPA has promulgated standards of performance are fossil fuel-fired steam generators, municipal incinerators, Portland cement plants, nitric acid plants, sulfuric acid plants, and motor vehicles.

The 1977 CAA amendments required the EPA to apply different levels of stringency to airborne emissions in areas that met the existing air quality standards (attainment areas) vs. those that did not (nonattainment areas). Furthermore, to ensure that pollution would not increase in attainment areas, the 1977 amendments incorporated a prevention of significant deterioration (PSD) requirement. New stationary sources in such areas were required to use the best available control technology (BACT). At the same time, the amendments required the EPA to take into account the costs of compliance. Existing sources in nonattainment areas were required to use reasonably available control technology (RACT), which represented a lesser level of control that could be achieved at lower cost.

One of the important changes in the 1990 CAA amendments was the separation of emission standards into several classes. These included risk-based standards designed to protect public health, technology-based standards requiring application of various levels of control technology, and technology-forcing standards designed to ensure that industries develop and apply the very best control technology. In many respects, these changes amplified the requirements mandated under the 1970 CAA amendments. At the same time, Congress mandated the regulation of 189 toxic air pollutants.

The 1990 CAA amendments also mandated further reductions in motor-vehicle emissions, as well as a 50% reduction in power-plant emissions of SO_2 and NO_X, and called for the establishment of a new permit system consolidating all applicable emission control requirements, and mandated a production phaseout by the year 2000 of the five most destructive ozone-depleting chemicals.

The traditional approach to mobile sources has been to require that pollution controls be incorporated into the product by the manufacturer. In contrast, the primary approach for limiting airborne emissions from stationary sources (for example, major manufacturing facilities) has been to apply a combination of controls, such as RACT or BACT, and to enforce the requirements through the granting of operating permits. To assure successful control, Congress mandated that each state develops an implementation plan describing how the federally specified standards would be met.

Among the new approaches incorporated into the 1990 CAA amendments was a provision that permits the buying and selling of air pollution emission allowances. The goal was to encourage those industries that can remove pollutants at minimal cost to sell their polluting allowances to industries whose costs were higher. Setting a limit on the total amount of pollution that can be released enables companies to trade their emission allowances at market prices. Reduced emissions have been achieved at a much lower overall cost than using any other approach, and the market for SO_2 allowances has functioned very well. Economic considerations also led Congress to mandate cost–benefit analyses under the 1990 CAA amendments. A retrospective cost–benefit analysis for the CAA for 1970–1990 has been completed (28) as has the first prospective analyses of the costs and benefits of the 1990 CAA amendments (1990–2010) (29). An Advisory Council on Clean Air Act Compliance Analysis was established to assist EPA with guidance on the conduct of these analyses and to provide peer review of the reports before their submission to the Congress. The findings are summarized in the next section.

V. Benefits and Costs of the CAA
A. Summary of EPA's Retrospective Report for 1970–1990
1. Study Design

Estimates of the benefits and costs of the CAA and its amendments were derived by examining the differences in economic, human health, and environmental outcomes under two alternative scenarios: a "control scenario" and a "no-control scenario." The control scenario reflected actual historical implementation of clean air programs, and was based largely on historical data. The no-control scenario was hypothetical, and reflected the assumption that no air pollution controls were established beyond those in place prior to enactment of the 1970 CAA amendments. Each of the two scenarios was evaluated by a sequence of economic, emissions, air quality, physical effect, economic valuation, and uncertainty models to measure the differences between the two scenarios in economic, human health, and environmental outcomes.

2. Direct Costs

To comply with the provisions of the CAA, businesses, consumers, and government entities all incurred higher costs for many goods and services. The higher costs were due primarily to requirements to install, operate, and maintain pollution abatement equipment. In addition, costs were incurred to design and implement regulations, monitor and report regulatory compliance, and in conducting research and development programs. The historical data on CAA compliance costs by year were adjusted both for inflation and for the value of long-term investments in equipment. The annual results yielded an estimate of approximately $ 523 billion for 1970–1990 direct expenditures.

3. Emissions

Emissions were substantially lower by 1990 under the control scenario than under the no-control scenario. SO_2 emissions were 40% lower, primarily due to utilities installing scrubbers and/or switching to lower sulfur fuels. NO_X emissions were 30% lower by 1990, mostly because of the installation of catalytic converters on highway vehicles. Volatile organic compound (VOC) emissions were 45% lower and CO emissions were 50% lower, also primarily due to motor vehicle emission controls. For PM, changes in air quality depend both on changes in emissions of primary particles and on changes in emissions of gaseous pollutants, such as SO_2 and NO_X, which can be converted to PM through chemical transformations in the atmosphere. Emissions of PM were 75% lower under the control scenario by 1990 than under the no-control scenario. This substantial difference was due primarily to vigorous efforts in the 1970s to reduce visible emissions from utility and industrial smokestacks. Lead (Pb) emissions for 1990 were reduced by about 99% from a no-control level of 237,000 tons to about 3000 tons under the control scenario. The vast majority of the difference in Pb emissions under the two scenarios was attributable to drastic reductions in the use of leaded gasoline. These reductions were achieved during a period in which population grew by 22.3% and the national economy grew by 70%.

4. Air Quality

The substantial reductions in air pollutant emissions attributable to the CAA translated into significantly improved air quality throughout the United States. For SO_2, NO_X, and CO, the improvements under the control scenario were assumed to be proportional to the estimated reduction in emissions. Reductions in ground-level O_3 were achieved through reductions in VOCs and NO_X. The differences in ambient O_3 concentrations estimated under the control scenario varied significantly by location, primarily because of local differences in the relative proportion of VOCs and NO_X, weather conditions, and specific precursor emissions reductions. On a national average basis, O_3 concentrations in 1990 were about 15% lower under the control scenario.

There are many pollutants that contribute to ambient concentrations of PM. While some fine particles are directly emitted by sources, the most important fine particle species are formed in the atmosphere through chemical conversion of gaseous pollutants, and are referred to as secondary particles, including: (1) sulfates, which derive primarily from SO_2 emissions; (2) nitrates, which derive primarily from NO_X emissions; and (3) organic aerosols, which can be directly emitted or can form from VOC emissions. Thus, controlling PM means controlling "air pollution" in a very broad sense. Reductions in SO_2, NO_X, VOCs, and directly emitted primary particles achieved by the CAA resulted in a national average reduction in PM_{10} of about 45% by 1990.

5. Physical Effects

The lower ambient concentrations of SO_2, NO_X, PM, CO, O_3, and Pb under the control scenario could be tied to a variety of human health, welfare, and ecological benefits. For some benefit categories, quantitative functions were available from the scientific literature that allowed estimation of the reduction in incidence of adverse effects. Examples of these categories include the human mortality and morbidity effects of a number of pollutants, the neurobehavioral effects among children caused by exposure to Pb, visibility impairment, and effects on yields for some agricultural products.

However, many benefit categories could not be quantified and/or monetized. In some cases, substantial scientific uncertainties prevailed regarding the existence and magnitude of adverse effects (e.g., the contribution of O_3 to air pollution-related mortality). In other cases, strong scientific evidence of an established effect existed, but data were too limited to support quantitative estimates of incidence reduction. Finally, there were effects for which there was sufficient information to estimate incidence reduction, but for which there were no available economic value measures; thus, reductions in adverse effects could not be expressed in monetary terms. Examples of this last category include relatively small pulmonary function decrements caused by acute exposures to O_3, and reduced time to onset of angina pain caused by CO exposure.

Table 3 provides a summary of the key differences in quantified human health outcomes that were estimated under the control and no-control scenarios. Results were presented as thousands of cases avoided in 1990 due to control of the pollutants listed in the table and reflect reductions estimated for the entire U.S. population living in the 48 contiguous states. Epidemiological findings about correlations between pollution and observed health effects were used to estimate changes in the number of health effects that would occur when pollution levels change. A range was presented along with the mean estimate for each effect, reflecting uncertainties that have been quantified in the underlying health effects literature.

Adverse human health effects of the CAA "criteria pollutants" dominated the quantitative effects estimates, because evidence of physical consequences was greatest for these pollutants. The CAA yielded other benefits that could not be quantified, including those associated with reductions in: (a) air toxics; (b) damage to cultural resources, buildings, and other materials; (c) adverse effects on wetland, forest, and aquatic ecosystems; and (d) a variety of additional human health and welfare effects of criteria pollutants. A list of these nonmonetized effects is presented in Table 4.

6. Economic Valuation

To compare or aggregate benefits across endpoints, the benefits had to be monetized. Assigning a monetary value to avoided incidences of each effect permits a summation, in terms of dollars, of monetized benefits realized allows that summation to be compared to the cost of implementing the CAA. Unit valuation estimates were derived from the economics literature in terms of dollars per case (or, in some cases, episode or symptom day) avoided for health effects, and dollars per unit of avoided damage for human welfare effects. The mean values of these ranges are shown in Table 5.

Combining the benefits with the cost estimates yielded the following analytical outcomes:

Table 3 Criteria Pollutant Health Benefits—Estimated Distributions of 1990 Incidences of Avoided Health Effects (In Thousands of Incidences Reduced) for the 48 State's Populations[a]

Endpoint	Pollutant(s)	Affected population	Annual effects avoided[b] (thousands)[a]			Unit
			5th percentile	Mean	95th percentile	
Premature mortality	PM[c]	30 and over	112	184	257	Cases
Premature mortality	Lead	All	7	22	54	Cases
Chronic bronchitis	PM	All	498	674	886	Cases
Lost IQ points	Lead	Children	7,440	10,400	13,000	Points
IQ less than 70	Lead	Children	31	45	60	Cases
Hypertension	Lead	Men 20–74	9,740	12,600	15,600	Cases
Coronary heart disease	Lead	40–74	0	22	64	Cases
Atherothrombotic brain infarction	Lead	40–74	0	4	15	Cases
Initial cerebrovascular accident	Lead	40–74	0	6	19	Cases
Hospital admissions						
All respiratory	PM andozone	All	75	89	103	Cases
Chronic obstructive pulmonary disease and pneumonia	PM andozone	Over 65	52	62	72	Cases
Ischemic heart disease	PM	Over 65	7	19	31	Cases
Congestive heart failure	PM and CO	65 and over	28	39	50	Cases
Other respiratory-related ailments						
Shortness of breath, days	PM	Children	14,800	68,000	133,000	Days

			5th percentile	Mean	95th percentile	
Acute bronchitis	PM	Children	0	8,700	21,600	Cases
Upper and lower respiratory symptom	PM	Children	5,400	9,500	13,400	Cases
Any of 19 acute symptoms	PM andozone	18–65	15,400	130,000	244,000	Cases
Asthma attacks	PM andozone	Asthmatics	170	850	1,520	Cases
Increase in respiratory illness	NO_2	All	4,840	9,800	14,000	Cases
Any symptom	SO_2	Asthmatics	26	264	706	Cases
Restricted activity and work loss days						
Minor restricted activity days	PM and ozone	18–65	107,000	125,000	143,000	Days
Work loss days	PM	18–65	19,400	22,600	25,600	Days

[a]The following additional human welfare effects were quantified directly in economic terms: household soiling damage, visibility impairment, decreased worker productivity, and agricultural yield changes.

[b]The 5th and 95th percentile outcomes represent the lower and upper bounds, respectively, of the 90% credible interval for each effects as estimated by uncertainty modeling. The mean is the arithmetic average of all estimates derived by the uncertainty modeling.

[c]In this analysis, PM is used as a proxy pollutant for all nonlead (Pb) criteria pollutants which may contribute to premature mortality.

Table 4 Central Estimates of Economic Value per Unit of Avoided Effect (In 1990 Dollars)

Endpoint	Pollutant	Valuation (Mean est.)
Mortality	PM and lead	$ 4,800,000 per case[a]
Chronic bronchitis	PM	$ 260,000 per case
IQ changes		
Lost IQ points	Lead	$ 3,000 per IQ point
IQ less than 70	Lead	$ 42,000 per case
Hypertension	Lead	$ 680 per case
Strokes[b]	Lead	$ 200,000 per case—males[c]
		$ 150,000 per case—females[c]
Coronary heart disease	Lead	$ 52,000 per case
Hospital admissions		
Ischemic heart disease	PM	$ 10,300 per case
Congestive heart failure	PM	$ 8,300 per case
COPD	PM and ozone	$ 8,100 per case
Pneumonia	PM and ozone	$ 7,900 per case
All respiratory	PM and ozone	$ 6,100 per case
Respiratory illness and symptoms		
Acute bronchitis	PM	$ 45 per case
Acute asthma	PM and ozone	$ 32 per case
Acute respiratory symptoms	PM, ozone, NO_2, and SO_2	$ 18 per case
Upper respiratory symptoms	PM	$ 19 per case
Lower respiratory symptoms	PM	$ 12 per case
Shortness of breath	PM	$ 5.30 per day
Work loss days	PM	$ 83 per day
Mild restricted activity days	PM and ozone	$ 38 per day
Welfare benefits		
Visibility	DeciView	$ 14 per unit change in DeciView
Household soiling	PM	$ 2.50 per household per PM_{10} change
Decreased worker productivity	Ozone	$ 1[d]
Agriculture (net surplus)	Ozone	Change in economic surplus

[a]Alternative results, based on assigning a value of $ 293,000 for each life-year lost are presented.
[b]Strokes are comprised of atherothrombotic brain infarctions and cerebrovascular accidents; both are estimated to have the same monetary value.
[c]The different valuations for stroke cases reflect differences in lost earnings between males and females.
[d]Decreased productivity valued as change in daily wages: $ 1 per worker per 10% decrease in ozone.

Table 5 Total Estimated Monetized Benefits by Endpoint Category for the 48 State's Populations for 1970–1990 Period (In Billions of 1990 Dollars)

Endpoint	Pollutant(s)	Present value		
		5th percentile	Mean	95th percentile
Mortality	PM	$2,369	$16,632	$40,597
Mortality	Lead	$121	$1,339	$3,910
Chronic bronchitis	PM	$409	$3,313	$10,401
IQ (lost IQ pts. + children w/IQ < 70)	Lead	$271	$399	$551
Hypertension	Lead	$77	$98	$120
Hospital admissions	PM, ozone, lead and CO	$27	$57	$120
Respiratory related symptoms restricted activity, and decreased productivity	PM, ozone, NO_2, and SO_2	$123	$182	$261
Soiling damage	PM	$6	$74	$192
Visibility	Particulates	$38	$54	$71
Agriculture (net surplus)	Ozone	$11	$23	$35

- The total monetized benefits of the CAA realized during the period from 1970 to 1990 ranged from $ 5.6 to 49.4 trillion, with a central estimate of $ 22.2 trillion.
- By comparison, the value of direct compliance expenditures over the same period equaled approximately $ 0.5 trillion.
- The central estimate of $ 22.2 trillion in benefits may be a significant underestimate, due to the exclusion of large numbers of benefits from the monetized benefit estimate (e.g., all air toxics effects, ecosystem effects, and numerous human health effects).

Clearly, even the lower bound estimate of monetized benefits substantially exceeds the costs of the historical CAA. An important implication of the results of this study was that a large proportion of the monetized benefits of the historical CAA were attributed to reductions of exposures to two pollutants: Pb and PM.

B. Summary of EPA's First Prospective Report, 1990–2010

The CAA Amendments of 1990 built upon the progress made by the original CAA of 1970 and its 1977 amendments in improving the nation's air quality. Because the 1990 amendments represent an incremental improvement to the nation's clean air program, the analysis summarized in the first prospective report was designed to estimate the costs and benefits of the 1990 amendments incremental to those assessed in the retrospective analysis.

1. Compliance Costs

Relative to the pre-CAAA case post-CAAA scenario, total annual compliance costs were approximately $ 21 billion higher by the year 2000, rising to $ 28 billion by the year 2010. Compliance with Title I (NAAQS) accounts for $ 14.5 billion by 2010, while compliance with mobile source emissions control provisions under Title II accounts for $ 9 billion annually. Provisions to control acid deposition and emissions of stratospheric O_3 depleting substances account for most of the remainder of the costs.

The EPA focussed its air quality modeling efforts on estimating the impact of emissions on ambient concentrations of O_3, PM_{10}, $PM_{2.5}$, SO_2, NO_X, and CO, and on acid deposition and visibility. The majority of the total monetized benefits were attributable to changes in PM concentrations and, more specifically, to the effect of these ambient air quality changes on avoidance of premature mortality.

The direct benefits of the air quality improvements estimated included reduced incidence of a number of criteria pollutant-related adverse human health effects, improvements in visibility, and avoided damage to agricultural crops. The estimated annual economic value of these benefits in the year 2010 ranged from $ 26 to 270 billion, in 1990 dollars, and had a central estimate, or mean, of $ 110 billion. As in the 1970–1990 retrospective study, the estimates did not include a number of other potentially important effects that could not be readily quantified and monetized.

2. Comparing Costs to Benefits

Based on the specific tools and techniques that were employed, EPA's primary estimate of the net benefit (benefits minus costs) over the entire 1990–2010 period of the additional criteria pollutant control programs incorporated in the post-CAAA case was $ 510 billion. These results, summarized in Table 6, indicate that the monetizable benefits alone exceeded the direct compliance costs by about four to one. For many of the factors contributing to this net benefit estimate, EPA was able to generate quantitative estimates of uncertainty. By statistically combining these uncertain estimates, it was able to develop a range of net benefit estimates which provided a partial indication of the overall uncertainty surrounding the central estimate of net benefits. This range, reflecting a 90% probability range around the mean, or central estimate, for 2010 was $ 30–$ 260 billion.

The estimates for Title VI (stratospheric O_3 controls) also indicate that cumulative benefits ($ 500 billion) well exceed cumulative costs ($ 27 billion). However, the time period of EPA's Title VI analysis (i.e., 175 years)

Table 6 Summary Comparison of Benefits and Costs (Estimates in Millions of 1990 $)[a]

	Titles I–V			Title VI	All titles
	Annual estimates 2000	2010	Present value estimate 1990–2010	Present value estimate 1990–2165	Total present value
Monetized direct costs					
Central	$19,000	$27,000	$180,000	$27,000	$210,000
Monetized direct benefits					
Low[b]	$16,000	$26,000	$160,000	$100,000	$260,000
Central	$71,000	$110,000	$690,000	$530,000	$1,200,000
High[b]	$160,000	$270,000	$1,600,000	$900,000	$2,500,000
Benefit/cost ratio					
Low[c]	Less than 1/1	Less than 1/1	Less than 1/1	Less than 4/1	1/1
Central	4/1	4/1	4/1	20/1	6/1
High[c]	More than 8/1	More than 10/1	More than 9/1	More than 33/1	12/1

[a]The cost estimates for this analysis are based on assumptions about future changes in factors such as consumption patterns, input costs, and technological innovation. We recognize that these assumptions introduce significant uncertainty into the cost results; however, the degree of uncertainty or bias associated with many of the key factors cannot be readily quantified. Thus, EPA was unable to present specific low and high cost estimates.

[b]Low and high benefits estimates are based on primary results and correspond to 5th and 95th percentile results from statistical uncertainty analysis, incorporating uncertainties in physical effects and valuation steps of benefits analysis. Other significant sources of uncertainty not reflected include the value of unquantified or unmonetized benefits that are not captured in the primary estimates and uncertainties in emmisions and air quality modeling.

[c]The low benefits/cost ratio reflects the ratio of the low benefits estimates to the central costs estimate, while the high ratio reflects the ratio of the high benefits estimates to the central costs estimate. Because we were unable to reliably quantify the uncertainty in cost estimates, we present the low estimate as "less than X", and the high estimate as "more than Y", where X and Y are the low and high benefit/cost ratios, respectively.

suggests that these estimates are very uncertain. Nonetheless, the conclusion that benefits well exceed costs holds even at EPA's primary low estimate of benefits (the low end of the 90% probability range, or $ 100 billion), and regardless of discount rate used to generate the cumulative estimates from the perspective of the present.

C. Need for Further Benefits and Cost Valuations

While the benefits attributed to the CAA overall were quite substantial in EPA's reports to Congress, as summarized above, and greatly exceeded the costs of the implementation of the CAA, it must be recognized that a dominant role in determining the benefits was played by PM, with most of that related to criteria pollutant-associated excess mortality as indexed by PM. The magnitude of the net benefit can dramatically change by using a valuation based on life-years lost instead of a $ 4.8 \times 10^6$ valuation on a premature death, or by using some other point valuation.

On both the benefit and cost sides of the comparisons, it must also be noted that EPA was unable to disaggregate the totals into those attributable to specific pollutants or titles in the act relating separately to individual criteria pollutants, air toxics, and ecological impacts of air pollution. Thus, the benefits of criteria air pollutant controls were, in effect, compared to all of the costs of air pollution control. In terms of the criteria pollutant control program, the subtraction of costs associated with the control of air toxics and acidic deposition would increase the benefit/cost ratio for the criteria pollutants. It would also, in all likelihood, result in a very low benefit/cost ratio for air toxics and acidic deposition control expenditures.

The council strongly recommended that EPA expand its analyses for its next prospective study of benefits and costs of the 1990 CAAA with respect to disaggregation of both costs and benefits. The major issue with respect to air toxics valuation is the current virtual absence of credible exposure–response relationships for carcinogenic chemicals. EPA could not rely on the reference concentrations and unit risk factors in its Integrated Risk Information System (IRIS) database for central estimates of exposure–response because of their highly conservative bases, generally involving multiple layers of relatively large safety factors. On the ecological and welfare issues, there is an extreme paucity of relevant peer-reviewed literature on either exposure–response relationships or economic valuation for damages or losses caused directly or indirectly by pollutant exposures.

VI. Unresolved Issues

While there is mounting evidence that excess daily mortality and morbidity are associated with short-term peaks in PM pollution, the public health implications of this evidence are not yet fully clear. Key questions remain, including:

- Which specific components of the fine particle fraction ($PM_{2.5}$) and coarse particle fraction of PM_{10} are most influential in producing the responses?
- Do the effects of the PM on respiratory disease mortality and morbidity depend on coexposure to irritant vapors, such as O_3, SO_2, and NO_2?
- Do the effects of the PM on cardiac disease mortality and morbidity depend on coexposure to CO?
- What influences do multiple-day pollution episode exposures have on daily responses and response lags?
- Does long-term chronic exposure predispose sensitive individuals being "harvested" on peak pollution days?
- How much of the excess daily mortality is associated with life-shortening measured in days or weeks vs. months, years, or decades?
- Can further epidemiological studies resolve these issues through refinements in analytical methodologies or through new studies using a broader array of air quality measures such as those now being generated by EPA's speciation site network?
- Can laboratory based inhalation exposure studies with human volunteers or laboratory animals resolve these issues? Short-term exposure studies using Concentrated Ambient Air Particle (CAPs) and some ultrafine aerosols at concentrations higher than those in ambient air have been informative in terms of measuring transient responses consistent with the development of adverse effects.
- Will adequate resources be made available to undertake the kinds of epidemiological and laboratory research that could answer these questions?

The findings of the previously discussed prospective cohort studies (16,17,24) indicate that mean lifespan shortening is of the order of 2 years, implying that many individuals in the population have lives shortened by many years, and that there is excess mortality associated with fine particle exposure greater than that implied by the cumulative results of the time-series studies of daily mortality.

In the absence of any generally accepted mechanistic basis to account for the epidemiological associations between ambient fine particles, on the one hand, and mortality, morbidity and functional effects, on the other, the causal role of PM remains questionable. However, essentially all attempts to discredit the associations on the basis of the effects being due to other environmental variables that may covary with PM have been unsuccessful. As shown in Fig. 7, the relative risk for daily mortality in relation to PM_{10} is remarkably consistent across communities that vary considerably in their peak concentrations of other criteria air pollutants. The possible confounding influence of adjustments to models to account for weather variables has also been found to be minimal (30,31).

While mechanistic understanding of processes by which ambient air PM causes human health effects remains quite limited, the credibility of ambient $PM_{2.5}$ as a cause of excess human mortality and morbidity has been enhanced by a series of inhalation studies involving exposures to CAPs. These studies have shown associations between ambient air PM and indices of cardiac function in both animals and humans. However, factors other than the mass concentration of $PM_{2.5}$ must be important, since the extent of the effects observed at a given concentration vary from day to day. This suggests that PM composition and/or surface activity are important. Many chemical transformations that occur in ambient air take place on the surfaces of airborne particles, and the products formed may account for the much closer associations between changes in health-related indices and particles of ambient origin than with particles of indoor origin. Biologically active components on the surface of fine particles may constitute only a very small fraction of the PM mass concentration.

In terms of identifying source categories that contribute heavily to the adverse effects of air pollution, research efforts are new focused the application of source-apportionment techniques. Such research may help resolve the temporal variations in biological responses and the relative impacts of PM attributable to major source categories, such as transportation, stationary sources, and wind-blown soil.

Several mechanistic pathways have been investigated that may link PM exposure with adverse health effects. Figure 10 highlights the complexity and interdependency of some of these pathways (5). The portal of entry for PM air pollution is the lung, and PM interactions with respiratory epithelium likely mediate a wide range of effects, as indicated by the central oval in Fig. 10. These include respiratory as well as systemic and cardiovascular effects. However, PM, or its reaction products, may stimulate airway sensory nerves, leading to changes in lung function and in autonomic tone, which influence cardiac function. Ultrafine particles by virtue of their extremely small size may enter pulmonary capillary blood and be rapidly transported to extrapulmonary tissues such as liver, bone marrow, and heart, with either direct or indirect effects on organ function.

Airway injury and inflammation is a well-known consequence of toxic inhalation exposures. The presence or absence of an inflammatory response is an important issue because inflammation may induce systemic effects, including an acute-phase response with increased blood viscosity and coagulability and possibly an increased risk for myocardial infarction in patients with severe coronary artery disease. In chronic respiratory diseases such as asthma and chronic obstructive pulmonary disease (COPD),

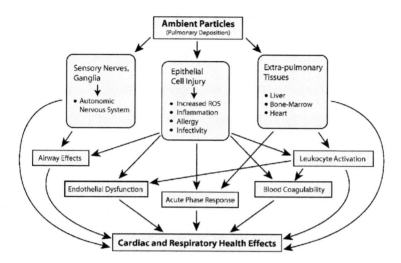

Figure 10   Hypotheses for health effects of PM.

inflammation is a key pathophysiologic feature. Since chronic, repeated inflammatory challenge of the airways may result in airway remodeling that leads to irreversible lung disease, inflammation may be involved in both acute and chronic effects.

Particulate matter generates reaction oxygen species (ROS), which provide proinflammatory stimuli to bronchial epithelial cells and macrophages. These cellular targets respond with cytokine and chemokine production, which can enhance the response to allergens. Particulate matter may therefore act as an adjuvant that strengthens the response of the immune system to environmental allergens. Hallmarks of allergic inflammation include increased immunoglobulin E (IgE) production, eosinophilic bronchial inflammation, airway hyperresponsiveness, and an increase of nitric oxide (NO) in exhaled air.

VII. Summary

While significant uncertainties remain concerning the biological mechanisms that can account for the adverse health effects that are significantly associated with human exposures to ambient air pollutants, the epidemiological and clinical evidence amassed in recent years has been consistent and coherent in linking exposures to health effects ranging from premature mortality through hospital admissions, function decrements and lost-time from work and school. The public health impacts and societal costs have been quite substantial, especially for PM and Pb, and regulatory actions taken to reduce exposures have been effective in minimizing health impacts and their costs to society.

References

1. Evelyn J. Fumifugium, or The Inconvenience of the Air and Smoke of London Dissipated; Together with some Remedies Humbly Proposed [Printed by W. Godbid for Gabriel Bedel and Thomas Collins, London]. 1661.
2. Ministry of Health. Mortality and Morbidity During the London Fog of December 1952. London: Her Majesty's Stationary Office 1954.
3. Firket J. Fog along the Meuse Valley. Trans Faraday Soc 1936; 32:1192–1197.
4. Schrenk HH, Heimann H, Clayton GD, Gafater WM. Air Pollution in Donora, Pennsylvania, Public Health Bulletin No. 306. Washington, DC: U.S. Government Printing Office, 1949.
5. Lippmann M, Frampton M, Schwartz J, Dockery D, Schlesinger R, Koutrakis P, Froines J, Nel A, Finkelstein J, Godleski J, Kaufman J, Koenig J, Larson T, Luchtel D, Liu S-JS, Oberdörster G, Peters A, Sarnat J, Sioutas C, Suh H, Sullivan J, Utell M, Wichmann E, Zelikoff J. The U.S. Environmental Protection Agency Particulate Matter Health Effects Research Centers Program: a midcourse report of status, progress, and plans. Environ Health Perspect 2003; 111:1074–1092.
6. Dhara R, Dhara VR. Bhopal—a case study of international disaster. Int J Occup Environ Health 1995; 1:58–69.
7. Anon. The effects of the fog on cattle in London. The Veterinarian. 1874; XLVII (no. 553):1–4.
8. Bell ML, Davis DL. Reassessment of the lethal London Fog of 1952: novel indicators of acute and chronic consequences of acute exposure to air pollution. Environ Health Perspect 2001; 109(suppl 3):389–394.
9. Commins BT, Waller RE. Determination of particulate acid in town air. Analyst 1963; 88:364–367.
10. Martin AE, Bradley WH. Mortality, fog and atmospheric pollution: an investigation during the winter of 1958–1959. Mon Bull Minist Health Public Health Lab Serv (BG) 1960; 19:56–73.
11. Lawther PJ. Compliance with the Clean Air Act: medical aspects. J Inst Fuel 1963; 36:341–344.
12. Ware JH, Thibodeau LA, Speizer FE, Colome S, Ferris BG Jr. Assessment of the health effects of atmospheric sulfur oxides and particulate matter: evidence from observational studies. Environ Health Perspect 1981; 41:255–276.
13. Lawther PJ, Waller RE, Henderson M. Air pollution and exacerbations of bronchitis. Thorax 1970; 25:525–539.
14. Holland WW, Reid DD. The urban factor in chronic bronchitis. Lancet 1965; 1:445–448.
15. Chinn S, Florey C, Du V, Baldwin IG, Gorgol M. The relation of mortality in England and Wales 1969–1973 to measurements of air pollution. J Epidemiol Commun Health 1981; 35:174–179.
16. Dockery DW, Pope CA III, Xu X, Spengler JD, Ware JH, Fay ME, Ferris BG Jr, Speizer FE. An association between air pollution and mortality in six U.S. cities. N Engl J Med 1993; 329:1753–1759.
17. Pope CA III, Thun MJ, Namboodiri M, Dockery DW, Evans JS, Speizer FE, Heath CW Jr. Particulate air pollution is a predictor of mortality in a prospective study of U.S. adults. Am J Respir Crit Care Med 1995; 151:669–674.

18. Dockery DW, Cunningham J, Damokosh AI, Neas LM, Spengler JD, Koutrakis P, Ware JH, Raizenne M, Speizer FE. Health effects of acid aerosols on North American children: respiratory symptoms. Environ Health Perspect 1996; 104:500–505.
19. Raizenne ME, Burnett RT, Stern B, Franklin CA, Spengler JD. Acute lung function responses to ambient acid aerosol exposures in children. Environ Health Perspect 1989; 79:179–185.
20. Krewski D, Barnett RJ, Goldberg MS, Hoover K, Siemiatycki J, Jerrett M, et al. Reanalysis of the Harvard Six Cities Study and the American Cancer Society Study of Particulate air Pollution and Mortality. Cambridge, MA: Health Effects Institute, 2000.
21. Abbey DE, Nishino N, McDonnell WF, Burchette RJ, Knutsen SF, Lawrence Beeson W, et al. Long-term inhalable particles and other air pollutants related to mortality in nonsmokers. Am J Respir Crit Care Med 1999; 159:373–382.
22. Lipfert FW, Perry HM Jr, Miller JP, Baty JD, Wyzga RE, Carmody SE. The Washington University-EPRI Veterans' cohort mortality study: preliminary results. Inhal Toxicol 2000; 12:41–73.
23. Laden F, Neas LM, Dockery DW, Schwartz J. Association of fine particulate matter from different sources with daily mortality in six U.S. cities. Environ Health Perspect 2000; 108:941–947.
24. Pope CA III, Burnett RT, Thun MJ, Calle EE, Krewski D, Ito K, et al. Lung cancer, cardiopulmonary mortality and long-term exposure to fine particulate air pollution. J Am Med Assoc 2002; 287:1132–1141.
25. Schwartz J. Harvesting and long term exposure effects in the relation between air pollution and mortality. Am J Epidemiol 2000; 151:440–448.
26. Gauderman WJ, Gilliland FD, Avol E, Vora H, Thomas DT, Rappaport E, Berhane K, Lurmann F, McConnell R, Stram D, Peters JM. Associations between air pollution and lung growth in southern California children. Am J Respir Crit Care Med 2002; 166:74–84.
27. Avol EL, Gauderman WJ, Tan SM, London SJ, Peters JM. Respiratory effects of relocating to areas of differing air pollution levels. Am J Respir Crit Care Med 2001; 164:2067–2072.
28. EPA. The Benefits and Costs of the Clean Air Act, 1970 to 1990. US Environmental Protection Agency, Washington, DC 20460, Oct 1997.
29. EPA. The Benefits and Costs of the Clean Air Act, 1990-2010. EPA-410-R-99-001. US Environmental Protection Agency, Washington, DC 20460, Nov 1999.
30. Samet JM, Zeger SL, Kelsall JE, Xu J, Kalkstein LS. Air pollution, weather, and mortality in Philadelphia. Report on Phase 1.B of the Particle Epidemiology Project. Cambridge, MA: Health Effects Institute, 1997:1973–1988.
31. Pope CA III, Kalkstein LS. Synoptic weather modeling and estimates of the exposure–response relationship between daily mortality and particulate air pollution. Environ Health Perspect 1996; 104:414–420.

Index